A Clinician's Survival Guide to District Nursing

A Clinician's Survival Guide to District Nursing

EDITORS

Dr NEESHA OOZAGEER GUNOWA, PhD, MSc, BSc (Hons), DN, RN, SFHEA, QN

Senior Lecturer and Community Pathway Lead
School of Health Sciences
The University of Surrey
Guildford
United Kingdom

MICHELLE McBRIDE, MSc, BSc (Hons), DN, RN, SFHEA, QN

Senior Lecturer
Nurse Education
University of Roehampton
London
United Kingdom

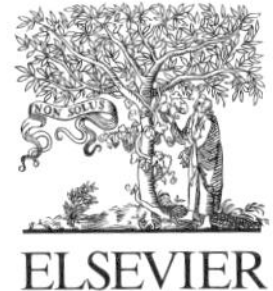

ELSEVIER

Notices

Practitioners and researchers must always rely on their own experience and knowledge in evaluating and using any information, methods, compounds or experiments described herein. Because of rapid advances in the medical sciences, in particular, independent verification of diagnoses and drug dosages should be made. To the fullest extent of the law, no responsibility is assumed by Elsevier, authors, editors or contributors for any injury and/or damage to persons or property as a matter of products liability, negligence or otherwise, or from any use or operation of any methods, products, instructions, or ideas contained in the material herein.

ISBN: 978-0-443-12481-5

Content Strategist: Robert Edwards
Content Project Manager: Shubham Dixit
Design: Matthew Limbert
Marketing Manager: Deborah Watkins

Printed in India

Last digit is the print number: 9 8 7 6 5 4 3 2 1

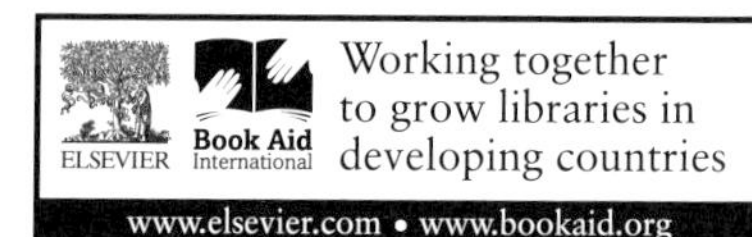

Special thanks to Dr Sam Sherrington, Dr Emma Pascale Blakey, the Queen's Nursing Institute and the Florence Nightingale Foundation who helped unite like-minded community nurses.

First and foremost, I want to express my deepest gratitude to my mum and dad, whose 'What's next' attitude has been a constant source of inspiration. Both of you have truly believed in my ability and never stopped supporting me. I could not have done it without you.

A special thank you to my striking husband, Vimal, whose ongoing support has been instrumental in the delivery of this book.

To Vihaan, my amazing son, who has shown me the importance of balance in life and reminded me to always make time for fun.

I am profoundly grateful to my supervisor and mentor, Professor Debra Jackson, who saw the potential in a young nurse starting her PhD journey in Oxford.

And last but by no means least, I extend my heartfelt thanks to all my incredible colleagues who made this book possible. Your support and collaboration have been invaluable.

Dr Neesha Oozageer Gunowa

Firstly, I would like to dedicate this book to my late mother Sheila, who always believed in my ability to succeed and without her support and dedication I would have never achieved all of my goals thus far.

To my family and friends who always 'adjusted' to my schedules and never complained when my mind was elsewhere!

A special thank you to my colleagues, near and far, who have been instrumental in the success of this book with contributions and morale boosting.

And finally, to all the community nurses out there who do the most amazing job, overcoming many barriers to ensure patients receive the best care.

Michelle McBride

FOREWORD

Written by experts in their field, this timely and ambitious book focuses on all aspects of District Nursing services, from the historical and policy context to the leadership, management and delivery of clinical services in local communities.

While the chapters are written mainly for a nursing audience working in services in England, there are many areas relevant to nurses working in community services throughout the UK. Indeed, many of the chapters, such as Chapter 4 (Autonomous Practice and Safe Ways of Working Alone), apply to all registered nurses serving their communities, regardless of the location of practice. Each one is skillfully authored by professionals with highly credible expertise and current knowledge of the immediate practical applicability of their subject.

The book captures the complexity of the District Nursing service, the skills, knowledge and day-to-day risk management required of the District Nurse team leader, and the central role of the service to the success of the entire health system.

The chapters are written in a way that permits the reader to select the area they wish to focus on, rather than expecting a linear read. This provides the reader with the opportunity to move between chapters as their interest and learning builds, with each chapter providing a standalone unit of study, reflection points and comprehensive reference lists.

The references provide the reader with signposting to more in-depth sources of information and research. For nurses new to working in the community this will be a valuable resource to which they will return many times and a springboard for further learning.

I anticipate that '*A Survival Guide to District Nursing*' will become core reading for student nurses too, experiencing the joy of learning about their community placement. It will be equally welcomed as core reading by nurses transitioning to a post with a District Nursing team, who are keen to develop and progress their careers in a service which holds the key to the agreed ambition of providing more care in people's homes and communities.

I congratulate the editors on bringing together such a comprehensive and varied range of experts and subjects, providing a guide which is both educational and a most enjoyable reading experience.

Dr Crystal Oldman CBE
Chief Executive
The Queen's Nursing Institute
London
United Kingdom

PREFACE

We are delighted to present this first edition of '*A Clinician's Survival Guide to District Nursing*' at a time when community nursing is evolving rapidly and the demand for high-quality, evidence-based care in the community has never been greater.

Through collaboration with nurses and other healthcare professionals who have generously offered their time for free, this book provides readers with a comprehensive insight into the District Nursing service, exploring the vast breadth and depth of skills required for this vital healthcare role. It delves into the complexities and nuances of working in a community setting, providing not only theoretical knowledge but also practical advice that can be applied in day-to-day practice. Readers will gain an understanding of the challenges and rewards of district nursing, learning how to navigate the unique aspects of patient care outside of a hospital environment. This book aims to equip new and experienced nurses with the tools and knowledge they need to excel in the field, fostering a deeper appreciation for district nurses' advanced and critical role in healthcare.

The book aims to provide a holistic overview of how community nursing fits into the wider structure of healthcare provision, and how it functions at both local and national levels, providing an insight into how policy influences care provision and how services are commissioned, recognising the importance of economic value. Furthermore, the chapters focus on the populations that community nurses would provide care for, with a focus on population health, public health and health promotion, recognising how some groups of people have poorer health outcomes and how to ensure that professional practice and the services we provide are inclusive, fair and respectful.

After reading the content, the readers should be able to appreciate the challenges of assessing patients in their own homes and the complexities of managing caseloads. This includes ensuring a safe and adequate skill mix, mitigating the risks of lone working and embedding discharge planning. All of this must be achieved whilst embracing innovations in healthcare, sustainability and the new digital age. Additionally, the focus on patient care is paramount. Readers will learn how to provide high-quality and safe practice for those with frailty, those needing nutritional support, or those requiring palliative care at home. The chapters also discuss common physical and mental health conditions and the challenges of meeting the needs of these patient groups while ensuring parity of esteem.

Throughout the book, the needs of the workforce and individual nurses are also considered, with suggestions for career and leadership development and guidance on how to establish a presence within research. Most importantly, there is guidance on self-care and ensuring one's own well-being, along with strategies for developing resilience to the challenges of working in the community.

The contributors have been brought together from a variety of backgrounds, including clinical practice, academia and senior leadership roles. Many of the authors are influencers and innovators in their fields, with long, sustained careers working within the community. Irrespective of their backgrounds, all these individuals share a passion for sharing their experiences and enhancing the learning of others.

Twelve years ago, we began dreaming about creating a community nursing book when we both transitioned from our day-to-day duties as district nurses to roles in academia. Despite our different geographical backgrounds within London, our shared passion for community nursing has always been a unifying force. This passion has remained steadfast and deeply ingrained in everything we do, even as we moved away from direct patient care. Throughout our academic careers, we have continually been inspired by the remarkable dedication and resilience of community nurses and Queen's Nurses. We saw a need for a comprehensive resource that could capture the essence of this profession, providing both practical guidance and a celebration of the unique challenges and triumphs that come with district nursing. Our goal was to create a book that would serve as a valuable tool for current and future nurses, ensuring they are well prepared and supported in their roles.

The idea for this book was born from countless discussions, reflections and a shared desire to give back to the community nursing field. We wanted to offer a resource that could bridge the gap between theory and practice, providing insights from our extensive experience, as well as that of our colleagues, while also addressing the evolving landscape of healthcare. Our hope is that this book will not only enhance the skills and knowledge of its readers but also reignite their passion for community nursing, keeping the heart of community care alive in every aspect of their professional journey.

District nursing has evolved significantly over the years, with nurses now being exposed to a wider array of clinical and technical tasks than ever before. A community nursing day is never the same; it can begin with administering insulin, cannulating a patient and administering intravenous drugs, all while managing a team and providing a shoulder to cry on for a bereaved relative. The skills of a community nurse cannot and will never be measurable solely within the context of science or social care. There is no other job where you might find yourself going into someone's house to carry out a nursing assessment, only to then offer social support by calling the vet because their pet iguana has not been responding. This unique blend of clinical expertise, emotional support and adaptability highlights the indispensable and multifaceted role of community nurses.

CONTRIBUTORS

Roseline Agyekum, BSc, MSc, PG Cert HCP, FHEA, CCN, RN
Lead Nurse, Clinical Practice and Education/Community Kidney Nurse Researcher
Renal Dialysis Unit
King's College Hospital
Senior Practitioner Lecturer
Adult Nursing
King's College London
London, United Kingdom

Katie Baichoo, BSc (Hons) RN, QN, PNA
Lead Triage Nurse
Planned/Unplanned Care
NMC
Rickmansworth, United Kingdom

Dr Helen Bosley, BSc (Hons), RN, RSCN, PhD
Nurse Consultant
Infection Prevention and Control
Oxford Health NHS Foundation Trust
Oxford, United Kingdom

Sue Brooks, BSc (Hons) Psychology with Nursing Studies, RN, PGCert in Education, Independent and Supplementary Prescriber, MSc Advanced Clinical Practice
Visiting Senior Lecturer
School of Health Sciences
University of Surrey
Guildford, United Kingdom

Sarah Brownlow, Dip in Health Studies, RN Degree in Professional Practice in Healthcare, PGDip in Community Specialist Practitioner, MSc Leadership in Healthcare
Clinical Service Manager
Adult Business Unit
Leeds Community Healthcare
Leeds, United Kingdom

Emma Budd, BSc, DipHE, PNA, QN
Clinical Lead
Procare Community Services
Guildford, United Kingdom

Alison Child, MSc, RN
Frontline Service Lead
Integrated Services
Your Healthcare CIC
Kington upon Thames, United Kingdom

Maria Cozens, BSc Nursing Intellectual Disability, BSc Nursing Mental Health, PGCE, MSc Nursing Research
Senior Lecturer – Mental Health Nursing
School of Life and Health Sciences
University of Roehampton
London, United Kingdom

Ann Marie Devitt, HD Nursing, SCPHN—Health Visiting BSc
Senior Lecturer – Adult Nursing
School of Life and Health Sciences
University of Roehampton
London, United Kingdom

Sandra Dilks, RGN, PGCE, BSc, MSc, SPPN, SFHEA
Senior Lecturer/Course Leader
Faculty of Education, Health and Wellbeing
University of Wolverhampton
Wolverhampton; External Examiner
University of Buckingham
Buckingham, United Kingdom

Linda Duggan, RN, BSc (Hons) Nursing, MSc, PG Dip DipHE District Nursing, District Nurse, Nurse Teacher
Lecturer in Adult Nursing
School of Nursing and Midwifery
University of Plymouth
Plymouth, United Kingdom

Siobhan Ebden, RN Adults and Children, Specialist Community Public Health Nurse (HV), MA Public Health, NMP
Community Nurse Fellow Alumni
CNO
NHS England
London, United Kingdom

Julia Fairhall, PGDip in Education, Community Specialist Practice Degree, MBA
Assistant Director of Nursing
Corporate Nursing
Sussex Community NHS Foundation Trust
Brighton, United Kingdom

Dr Jemell Geraghty, RGN, BN, MSc, FHEA, DHRes
Lecturer
Adult Nursing—Faculty of Nursing Midwifery and Palliative Care
King's College London
London, United Kingdom
Nurse Consultant Tissue Viability
Ad Integrum Vascular and Wound Care
Royal Tunbridge Wells, United Kingdom

Lincoln Gombedza, BSc, MSc
Learning Disability Nurse
North Staffordshire Combined Healthcare NHS Trust
Stoke-on-Trent, United Kingdom

Dr Richard Green, PhD
Future Fellow
School of Health Sciences
University of Surrey
Guildford, United Kingdom

Prof Sue Green, RN, BSc, PGCert, MedSci, PhD
Professor and Head of Department of Nursing Science
Faculty of Health & Social Sciences
Bournemouth University
Bournemouth, United Kingdom

Prof Vanessa Heaslip, RN, DipHE, BSc (Hons), MA, PhD, DN
Professor of Nursing and Healthcare Equity
Nursing and Midwifery
University of Salford
Salford, United Kingdom
Adjunct Professor Public Health
Social Work
University of Stavanger
Stavanger, Norway

Karen Heggs, BSc (Hons), MA, PGCert, PGDip
Director of Nursing and Midwifery
School of Health and Society
University of Salford
Manchester, United Kingdom

Dr Nathan Illman, DClinPsy, PhD
Clinical Psychologist
Nurse Wellbeing Mission
Brighton, United Kingdom

Kumbi Kariwo, BSc in Health, Dip in Learning Disability Nursing
Health Inequalities Lead
Equality and Inclusion, Medical Directorate
Birmingham Community Healthcare Trust
Birmingham, United Kingdom

Fiona Kaye, BSc (Hons), RN, PNA
Student District Nurse
HCRG Care Group
Surrey and North East Hants and Farnham Adult Community Services
Farnham, United Kingdom

Cliff Kilgore, BSc (Hons) Advanced Practice, MA Advanced Clinical Practice
Consultant Practitioner Older People
Community Services
Bournemouth University
Bournemouth, United Kingdom

Caroline Knott, RGN, BSc, QN
Clinical Safety Officer
Information Technology and Finance
Kent Community NHS Foundation Trust
Ashford, United Kingdom

Janine Lane, BSc (DN), MSc, RGN
Consultant Nurse
Dementia, Frailty and Care Homes
Central London Community Healthcare Trust
Morden, United Kingdom

Heather Lane, BSc (Hons), PGCE, RNC, CCN, QN
Lecturer and Pathway Lead for Community Children's Nursing (CCN) SPQ Programme
Faculty of Health and Medical Sciences
University of Surrey
Guildford, United Kingdom

Hannah Little, BA (Hons), MSc
Assistant Chief Nursing Officer – Cancer Services
North Bristol NHS Foundation Trust
Bristol, United Kingdom

Ashley Luchmun, BA, PGCert Ed, PG Dip, MA Ed
Senior Lecturer and Placement Lead
School of Health Sciences
London Metropolitan University
London, United Kingdom

Dr Kirsty Marshall, PhD
Senior Lecturer
Health and Society
University of Salford
Salford, United Kingdom

Paul McAleer, QN, BSc, MSc, RNLD, PGCHET, FHEA
Lecturer
School of Nursing and Midwifery
Queen's University
Belfast, United Kingdom

Michelle McBride, MSc, BSc (Hons), DN, RN, SFHEA, QN
Senior Lecturer
Nurse Education
University of Roehampton
London, United Kingdom

Sifiso Mguni, RGN, PostGradDip, BSc (PubH), Exc MSc
Macmillan Palliative and End of Life Care Transformation Lead
NHS Mid and South Essex Integrated Care Board
Basildon, United Kingdom

Lesley Mills, BA (Hons), DipHE, RN, QN, MPhil
Consultant Nurse
Diabetes Centre
Warrington and Halton Teaching Hospitals NHS Foundation Trust
Warrington, United Kingdom

Prof Caroline Nicholson, BSc (Hons), MSc, PhD, RGN FEHA
Professor of Palliative Care and Ageing
School of Health Sciences
University of Surrey
Guildford, United Kingdom

Caroline Ogunsola, MSc, BSc (Hons), DMS, RN, SPQDN, QN, MIHM, MNDNN
Professional Development Lead Nurse & Trust Lead Governor
Lead for Non Medical Prescribing (NMP) for CHS & Pry Care
Strategic Trust Lead for International Recruitment;
Trust Lead for Professional Nurse Advocate (PNA)
East London NHS Foundation Trust
Mile End Hospital
London, United Kingdom

Dr Neesha Oozageer Gunowa, PhD, MSc, BSc (Hons), DN, RN, SFHEA, QN
Senior Lecturer and Community Pathway Lead
School of Health Sciences
The University of Surrey
Guildford, United Kingdom

Gabbie Parham, BA (Hons) Adult Nursing, PGDip Gerontology, Adv Dip Community Nursing in the Home (District Nursing), RN, QN
Senior Matron for Community Nursing
Planned and Preventative Care
Oxford Health NHS Foundation Trust
Oxfordshire, United Kingdom

Dr Jonathan Parker, BA (Hons), MA, PhD
Professor of Society and Social Welfare
Social Sciences and Social Work
Bournemouth University
Bournemouth, United Kingdom
Professor Emeritus
Social Work
University of Stavanger
Stavanger, Norway

Alyson Price, BA (Hons) Psychology, DipHE (Mental Health Nursing), PGCE, PGCert (Research Methods)FHEA
Senior Lecturer – Mental Health Nursing
School of Life and Health Sciences
University of Roehampton
London, United Kingdom

Paulette Ragan, RN, BA (Hons), FHEA, NMP, PGCE (PracEd)
Senior Lecturer
Nursing, School of Life and Health Sciences
University of Roehampton
Croydon University Centre
Croydon, United Kingdom

Anna Roberts, RGN, NDNCert, Dip PP
District Nurse Team Leader
Community Nursing
Betsi Cadwaladr University Health Board
Bangor, United Kingdom

Katie Romanillos, BSc (Hons) Adult Nursing, BSc (Hons) Specialist Practice Qualification in District Nursing
Clinical Lead District Nurse
District Nursing
Dorset HealthCare University NHS Foundation Trust
Sherborne, United Kingdom

Samantha Rose, Bsc (Hons) in Adult Nursing, PGDip Specialist in Community Nursing
Adult Nursing Lecturer
Health and Society
University of Salford
Manchester, United Kingdom

Kendra Schneller, MBE
Nurse Practitioner - Homeless and HIU
Guy's and St Thomas' NHS Foundation Trust
London, United Kingdom

Jacqui Scrace, RN Child, BSc (Hons), MA, QN
Assistant Director of Nursing for Children and Young People
South West Region
NHS England
Southampton, United Kingdom

Karen Storey, RN, MSc, QN
ILM Level 7 Executive Coach and Mentor
Axminster Devon, United Kingdom

Charlotte Sumnall, MSc, PGCert (Older Person's Fellowship), BSc (SPQ- District Nurse), DipHE (Adult RGN)
Community Lead Nurse for Safety & Quality
Royal Devon University Healthcare NHS Foundation Trust
North Devon District Hospital
Barnstaple, United Kingdom

Jonathan Taylor, BSc Adult Nursing Degree, Foundation Degree in Health and Social Care
Clinical Audit and Quality Improvement Facilitator
The Royal Marsden NHS Foundation Trust
Woking, United Kingdom

Rob Taylor-Ball, BSc, MSc
Senior Advanced Nurse Practitioner
Kings Park Hospital
Dorset HealthCare University NHS Foundation Trust
Bournemouth, United Kingdom

Anthea Thorpe, BSc, BA (Hons), RN, QN
Head of Clinical Support Team
NHS Blood and Transplant
Southampton, United Kingdom

Hayley Thrumble, PGDip, BSc (Hons), DN, RN
Lecturer in Clinical Skills and Simulation
University of Roehampton
Croydon, United Kingdom

Lee Tomlinson, Master of Clinical Research, BSc Professional Practice in Clinical Nursing Critical Care, Dip HE Adult Nursing
Associate Director of Nursing
Clinical Care and Quality
Kent Community Health NHS Foundation Trust
Ashford, United Kingdom

Samantha Wakefield, BA (Hons), PGDip, RN, DN, PGCE
Lecturer in Community Nursing (Specialist Practice Pathway—District Nursing)
School of Health Sciences
University of Surrey
Guildford, United Kingdom

AnnMarie Whyte, SPDN, BSc (Hons), PGCert
Professional Lead District Nurse
Community Nursing
Kent Community Health, NHS Foundation Trust
Sevenoaks, United Kingdom

Emily Winter, BSc, QN
Professional Lead for Education
Adult Community Nursing
Procare Community Services
Guildford and Waverley, United Kingdom

CONTENTS

CHAPTER 1

The Role of Community and District Nurses

Michelle McBride ■ Cliff Kilgore ■ Neesha Oozageer Gunowa

LEARNING OUTCOMES

After reading this chapter you should be able to:

- Understand the development of the community and district nurse role
- Critically explore the concepts of care delivered by nurses working in the community
- Recognise district nursing as a career choice
- Comprehend the nature of transitioning to community nursing

1.1 Introduction

DEFINITIONS

Community Nursing: Community nursing encompasses a range of healthcare services provided to individuals and families within their homes and communities. It involves promoting health, preventing illness and managing chronic conditions.

District Nursing: District nursing is a specialised field within community nursing that focuses on providing comprehensive care at an advanced-level to individuals with complex health needs. District nurses are highly skilled specialist practitioners who are appropriately prepared through the Specialist Practice Qualification (District Nursing) often working in specific geographic areas, forming deep connections while leading and managing a team of community nurses.

Community and district nurses play a pivotal role in the healthcare system, serving as a bridge between hospitals and the communities they serve. This chapter explores the multifaceted responsibilities and significant impact that community and district nurses have on the overall well-being of individuals and communities as well as offers support to nurses considering a career in the community.

The National Health Service (NHS) continues to face increasing demands because of the ageing population, the rising numbers of people living with multiple long-term chronic conditions alongside a reduction in funding and recruitment and retention issues. Although the NHS Long Term Plan (NHS England, 2019) identified the need for investment into community and primary care services to support the increasing demands, district nurses have historically been the primary providers of care in the community.

BOX 1.1 ■ Some Key Responsibilities and Functions of a Community Nurse

- Health promotion and education
- Chronic disease management
- Wound care
- Medication management
- Home health services, which includes home visits to assess patients' needs, monitor their health status and coordinate care with other healthcare professionals
- Palliative and end-of-life care
- Coordination of care
- Health equity and social justice
- Emergency response and crisis intervention

By completing further study and expanding their advanced level skills and scope of practice, district nurses have become specialists in holistic care by undertaking effective patient assessments in a variety of community settings often ensuring patients can remain in their own homes. The development and expansion of skills enable the NHS and community providers to offer a service that is flexible, proactive and individualised to meet the needs of the patient. Furthermore, the future of the NHS continues to place district nurses at the forefront of healthcare with a new ambitious highly anticipated workforce plan which will see training places increase by more than 150% by 2031/32 (NHS England, 2023).

> *District nurses are the air traffic control of healthcare – cut the numbers and you might expect more plane crashes or not being able to take off at all. It's a risk to all of us, we're more likely to need nursing care in our lives than any other kind of care.*
>
> – PROFESSOR ALISON O'LEARY

No day in the life of a community nurse working in a district nursing team is the same. Overall, the role of a community nurse is multifaceted, dynamic and evolving, encompassing a wide range of responsibilities aimed at promoting health, preventing illness and improving the quality of life for individuals and communities in diverse settings. Through their expertise, compassion and dedication, community nurses play a vital role in advancing public health and wellness initiatives and addressing the healthcare needs of underserved populations. In Box 1.1, some key responsibilities and functions of a community nurse have been included.

1.2 The Role of Community Nurses in Care Homes

The role of the community nurse in a residential care home setting can vary depending on the specific needs of each resident's mental, physical and emotional health. However, it is important to recognise that community nurses play a vital role in providing comprehensive healthcare services to support people living in care homes. Individualised care plans are developed to address the specific needs and preferences of each resident considering factors such as nutrition, mobility, medication management, wound care and personal care. These should always be developed in partnership with the professional staff based within care homes and with the patient themselves.

Enhanced health in care homes (NHS England, 2020) is an ambition to strengthen the NHS support for people who live and work in care homes. This should mean that people living in care homes should receive the same level of healthcare as if they were living in their own homes and it is recognised that community nursing has some significant part to play in this. As well as providing individualised treatments, there is a need for community nurses to be involved in multidisciplinary meetings and planned holistic assessments after admission to a care home. The overall model for enhanced health in care homes moves away from previous traditional reactive models of care delivery and places greater emphasis on proactive care, centred on the needs of an individual (NHS England, 2020). Specialist nurses with extended skills may even be required to provide a weekly 'home' round to prioritise needs and provide planning for anticipatory care and for some will be named clinical leads for care homes (Vellani et al., 2021).

DEFINITION OF TERMS

'Nursing homes' and 'care homes' are terms often used interchangeably, but they can have different connotations depending on funding streams. Both the care that people receive and the premises are regulated by the Care Quality Commission.

Care home with nursing services: A nursing home typically provides more intensive medical care and support; nursing homes are designed for individuals who require round-the-clock nursing care and assistance with activities of daily living due to chronic illness, disability or frailty. People may live in the service for short or long periods. For many people, it is their sole place of residence and so it becomes their home, although they do not legally own or rent it.

Care home services without nursing (e.g., residential care home): Residents of care homes may have varying levels of independence and may not require skilled nursing care on a daily basis. Care homes without nursing often focus on promoting independence, socialisation and quality of life for residents while providing a supportive and safe environment.

REFLECTION

- District nursing teams do not generally visit nursing homes due to funding streams however there are some exceptions. Consider the care homes in your local area, do they provide nursing care?

The role of the community nurse in health monitoring is fundamental for evaluating the effectiveness of healthcare interventions and identifying areas for improvement for care home residents. Nurses actively participate in monitoring and assessing the health outcomes of individuals employing standardised tools and measures to quantify and evaluate improvement reference. Progress tracking with comparative pre- and postintervention data to identify disparities is used to assess whether desired outcomes have been achieved reference. Analysis of these data is used to recognise variations in outcomes among different demographic populations, such as gender, ethnicity or socio-economic status. This evaluation helps to identify effective strategies for future use and improvement.

Collaborations with the wider multidisciplinary team, such as medical staff, therapists, social workers and carers, assist in obtaining a comprehensive perspective and ensure that multiple perspectives and expertise are considered. This, in turn, supports quality improvements in patient care that is supportive of all disciplines and holds the patient at the centre (NHS England, 2020). Promotion of patient education and self-management, including ideas on lifestyle modification, helps to empower individuals to take control of their health and encourages shared care decision-making and improves overall engagement in care.

It is often recognised that in a modern care system, many older people living in care homes are approaching the end of their life (Office for National Statistics, 2021). This means that there is a need for community nurses to understand a structured approach to end-of-life care, with the Gold Standard Framework being widely used in care homes in the UK (British Geriatric Society, 2020). The idea of a structured framework for end-of-life care matches the aims of enhancing health in care homes with the role of community nursing potentially providing professional advice and guidance to the staff based in care homes.

Overall, the community nurse in the care home plays a pivotal role in delivering person-centred care, promoting resident's well-being and ensuring their health needs are met effectively within the care environment.

1.3 History of District Nursing

The history of district nursing focuses on compassion, innovation and the evolution of healthcare delivery. The concept of district nursing emerged in the 19th century, and its development has been closely linked to societal changes, advances in nursing education and the recognition of the importance of community-based care. The roots of district nursing can be traced back to the pioneering efforts of key individuals and the social reform movements of the time including Florence Nightingale.

The history of district nursing reflects a continuous evolution driven by the commitment to providing quality care within the community. From its beginnings in the 19th century to its present-day adaptation to contemporary healthcare challenges, district nursing remains an integral part of the healthcare landscape, embodying the principles of compassion and community-based care (QNI Heritage, 2020).

1.4 Policy and District Nursing

Policy plays a crucial role in shaping the landscape of district nursing, influencing the delivery of healthcare services, the scope of practice for nurses and the overall quality of care provided in the community. Various policies at local, national and international levels impact district nursing which focus on the topics included in Box 1.2.

Policy considerations are integral to the effective functioning and advancement of district nursing. Policies shape the regulatory environment, resource allocation and the

BOX 1.2 ■ Key Policy Areas Affecting District Nursing

- Healthcare funding and resource allocation
- Legislation and scope of practice
- Integrated care and interprofessional collaboration
- Telehealth and technology integration
- Public health and preventive care initiatives
- Ageing population and long-term care policies
- Quality improvement and performance metrics

TABLE 1.1 **Misconceptions**

Misconceptions Regarding Community nursing	Counterargument
You need 1 year on a hospital based ward before joining the community	This is not essential. Newly qualified nurses can go straight into the community and receive preceptorship to help them adjust to their new role and consolidate their knowledge and skills. They do, however, need the confidence to be a lone worker.
Working in the community deskills you	This is not true. The role of the community nurse involves many advanced nursing skills and training is provided to support achieving these competencies.
District nursing is where you go to retire	This is not true. The community nursing workforce is mixed in age range and is not a physically easier role than working in a hospital environment. You need to be fit and agile and many nurses start progressive advanced nurse careers within the community setting.
Career progression is difficult	Nurses working in the community can often progress faster than their hospital counterparts with fast-track programmes available in some areas, and opportunities for additional training to qualify as a District Nurse or Advanced Nurse Practitioners in their chosen field.
District nursing is not real nursing	This is not true. Nursing in the community, in patients' homes is where you can provide the most holistic, person-centred care possible. Often caring for very complex, acutely unwell individuals and their families when they are most vulnerable, community nurses can have an enormous impact on patient experience.

overall framework within which district nurses operate, influencing their ability to provide comprehensive and patient-centred care in community settings.

1.5 Nurse Education in the Community

As explained in Table 1.1, both community and district nurses work in the community. However, to be recognised and practice as a district nurse, even though the title is not protected, registered nurses must undergo specialised training and attain specific qualifications. The postgraduate specialist practice qualification in district nursing (SPQDN) is a recognised credential that signifies a nurse's advanced knowledge, skills and competence in the field of district nursing. This qualification is typically obtained through formal education, training and assessment and it allows nurses to specialise in providing healthcare services within the community, often focusing on home-based care and health promotion. The SPQDN equips nurses with the knowledge and skills needed to address the diverse and complex healthcare needs of individuals and families in their homes, contributing to the overall improvement of community health outcomes. Advanced practice in district nursing refers to a level of nursing practice that extends beyond basic or general nursing roles. It involves nurses taking on advanced responsibilities, often including clinical leadership, advanced assessment, diagnosis and the management of complex health conditions within the community or home setting. Advanced practice developed within the SPQDN enables nurses to have expanded roles that allow them to provide a higher level of care and contribute to the development and improvement of community healthcare services.

1.6 District Nursing as a Career Choice

Many student nurses choose the community for their first post as soon as they graduate from their university, particularly if they have been allocated there for their final placement (Phillips, 2014). Others may commence their career pathways in a hospital environment and then transition soon after when they have consolidated their skills and increased their confidence. However, there are still some misconceptions regarding community nursing as an appropriate newly registered nurse role that require addressing (see Table 1.1).

As Phillips (2014) suggests, we should embrace novice nurses in the community and indeed prepare students during their placement for registered practice there, although one of the limitations is that not all preregistration nurses have adequate community placements. For student nurses to be inspired to take a post in the community, they need to gain a wider range of learning experiences. As the QNI (2021) indicate, excellent placement opportunities have never been more necessary, with learning and support being essential (Wareing et al., 2018). Many student nurses are not aware of the flexible and dynamic career pathways available within the community setting (QNI, 2021). To influence career choices after qualifying, there have been recent improvements in this area whereby commitments have been made to grow preregistration clinical placement capacity to provide more high-quality learning experiences (Health Education England (HEE), 2020). One must also be mindful that assisting with the transition to community nursing will also facilitate workforce development and reduce healthcare pressure (Chamberlain et al., 2020).

For those that have been inspired, once qualified, that transition into the community is not always easy. Being a guest in a patient's home and being exposed to their lifestyle choices is often a challenge, and at times, it is difficult to be nonjudgemental and be able to deliver nursing care safely in an environment that may not be designed for that purpose (QNI, 2016). There are additional issues to consider when care is being delivered in a home environment which may include types of housing, environments and facilities available that nurses may have not previously considered if they have not worked in a community setting (QNI, 2016).

Community nurses must learn to develop positive relationships with their patients and their families, which are different to inpatient settings. Time is needed to build trust and get to know the individual needs. These relationships are unique and require professional boundaries that will protect both the nurse and the patient (QNI, 2016). Effective working in the community is built on communication and established partnerships; this applies to patients and their families but also the teams that nurses work in.

1.7 Career Transition Into the Community

It has been suggested that both clinical support and educational support should be included in a transition programme, and that orientation should also include an introduction to broader community issues and a structured approach to ongoing mentoring (Chamberlain et al., 2020). Nurses within the community need to be critical thinkers and the support needs to be in place to facilitate this with a focus on personal and professional safety. Hampson et al. (2017) have also recognised that preceptorship will be beneficial, both professionally and personally, for transitioning staff and will engender competence and confidence. A period of preceptorship support is beneficial to staff professionally and personally. Preceptees have reported they feel valued, and that the preceptorship process engenders confidence and competence.

There has been some research relating to developing oneself in the role of a nurse within the community setting, and the notion of developing a sense of belonging within that environment (Chamberlain et al., 2020). Both Harvey et al. (2019) and Chamberlain et al. (2020) concur that there are formal and informal processes that occur during this transition and that this sense of belonging is paramount, which embraces embedding oneself in the culture and being accepted in the team, which is essential for optimum practice and staff retention. Often working in the community after qualifying or moving from a hospital setting evokes a sense of being a 'novice' or 'imposter syndrome' which can often appear at times as one progresses through their career (John, 2019). As Harvey et al. (2019) have identified, there is also often a sense of being a 'generalist' but needing to be a 'specialist' which compounds the degree of discomfort. They also suggested that transitioning individuals need time to adapt, and that often relates to facing the challenges of becoming a sole practitioner and the isolation of being a lone worker (QNI, 2016). An ideal transition experience requires an individualised approach where the nurse can progress at their own pace and socialise adequately; the need for robust preceptorships is paramount and can reduce occupational distress (Darvill et al., 2014; Lea & Cruickshank, 2017). In addition, this is a vulnerable time when it is easy to experience low motivation and unnecessary conflict, which can be avoided with a nurturing environment (Lea & Cruickshank, 2017). It has also been recognised that whilst nurses might leave their university with a high level of knowledge and motivation, when faced with the resource issues and frustrations of practice, it is often easy to become demoralised (QNI, 2016).

1.8 Conclusion

This chapter delves into the critical role of community and district nurses in modern healthcare, serving as a vital link between hospitals and local communities. It explores their diverse responsibilities and profound impact on individual and community wellbeing, offering insights for those considering a career in community nursing. Despite the NHS facing escalating demands and resource challenges, district nurses remain central to community care. Their advanced skills enable holistic care delivery, empowering patients to stay in their homes and adapting to evolving healthcare needs. With a workforce expansion plan underway, district nurses are poised to meet future healthcare challenges head-on.

References

Braveman, P., & Gottlieb, L. (2014). The social determinants of health: It's time to consider the causes of the causes. *Public Health Reports*, *129*(Suppl 2), 19–31.

British Geriatric Society. (2020). *End of life care in frailty: Care homes*. Available at: https://www.bgs.org.uk/resources/end-of-life-care-in-frailty-care-homes.

Chamberlain, D., Harvey, C., Hegney, D., Tsai, L., Mclellan, S., Sobolewska, A., Wake, T. (2020). Facilitating an early career transition pathway to community nursing: A Delphi policy study. *Nursing Open* (7), 100–126. https://doi-org.roe.idm.oclc.org/10.1002/nop2.355.

Darvill, N., Fallon, D., & Livesley, J. (2014). A different world?: The transition experiences of newly qualified children's nurses taking up first destination posts within children's community nursing teams in England. *Issues in Comprehensive Pediatric Nursing*, *37*(1), 6–24.

Hampson, J., Gunning, H., Nicholson, L., Hegney, D., Gee, C., Jay, D., & Sheppard, G. (2017). Role of clinical practice educators in an integrated community and mental health NHS foundation trust. *Nursing Standard*, *32*(7), 49–55.

Harvey, C., Hegney, D., Sobolewska, A., Chamberlain, D., Wood, E., Wirihana, L., Wake, T. (2019). Developing a community-based nursing and midwifery career pathway – a narrative systematic review. *PLoS ONE*, *14*(3).

Health Education England. (2020). *Community and district nursing*. Health Education England. https://hee.nhs.uk.

John, S. (2019). Imposter syndrome: Why some of us doubt our competence. *Nursing Times*, *115*(2), 23–24 [online].

Lea, J., & Cruickshank, M. (2017). The role of rural nurse managers in supporting new graduate nurses in rural practice. *Journal of Nursing Management*, *25*, 176–183.

NHS England. (2019). *The NHS long term plan*. Available at: www.longtermplan.nhs.uk/publication/nhs-long-term-plan.

NHS, England. (2020). *Enhanced health in care homes*. https://www.england.nhs.uk/community-health-services/ehch/.

NHS England. (2023). *NHS long term workforce plan*. Available at: https://www.england.nhs.uk/publication/nhs-long-term-workforce-plan/.

Office for National Statistics. (2021). *Life expectancy in care homes, England and Wales: 2011 to 2012*. (Accessed internet 10/07/2023).

Phillips, J. (2014). Helping community-based students on a final consolidation placement make the transition to registered practice. *British Journal of Community Nursing*, *19*(7), 352–619.

QNI. (2016). *Transition to district nursing service*. https://www.qni.org.uk/wp-content/uploads/2017/01/Transition-to-District-Nursing.pdf.

QNI. (2021). *Pre-registration community nursing placements survey report*. London: QNI.

QNI Heritage (2020) History of District nursing. Available from: https://qniheritage.org.uk/ (Accessed on 16th August 2024).

Vellani, S., Boscart, V., Escrig-Pinol, A., Cumal, A., Krassikova, A., Sidani, S., McGilton, K. (2021). Complexity of nurse practitioners' role in facilitating a dignified death for long-term care home residents during the COVID-19 pandemic. *Journal of Personalised Medicine*, *11*(5), 433.

Wareing, M., Taylor, R., Wilson, A., & Sharples, A. (2018). Impact of clinical placements on graduates' choice of first staff-nurse post. *British Journal of Nursing*, *27*(20), 1180–1185.

CHAPTER 2

Community Nursing and System Working

Sarah Brownlow · Siobhan Ebden

LEARNING OUTCOMES

After reading this chapter you should be able to:

- Gain knowledge of the structure, organisation and functioning of healthcare systems at local and national levels
- Understand the policy context around system working and integration
- Recognise how community nurses can influence commissioning

2.1 Introduction

Both the National Health Service (NHS) Long Term Plan (2019) and the NHS Constitution (2023) emphasise the need for collaboration, joined-up working and coordinated care. This needs to take place across organisational boundaries in partnership with others, including local authorities and voluntary organisations with a commitment to provide the best value for money.

Collaboration and working across organisational boundaries can only be effectively achieved through system working, which is also a key enabler of integration. The changes made by the development of integrated care systems (ICSs) will have a lasting impact on how services are commissioned (bought) with a greater emphasis placed on professionals working together. Historically, commissioning has focused on competition but the recent changes in health policy move this toward collaboration (Bramwell et al., 2023).

This chapter will define key terms such as commissioning and how the changes impact community nursing. It will provide an overview of system working and why integration can be seen as a key enabler to this, whilst appreciating and understanding the changes made at a system level and how these impact the care delivered and the experience for the patient.

REFLECTION

- What do you understand by the terms 'system working', 'integration' and 'commissioning'?
- Consider also how much of this knowledge is necessary to you as you provide care in the community.

Integrated care has been the backbone of community services for many years; it remains the way of effective care provision and is not a new idea. However, the many changes in policy, especially the recent development of ICSs, can leave the community nurse feeling confused; when many terms are used to describe similar concepts, it can be hard to understand what has changed and why. There is a plethora of guidance and policies relating to integrated care and integration, and often the terms, along with collaboration, are used interchangeably but relate to the same concept (Timmins, 2019).

Integrated care is defined as the coordination of care delivered through joint health and care services (Scobie, 2021). Buckingham et al. (2023) discuss that integration is demonstrated by interlinking systems, processes and behaviours that impact how professionals and teams work together. The outcome of this is coordinated services with patient needs at the centre and perhaps this is the most helpful definition for community nurses.

As integration is examined, it is useful to understand that this can be viewed through two different lenses. One lens focuses on the structure of organisations at a system level, the relationships across organisational boundaries and the development and delivery of care within the ICS. The other lens focuses on what happens at the point of care delivery, the working together between multiple professionals to deliver effective high-quality care to patients and their families. This chapter will cover the viewpoints of both lenses, offering an understanding of how a community nurse can work within the larger system and how care can be delivered effectively in an integrated way within and across teams.

2.2 Background

The delivery of care through integration has long been key to effective community nursing, with professionals across the multidisciplinary team working together to provide effective care. It is useful to understand the historical background of health policy and the effects on community care provision to appreciate the current position and context of community services. There are two keywords used within this section and it is beneficial to understand what they mean.

DEFINITIONS

Collaboration: Collaboration is defined as 'two or more people working together to create or achieve the same thing' (*Cambridge Dictionary*, 2023).

Commissioning: Commissioning is defined as 'assessing need, purchasing and monitoring the services' (Wenzel et al., 2023).

2.2.1 COLLABORATION

Community nurses have worked in collaborative joined-up ways for many years. This can be seen within palliative care where community nursing teams and multiprofessionals work together for effective care provision (NHS England, 2022a). All community nurses will have examples of where care provision has benefited from integrated and collaborative working; however, not all staff have good examples to share. Over time, health policy has evolved to reflect changing demographics, disease progression, demands of the population, technology and the increasing challenges presented financially (Buckingham et al., 2023). The need for integrated ways of working and collaboration has increased whilst at the same time the role of community care has become more prominent (Bramwell et al., 2023). Health and social care policy has driven the move towards joined-up, collaborative integrated services and places community services centrally. This is a move away from policies that previously focused on competition to policies that currently focus on collaboration and working together (Bramwell et al., 2023).

Bramwell et al. (2023) conclude their research on the history of district nursing with a desire for more integrated community-based care but recognise that the impact on community nursing services is rarely the focus of policy, nor is a consideration made of how, what and where services are delivered.

2.2.2 COMMISSIONING

Services continue to be commissioned in outdated ways on historical data and in block contracts as part of the whole of community services (The Royal College of Nursing (RCN) and Queen's Nursing Institute (QNI), 2019; Wenzel et al., 2023). The assumption of this way of working is the provision of a service that can meet multiple and varied needs of anyone with an acute health need through to long-term chronic conditions management. However, without sufficient planning and the capacity to truly understand the nature, scale and complexity of the district nurse's daily caseload, this way of working cannot be successfully achieved (Bramwell et al., 2023).

Since the publication of *The NHS Plan* (Department of Health (DH), 2000), there has been increased emphasis on modernising the NHS, joining up services and increasing multidisciplinary working. There was a need for a redesign of the whole care system focusing on a move toward community health services with localised commissioning of services. The commissioning of health services has been subject to many changes since the inception of the NHS in 1948, with many of these changes impacting directly on community service provision.

The NHS Plan (DH, 2000) saw the formation of Primary Care Trusts, where commissioning and service provision were combined into the same organisations covering local geography, but The Next Stage Review (Department of Health and Social Care, 2008) repealed these arrangements with commissioning and provision separated into different organisations again, as it was recognised at this time that this had in fact led to a conflict of interest. *Transforming Community Services: Enabling New Patterns of Provision* (DH, 2009) was instrumental in these changes. This change also led to some community organisations being established as independent social enterprises, many of which remain today.

The Health and Social Care Act (2012) established more than 200 clinical commissioning groups (CCGs). The CCGs were groups of general practitioners (GPs) and additional staff charged with purchasing and monitoring care provision for a geographical area. All CCGs were of variable size and covered different population areas, and many struggled with GP recruitment, managing their financial resources and overall governance: this led to disparity in provision, with little focus on preventive health (Grant Thornton, 2018).

The Queen's Nursing Institute (QNI, 2014) emphasised that despite the changes made by policy, thus far community nursing teams and district nurses needed a place at the table and needed to increase their visibility and actively shape national policy.

The Five Year Forward View (NHS England, 2014) and the NHS Long Term Plan (NHS England, 2019) then moved investment from hospital-based toward community-based services, thus bringing care closer to home. This has been achieved through collaboration between professionals and teams and paves the way towards ICSs, improving integration and care delivery in the community. These policies whilst still being rolled out have not yet produced the desired impact, with Buckingham et al. (2023) pointing out that much of this was rhetoric, with a focus remaining on hospital care provision and fragmented systems.

2.3 Recent Policy Context

Since 2000 there have been a plethora of different health and social care policies; many have the same aims and goals of moving care closer to home with more dependence on multidisciplinary working. Integrated working has long been desired, but the achievement of this varies. Integrated care can be seen as the driver to delivering care closer to home whilst achieving improved patient engagement, experience and reducing cost and demand. The development of ICSs in 2022 (The Health and Care Act, 2022) has led to the existing NHS budget being devolved to larger geographical areas with an increasing focus on population health including preventative care.

Many policies have the potential to raise the profile of community nurses, expand their clinical skill set and position them as central to the development of care close to home. The development of ICSs provides community nurses with means to shape policy for their patient population, working through their place-based partnerships and neighbourhoods (Naylor & Charles, 2022). ICSs bring together health and social care partners with given responsibility for the population's health within an area and this can place community nurses central to care provision locally. Community and district nurses have a better understanding of their populations' needs and are familiar with working within their area whilst understanding other services and organisations (The Royal College of Nursing and Queen's Nursing Institute, 2019).

2.4 Integrated Care Systems

Fig. 2.1 demonstrates the potential agencies and people involved in the care of an older individual. The infographic shows how these organisations are connected and where they are in the wider system.

The Health and Care Act (2022) placed integrated care on a statutory (legal) footing with legislation confirming the role of ICSs in the commissioning and delivery of services in specific area focused localities. There are 42 ICSs across England; all are partnerships of health and care organisations that come together to plan and deliver joined-up services and to improve the health of people who live in their area.

All ICSs are to achieve the same four aims:

- Improve outcomes in population health and healthcare
- Tackle inequalities in outcomes, experience and access
- Enhance productivity and value for money
- Help the NHS support broader social and economic development

ICSs are several organisations brought together with different functions but all working towards these same aims. Each ICS has its own governance structures and is designed to focus on local needs through collaborative working. Whilst ICSs are still in their infancy and will change and evolve over time, there are certain specific structures in place across them all. It is helpful to understand these structures in order to work effectively and promote services and patient care.

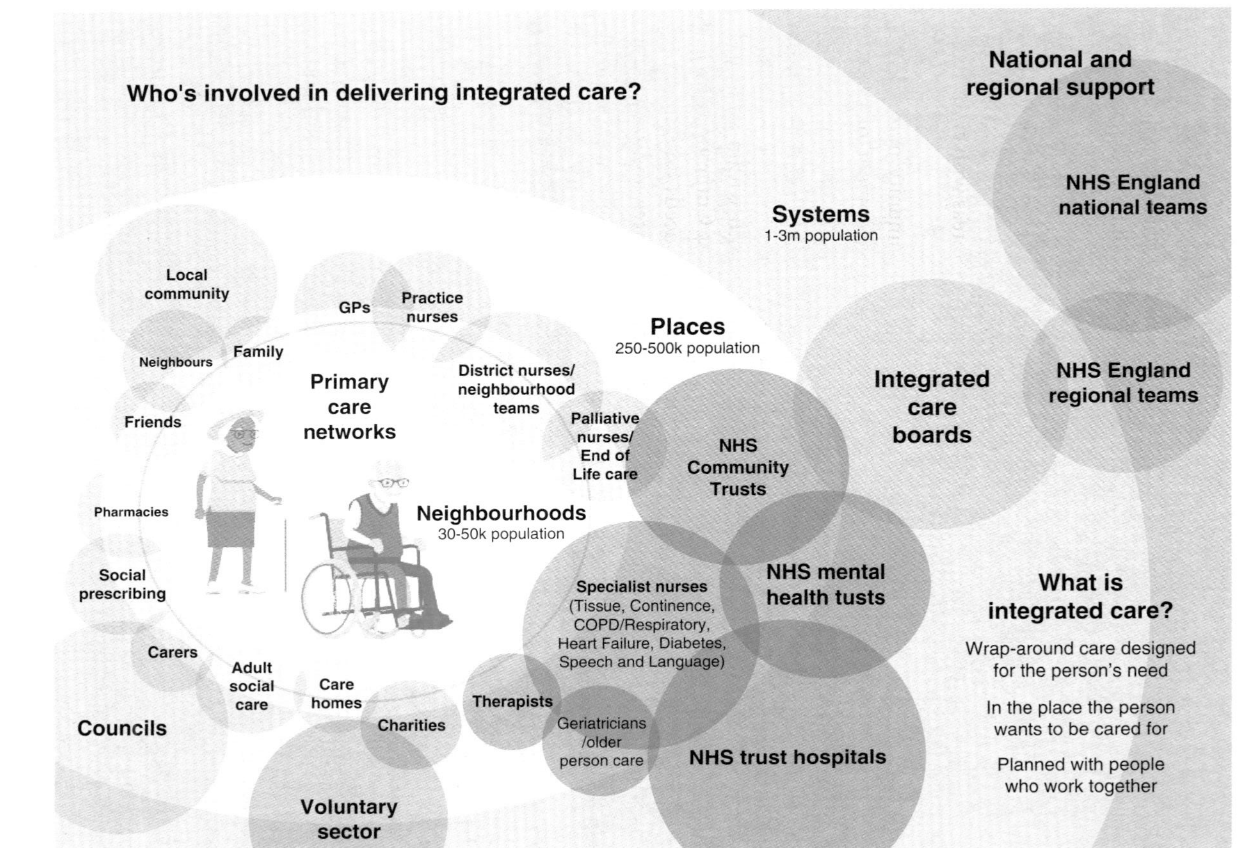

Fig. 2.1 Who is involved in delivering integrated care?

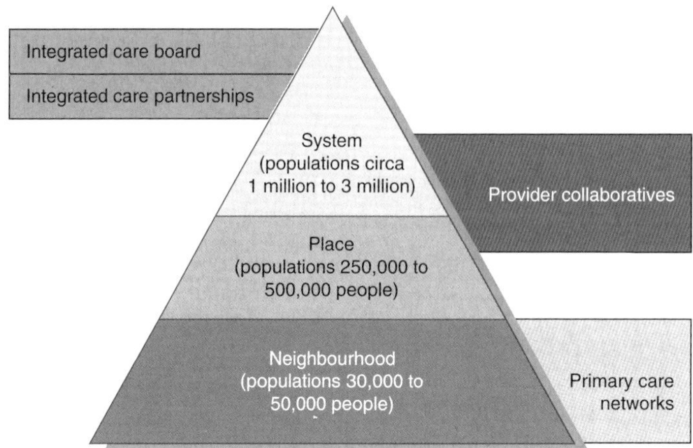

Fig. 2.2 How does it all fit together?

Fig. 2.2 demonstrates the different areas of the ICS with *subsections* working at different levels. These structures can be confusing, and it is useful to understand the purpose of each area. The system level provides strategic leadership across the whole population of the ICS with the Integrated Care Board (ICB) governing this space and developing a single plan overseeing operational and long-term priorities. The ICB is a statutory body that brings together local NHS organisations focused on improving health and care with Integrated Care Partnerships developed as an alliance of organisations including the local authority. The ICB takes on the commissioning responsibilities of the ICS. Provider collaboratives sit across the place and system level. These collaboratives join up services between places and within the local place area, for example, primary care, hospitals, community and social care. Often, they have natural geographies or council boundaries. Finally, the neighbourhood level is seen as the cornerstone to integrated care as they are at the local level. These are individuals and teams working closely together across boundaries, for example, care homes, primary care networks (PCNs), community and mental health teams and voluntary services. The focus at this level of the ICS is multidisciplinary collaborative working between professionals and organisations.

It is worth noting at this point that provider collaboratives and neighbourhoods are individual separate organisations working together. They do not belong to the same organisation, and this is the premise that good integration is built upon. Effective integration relies on strong personal relationships, not necessarily contractual partnerships.

REFLECTION

- Many board meetings and subsequent minutes can be accessed on the internet; try to access these to understand what happens locally in your system.

2.5 The Role of the Community Nurse in Commissioning

The King's Fund (Charles, 2022) and Health Foundation (Dunn et al., 2022) discuss integration at length, and additional learning can be sought from these sources.

BOX 2.1 ■ Ways in Which Community Nurses Can Get Involved with Integration

- Shadow senior staff and understand local systems
- Maximise opportunities to influence
- Share existing knowledge of populations and communities and showcase what your service/team does well
- Understand where your own service can proactively develop
- Look for ways to shape priorities and plans
- Maximise opportunities to work in collaboration with others
- Look to be an equal partner in local developments
- Leading innovation after maximising opportunities to influence

However, so far, there has been minimal discussion about the role of community nurses within these systems and how they can work effectively. This could be considered as a missed opportunity at a statutory level (policy), which means that community nursing does need to use its voice in other ways (Bramwell et al., 2023).

The role of the community nurse in an ICS can be varied, from sharing board stories of examples of integrated care to active involvement in specific working groups. At the neighbourhood level, community nurses can demonstrate and deliver integrated care by working alongside other professionals including the voluntary sector to deliver patient care. Active involvement in PCNs (groups of GPs working together with local providers of health, social care and voluntary services) can strengthen working relationships and collaboration with others whilst maintaining a focus on their own patient population.

It is imperative that community nurses understand the policy that directly affects their work so that they can understand how to influence this space, understand the significance behind the recent policy changes and understand where they 'fit' into the system. There is increasing focus on care delivered in the community setting and it is important that community nurses are influencing these plans. Coxon (2017) suggests that the community nursing role is vital to drive forward change in integration. Furthermore, community nurses understand their populations and areas and have the local expertise needed to work effectively within their neighbourhood and places (Box 2.1).

Wain (2022) researched integrated health and care in the community setting from a workforce perspective, based on the lived experience of staff and the findings demonstrated four themes that were necessary for effective integration, summarised under four headings.

- Insight of integrated care and its links to collaborative working. The finding suggest that people had differing viewpoints, and this impacted on their experience.
- The terms 'integration' and 'collaboration' were used interchangeably, leading to a degree of confusion, perceptions and experiences related to professional identity and cultural differences across professions and organisations.
- The impact of workforce engagement with colocation is seen as vital in terms of success.
- Standardised processes and systems improved staff experience.

Wain (2022) highlights that collaborative working, staff engagement, culture and organisational structures are key to the success of integrated care. This is relevant both within systems and individual teams at the neighbourhood level. The Nuffield Trust summarises the key issues determining that 'Integration will only improve if people who deliver services do something different as part of their day jobs' (Buckingham et al., 2023, p. 2). This means that community staff need to explore and make use of opportunities to work collaboratively with others in different ways, not necessarily recruiting staff to deliver this work. It is only when community nurses take control and actively work towards this, can sustainable change be made that follows policy. As community nurses, it is within their power to make a change for their own patient population and for their teams.

There are many challenges presented by the formation of the ICS. These can be seen as culture and associated behaviours, power dynamics, organisation complexity and duplication and resource constraints, which can make change challenging (Buckingham et al., 2023). It is difficult in this arena to define measures and evaluate outcomes, especially when looking at the four aims of the ICS as these are long-term targets and results may take many years to be evidenced (Buckingham et al., 2023). Many of these challenges are also relevant to the delivery of integrated care in teams, and therefore it is important to find ways to mitigate these risks.

Thinking differently within these systems is crucial and staff need a system thinking mindset. Systems thinking recognises the need to build relationships, understand multiple perspectives and have the ability to frame situations appropriately (O'Donnell, 2023). In an era of complexity, where the answers to the challenges that are faced are not simple, it requires an ability to think differently and form diverse relationships. These challenges may be viewed differently by others and the responses needed may be varied and complex themselves. Adapting leadership in this way helps to understand the need to work closely with people, understand the issues from multiple viewpoints and work across several different boundaries. Developing these skills alongside an ability to walk in others' shoes and an ability to persuade others towards change are vital skills that community nurses need to develop (Wenzel et al., 2023).

2.6 Conclusion

In conclusion, good integration for community nurses is about understanding the structures, understanding how to influence and actively build relationships at many different levels. The key skills needed are good relationships, active listening, compassion, empathy and an ability to work with others. Collaboration has been discussed many times within this chapter; it is pivotal to effective integration both at a system level and on the ground care delivery.

Working in isolation is often seen as easier than collaboration and integration particularly at times of high demand community nursing cultures and behaviours support working in isolation. This therefore requires community nurses to work hard to develop relationships, demonstrate good listening skills, recognise professional identity and work with this proactively whilst developing leadership along with a desire to work in new ways. It is imperative that community nurses look for new innovative ways to work with others and at times put aside professional boundaries and professional identity for the sake of delivering high-quality effective healthcare to patients and population alongside others.

Community nurses are well placed to work effectively at the neighbourhood level with their key partners and need to grasp this opportunity to develop themselves and their services in line with the aims of integrated care. The changing needs of society, the finite financial resources and the increasing role of the private and third sector mean that the only way that healthcare provision will move forward for the whole population is through collaboration and innovation.

The task of community nurses is to lead by example, build collaborative relationships with others, understand local systems and look for ways to be involved. By demonstrating good integration within teams and striving to become key partners, community nurses can exercise good leadership and role model behaviours.

References

Bramwell, D., Checkland, K., Shields, J., & Allen, P. (2023). *Community nursing services in England. An historical policy analysis*. Open Access Palgrave Macmillan.

Buckingham, H., Reed, S., Kumpunen, S., & Lewis, R. (2023). *People, partnerships and place: How can ICSs turn the rhetoric into reality?* Nuffield Trust. Available at: https://www.nuffieldtrust.org.uk/research/people-partnerships-and-place-how-can-icss-turn-the-rhetoric-into-reality.

Cambridge Dictionary. (2023). Collaboration definition. Available at: https://dictionary.cambridge.org/dictionary/english/collaboration.

Charles, A. (2022). *Integrated care systems explained*. The King's Fund. Available at: https://www-.kingsfund.org.uk/publications/integrated-care-systems-explained. [Accessed 20 March 2023].

Coxon, G. (2017). Health and social care integration for older people. *Nursing in Practice*. 13 June 2017.

Department of Health. (2000). *The NHS Plan: A plan for investment. A plan for reform*. HMSO.

Department of Health. (2009). *Transforming community services: Enabling new patterns of provision*. Transforming Community Services Team, Department of Health.

Department of Health and Social Care. (2008). *High quality care for all: NHS next stage review final report*. Available at: https://www.gov.uk/government/publications/high-quality-care-for-all-nhs-next-stage-review-final-report.

Dunn, P., Fraser, C., Williamson, S., & Alderwick, H. (2022). *Integrated care systems: What do they look like?*. Available at: https://www.health.org.uk/publications/long-reads/integrated-care-systems-what-do-they-look-like. [Accessed 20 March 2023].

Grant Thornton. (2018). *CCGs – the key issues impacting NHS England*. Available at: https://www.grantthornton.co.uk/insights/ccgs-the-key-issues-impacting nhs-england/.

Health and Care Act 2022 c.31 Health and Care Act 2022 (legislation.gov.uk) UK Public General Acts. https://www.legislation.gov.uk/ukpga/2022/31/contents.

Naylor, C., & Charles, A. (2022). *Place-based partnerships explained*. The King's Fund. Available at: https://www.kingsfund.org.uk/publications/place-based-partnerships-explained.

NHS England. (2014). *NHS Five Year Forward View*. Available at: https://www.england.nhs.uk/publication/nhs-five-year-forward-view/.

NHS England. (2019). *The NHS Long Term Plan*. Available at: https://www.longtermplan.nhs.uk/.

NHS England. (2022a). *Understanding integrated care systems for community nurses*. NHS England.

NHS England. (2022b). *Palliative and end of life care*. Available at: https://www.england.nhs.uk/wp-content/uploads/2022/07/Palliative-and-End-of-Life-Care-Statutory-Guidance-for-Integrated-Care-Boards-ICBs-September-2022.pdf.

O'Donnell, J. (2023). *Developing a systems thinking lens for collective leadership*. Collective Leadership for Scotland.

Queen's Nursing Institute. (2014). *2020 Vision 5 years on: Reassessing the future of district Nursing*. Queen's Nursing Institute.

Scobie, S. (2021). *Integrated care explained*. Nuffield Trust. Available at: https://www.nuffieldtrust.org.uk/resource/integrated-care-explained#:~:text=Clinical%20integration%20involves%20the%20coordination,protocols%20across%20boundaries%20of%20care.

The NHS Constitution. (August 2023). https://www.gov.uk/government/publications/the-nhs-constitution-for-england/the-nhs-constitution-for-england.

The Royal College of Nursing and Queen's Nursing Institute. (2019). *Outstanding models of district nursing*. Available at: https://qni.org.uk/explore-qni/policy-campaigns/outstanding-models-of-district-nursing/.

Timmins, N. (2019). *Leading for integrated care*. Available at: https://www.kingsfund.org.uk/sites/default/files/2019-11/leading-integrated-care-summary.pdf.

Wain, L. (2022). Does integrated health and care in community deliver its vision? A workforce perspective. *Journal of Integrated Care*, *29*(2), 170–184 2021.

Wenzel, L., Robertson, R., & Wickens, C. (2023). *What is commissioning and how is it changing?* The King's Fund. Available at: https://www.kingsfund.org.uk/publications/what-commissioning-and-how-it-changing.

CHAPTER 3

Economic Value of Community Nursing

Sifiso Mguni ■ Charlotte Sumnall

LEARNING OUTCOMES

After reading this chapter you should be able to:

- Understand how community nursing services are commissioned
- Appreciate the importance of economic value in community nursing
- Recognise the difference between articulating community nursing value and demonstrating their value

3.1 Introduction

Traditionally, community nursing services have been commissioned based on general practitioner (GP) registered population and block contracts, mainly due to a lack of data and quality metrics. The consequence of this payment method has resulted in providers not being accurately rewarded for the work they undertake. Recently integrated care systems have been formed, which are made up of integrated care partnerships (ICPs) and integrated care boards (ICBs). The ICB is responsible for commissioning most NHS services for their populations to meet local needs, providing the ICBs with an opportunity for a collaborative approach to planning and improving services. It has been acknowledged that commissioning should move towards a population health-based approach, aiming to better tackle health inequalities in their local area (Evans, 2015; Wenzel et al., 2023). This can be achieved through outcome-based commissioning, which focuses on local needs and prevention, centred on what matters to the person through the personalised care agenda.

Community nurses in England account for one-fifth of the total NHS community services workforce yet is often described as the silent workforce, often invisible, misunderstood and work unassumingly (Stevens et al., 2021). The Healthcare Financial Management Association (HFMA, 2022) explains that community nurses struggle to demonstrate value to their system partners and articulate and measure patient outcomes, all presenting a challenge to secure investment into community nursing services.

DEFINITION

Economic value: Professor Robert Kaplan and Professor Michael Porter define value as the outcomes that matter to patients, and the costs of achieving those outcomes frequently referred to as technical value (Fig. 3.1) (Kaplan, 2015).

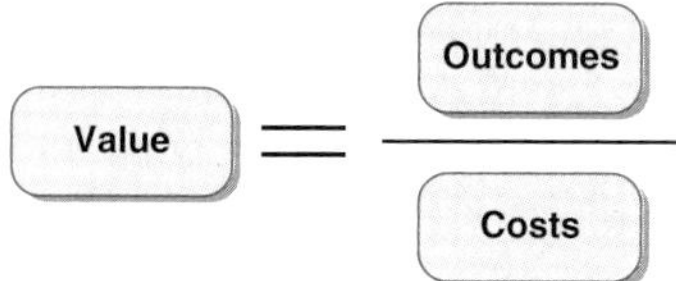

Outcomes are the full set of patient outcomes over the patient pathway
Costs are the total costs of resources used to care for a patient over the patient pathway

Fig. 3.1 The value equation. (From Kaplan, R. (2015). *Costing and the pursuit of value in healthcare.* Healthcare Financial Management Association (HMFA).)

BOX 3.1 ■ Triple Value

Professor Sir Muir Gray describes three dimensions of value:

Personal Value

Improving the outcomes that matter to an individual for a given amount of resources used not only by the health system but also by the individual and their family, recognising that the experience of care is a critical element

Technical Value

Optimising the use of resources to achieve the best possible outcomes for people being treated within a given pathway or process

Population Value

Investing resources more wisely within a health system to optimise the outcomes for the population for which the health system is responsible

(From HFMA (2019) Joint working vital for sustainability. Blog by Professor Sir Muir Gray CBE. Available from https://www.hfma.org.uk/system/files/what-finance-data-is-required-to-drive-value-at-a-population-level.pdf.)

Modern healthcare across the world is struggling to meet the demands of the population shift and is not growing fast enough. Health economists argue that the focus of healthcare needs to shift to value, explaining the triple value elements: personal, technical and population value (Box 3.1). Value-based healthcare focuses on increasing value through the resources available for a specific population group to achieve specific outcomes. Value-based healthcare moves away from the current model which looks at improvements from a quality, safety and productivity perspective (HFMA, 2019).

Consideration is needed on how accessible these value definitions are, what they mean to community nurses and how they affect the services and population they serve. Buffet (2020) suggests quite simply that 'price is what you pay, value is what you get'. Historically, the commissioning of community nursing has not provided a sustainable service, instead having separate funding streams between primary and community care, which has led to a lack of flexibility to shift funding that could support the delivery of care at home (McDermott et al., 2018).

When discussing the value of a service or pathway in healthcare, it is imperative not to just consider the financial costs but to include the impact a service or pathway may have on that population group, including their well-being. Patient outcomes must be measured to evidence other indirect benefits and consequences that those services or pathways provide. Patient outcome measures report a patient's health status or health-related quality of life and they indicate the outcomes or quality of care delivered to NHS patients (Bell, 2023).

According to Jones et al. (2016), clinicians have a responsibility to be economically literate and measure experiences and outcomes, not only asking their patients about their experience of the service but asking how the service has improved their quality of life. The interventions and outcomes will shift the clinician from a task-orientated service towards an outcome-based service with a personalised approach where together the clinician and patient plan their care outcomes. Clinicians working in the community and primary care settings have a proactive and health education approach throughout the patient's journey. They need to better evidence this if they are making the shift of care closer to home, by demonstrating where resources need to be allocated across the NHS to increase proactive, personalised care.

However, an added complexity across community and primary care services is due to patient inequalities and social demographics in how population groups can be better treated and managed, so the importance of measuring patients' outcomes and cost efficiencies for the communities we serve is paramount (Welton & Harper, 2016). This demonstrates the importance for community nurses to have some understanding of economic assessment terminology and the need to evidence innovation, improved performances, productivity and value, demonstrating the benefits of interprofessional working across health and social care. In Box 3.2, some methods of economic assessments are explained.

3.2 Demonstrating the Value of Community Nursing

Community nurses are often focused on clinical tasks and sometimes do not capture all the patient outcomes that could support and further demonstrate their economic value, such as visiting a patient to administer insulin would be the clinical task, however, longer-term outcomes for the patient may include diabetes management, health promotion or psychosocial support, which is not always evidenced. A focus group report (Cummins et al., 2022) highlights that nurses struggled with articulating the nontangible aspects of their job, the psychosocial aspect of the patient's needs that may not necessarily be captured as they document and outcome their visits. The short, medium and long-term economic value of the visit is not always captured or measured in a way that allows their nursing care to be appropriately costed or understood.

As part of an NHS England project with NHS Horizons (Mguni et al., 2023), patient process mapping and personas were designed and developed. A persona is a fictional character created to represent a group of users, typically patients or staff groups. The development of personas involves careful psychographic analysis of data and interviews with users to understand the values, attitudes and beliefs that drive their behaviour. The aim was to encourage and provoke discussion about service provision, supporting teams to identify opportunities for service improvement, articulate the economic value added by community nursing and consider service provision at a system level. Two case studies from the persona's facilitation pack provide an example of how community nurses could demonstrate their value and consider if services meet the needs of our local population (Case Study 3.1 and Case Study 3.2).

CASE STUDY 3.1 Part 1

Bob has advanced dementia and lives with his wife Anne, who is his main carer. Bob has bouts of confusion and distress and has an indwelling catheter which is supported by his local community nursing team. Anne has an extensive mental health history and is known to the mental health team as having a history of suicidal thoughts. Bob has an advanced care plan which expressed his wishes to live and die at home, and specifically stating his and Anne's wish to live together in their own home, and for Anne to be given the additional support she needs when Bob can no longer support her.

Questions to consider:

- How would we assess the impact on Anne?
- How can we avoid hospital admission for Bob in the future?
- How closely do our services communicate about patients who are also carers like Anne?
- What charity or voluntary services do you have in your locality to support Anne as Bob's carer?

BOX 3.2 ■ Methods of Economic Assessments

- Cost–benefit analysis

Compares the costs and benefits of an intervention, where both are expressed in monetary units.

- Cost-effectiveness analysis

Examines both the costs and health outcomes of one or more interventions. It compares an intervention to another intervention (or the status quo) by estimating how much it costs to gain a unit of a health outcome, like a life year gained or a death prevented.

- Cost utility analysis

Is one type of economic evaluation that can help you compare the costs and effects of alternative interventions. Cost utility analysis measures health effects in terms of both quantity (life years) and quality of life.

- Cost minimisation analysis

A financial strategy that aims to achieve the most cost-effective way of delivering goods and services to the required level of quality. It is important to remember that cost minimisation is not about reducing quality or short-changing customers; it always remains important to meet customer needs.

- Cost-consequence analysis

This is a form of economic evaluation in which the outcomes (of which a variety of measures are normally presented) are reported separately from costs.

- Cost-avoidance analysis

The preservation of existing spending to prevent price increases due to inflation, economics or the rising costs of products or services. An example of cost avoidance is when a company purchases an extended equipment warranty to limit maintenance costs or out-of-pocket expenses.

- Social return on investment (SROI)

SROI is a method for measuring values that are not traditionally reflected in financial statements, including social, economic and environmental factors. They can identify how effectively a company uses its capital and other resources to create value for the community. SROI is a systematic way of incorporating social, environmental, economic and other values into decision-making processes.

- Cost feasibility

Analysis compares total cost to available budget; no direct assessment of effectiveness.

(From Turner, H.C., Archer, R.A., Downey, L.E., Isaranuwatchai, W., Chalkidou, K., Jit, M. and Teerawattananon, Y. (2021). An introduction to the main types of economic evaluations used for informing priority setting and resource allocation in healthcare: Key features, uses, and limitations. *Frontiers in Public Health*, 9.)

The true art of community nursing is having a good understanding of not only your patients but all the psychosocial aspects of their daily lives, thus demonstrating the importance of not only 'what matters to me' but what may impact their wider family, friends and support system (NHS England, 2023).

CASE STUDY 3.1 Part 2

Six months later:

Bob's dementia has advanced. Anne now takes care of Bob all day, expressing that she manages ok, but can no longer leave him alone at home, making it difficult to get to the shops and see her friends. Anne demonstrates her fear during the winter months, that one of them may become unwell and be admitted into hospital, more importantly feeling scared one of them may not come home if admitted.

Questions to consider:

- If Bob developed a urinary infection, how could this be managed at home?
- What would be the impact on Anne's mental health as Bob was her main carer previously?
- How would an advanced care plan be established and shared between services for a patient like Bob; are there clear roles and responsibilities in how this information is shared?

This case study (Case Study 3.1) demonstrates how community nurses can support the Ageing Well at home agenda, and if patients are supported appropriately at home, they can avoid hospital admissions (NHS England, 2019). To generate more funding, community nurses need to be able to articulate their value and expertise in new and existing patient pathways and services. This should include evidence of patient-reported outcome measures, where the quality of life and respecting the wishes of patients and their families are paramount for good quality community nursing services. To demonstrate the value of patient pathways such as hospital avoidance with virtual wards or urgent community response services, it is important to provide patient case studies that can show commissioners and ICB leaders examples of where the service has had a direct impact. This should address how community nurses can support patients appropriately at home to avoid hospital admissions and hospital deconditioning as well as enabling the Ageing Well at home agenda by bringing together other services that support patients.

The RCN's (2020) Demonstrating Value programme has supported frontline clinicians with the skills, tools and techniques to secure funding and support ongoing development for their service. They show how the principles of economic assessments can be implemented to demonstrate value. For example, a childhood bereavement support service was able to evidence the short, medium and long-term impacts of bereavement, and how the service could mitigate the negative outcomes through providing early intervention; the economic assessment method they used was cost-avoidance analysis, which looked at avoided spend, not a decreased spend.

Community nurses are able to provide continuity of care, which is essential for patients, as they can build trust, rapport and relationships with them; having consistency means they do not need to keep repeating their story or health needs to different teams. However, the importance of district nurses should be highlighted, as they have a thorough understanding of particular health conditions and have expert knowledge (HealthWatch, 2022). District nurses and specialist nurses working in the community could be better integrated and joined up across the NHS and other independent providers, such as hospices, to enable a more holistic and personalised care approach to providing care in the community.

CASE STUDY 3.2

Yolanda has been receiving treatment for metastatic breast cancer but has recently declined further treatment in favour of palliative care. She lives with her son Kofi and partner Gareth. District nurses provide support visits for her central venous line during treatment and will maintain visits as her diagnosis becomes palliative.

Questions to consider:

- How joined up are your cancer services to coordinate Yolanda's care?
- How might Yolanda's needs evolve over time and how would your provider respond?
- What funding might be available to Yolanda and how could your provider support her in applying for and making use of the funding?

3.3 Patient-Reported Outcomes in Community Nursing

Use of patient-reported outcomes is not a new concept, yet it is often not utilised in adult nursing, particularly District nursing in the community. The Cummins et al. (2022) report described how children's and palliative care services are more likely to discuss patient-reported outcomes measures, patient-reported experience measures and quality of life measures; however, those outcome measures were not always documented in the patient's electronic records, therefore demonstrating those impacts remains a challenge. The report demonstrated how across mental health services, these methods are used frequently as they might be the only way to measure or demonstrate impact and improved outcomes for their patients. A person's physical illness is not always in isolation, frequently, there are mental and psychological challenges and multiple long-term conditions. A person needs to be assessed from a holistic approach, and not only the patient's health and well-being should be measured, but also the impact the service has had on their personal experience and improved quality of life. An example of this would be to review the outcome measure for a patient who is at the end of their life; the outcome is not the reversal of death but the patient and family feeling that they were well supported in the journey. The measure of effective care would need to be measured on outcome measures looking at experience and quality of life even if death was the expected outcome.

District nurses who are better skilled and trained with improved economic literacy can use those skills to improve how they measure outcomes in care as well as carry out community needs assessments and more importantly that these outcomes are linked to the commissioning of services. This will ensure that community nurses are able to demonstrate their value through improved business cases and strategy planning for community services. Improved patient-reported outcome measures will provide credible evidence and help all relevant stakeholders comprehend the complexity of district nursing services (Skinner, 2018).

3.4 Conclusion

The current changes across the NHS are bringing forward a renewed focus on community nursing and care closer to home as well as greater investment in community services. It is therefore crucial that economic evaluations provide evidence of the impact of interventions and models of care, comparing both cost and patient outcomes. Community nurses must demonstrate the benefits of their speciality by identifying and capturing outcomes using different approaches. By investing in community nursing, policymakers, healthcare organisations and communities can create a more sustainable and economically resilient healthcare system that prioritises preventive care, improves health outcomes and enhances overall well-being.

References

Bell, G. (2023). *Patient reported outcome measures (PROMs)*. NHS England.

Buffet, W. (2020). Price is what you pay, value is what you get. *The Escape Artist*.

Cummins, L., Ettinger, J., Ricci-Pacifici, L., Mguni, S., & Sumnall, C. (2022). *Understanding and articulating the 'economic value' of community nursing*. Health Economics Unit and NHS England.

Evans, K. (2015). *Framework for commissioning community nursing*. NHS England. https://www.england.nhs.uk/wp-content/uploads/2015/10/Framework-for-commissioning-community-nursing.pdf.

HealthWatch. (2022). *Value of community nursing: engagement with patients, carers and families across the east of England*. HealthWatch & NHS England. Available from https://www.healthwatchbedfordborough.co.uk/sites/healthwatchbedfordborough.co.uk/files/East%20of%20England%20Community%20Nursing%20Engagement%20Report%20FINAL_0.pdf.

HFMA. (2019). Joint working vital for sustainability. *Blog by Professor Sir Muir Gray CBE*. Available from https://www.hfma.org.uk/system/files/what-finance-data-is-required-to-drive-value-at-a-population-level.pdf.

HFMA. (2022). *Measuring the Economic Value of Community Nursing: Scoping the Challenge*. Healthcare Financial Management Association (HMFA).

Jones, T. L. (2016). What nurses do during time scarcity—and why. *The Journal of Nursing Administration*, *46*(9), 449–454.

Kaplan, R. (2015). *Costing and the pursuit of value in healthcare*. Healthcare Financial Management Association (HMFA).

McDermott, I., Warwick-Giles, L., Gore, O., Moran, V., Bramwell, D., Coleman, A., & Checkland, K. (2018). Understanding primary care co-commissioning: Uptake, development, and impacts. *Final report. PRUComm*. https://prucomm.ac.uk/assets/uploads/blog/2018/03/PCCC-final-report-v11-final.pdf.

Mguni, S., Sumnall, C., Sheilds, C., & Johal, R. (2023). *Community currencies. Personas. Facilitation pack*. NHS Horizons. Available from: https://horizonsnhs.com/programmes-ofwork/personas/#:~:text=What%20are%20personas%3F,beliefs%20that%20drive%20their%20behaviour.

NHS England. (2019). *NHS long term plan*. NHS England. Available at: https://www.longterm-plan.nhs.uk/.

NHS England. (2023). *Personalised care*. NHS England. Available from: https://www.england.nhs.uk/personalisedcare/.

RCN. (2020). *Case studies demonstrating the value of nursing*. Royal College of Nursing. Available from: https://www.rcn.org.uk/Professional-Development/research-and-innovation/Innovation-in-nursing/Case-studies-demonstrating-the-value-of-nursing.

Skinner, R. (2018). *Quality impact assessment policy*. NHS Herefordshire & Worcestershire CCG.

Stevens, E., Price, E., & Walker, E. (2021). Making the mundane remarkable: An ethnography of the 'dignity encounter' in community district nursing. *Ageing and Society*, *1*(23).

Turner, H. C., Archer, R. A., Downey, L. E., Isaranuwatchai, W., Chalkidou, K., Jit, M., et al. (2021). An introduction to the main types of economic evaluations used for informing priority setting and resource allocation in healthcare: Key features, uses, and limitations. *Frontiers in Public Health*, 9:722927.

Welton, J., & Harper, E. (2016). Measuring nursing care value. *Nursing Economics*, *34*(1), 7–14.

Wenzel, L., Robertson, R., & Wickens, C. (2023). *What is commissioning and how is it changing*. King's Fund.

CHAPTER 4

Autonomous Practice and Safe Ways of Working Alone

Cliff Kilgore ■ Rob Taylor-Ball

LEARNING OUTCOMES

After reading this chapter you should be able to:

- Understand the skill of autonomous practice
- Recognise the link between the ability to think critically, analyse complex situations and solve problems autonomously
- Comprehend safe ways of working alone, particularly in a community setting

4.1 Introduction

Community nurses are an integral part of the NHS workforce and are key to delivering the ambition to increase care in the community; the success of the NHS Long Term Plan (2019) depends on strong community nursing. Their expert leadership, clinical skills and knowledge enable them to support people in managing their health needs and maximise independence.

Throughout this chapter, consideration will be given to understanding autonomy as a skill and exploring safe ways of working alone.

4.2 Autonomous Practice as a Skill

Professional autonomy in nursing means having the freedom and authority to make decisions within the practitioner's own knowledge (Pursio et al., 2021). Understanding autonomy is an important factor within community nursing as the nurse is often required to take charge in situations where they are responsible. However, autonomous practice is something that needs to be developed over time and may require the community nurse to develop different levels of autonomy through continuous professional development.

There is a need for community nurses to have confidence in their ability during clinical interventions and to focus learning on obtaining clinical acumen. This enables a nurse to develop autonomous practice as a skill that takes them beyond standard practice and empowers a community nurse to make decisions regarding a patient's care without direct supervision or oversight (Oshodi et al., 2019). This development occurs over time with the advancement of critical thinking but can be enhanced with additional skills and knowledge.

4.3 Autonomy and Critical Thinking Skills

The drive for evidence-based practice has increased the need to understand decision-making in healthcare (Majid et al., 2011). In addition to this, clinical practice has evolved with the expectation that a nurse should have the knowledge and experience to correctly identify patient problems and make appropriate decisions that may affect an older patient's well-being (Wolf, 2012). This is more evident in community nursing where the nurse will likely be isolated from colleagues.

Nurses make decisions about patient care every day but probably do not think too much about the complex processes that result in appropriate conclusions. Rutter and Brown (2013) suggest that appraising the situation through standards of analysis is important, but judgment also plays a part. The deductive argument says that a premise is only acceptable if the judgment can be adequately defended. In practice, this means reaching a conclusion that has a good argument, can be supported by expert views and does not contradict the evidence. Many nurses are aware of evidence-based practice and would consider this the cornerstone of their practice. However, it is the idea that evidence-based practice and critical thinking are so closely related that they are most crucial for any patient intervention thus suggesting that critical thinking is based on sound knowledge and learning gained through education (Bate et al., 2012). Therefore developing critical thinking helps to build clinical autonomy, which leads to enhanced patient care and subsequently to greater professional satisfaction.

Decision-making in nursing is seen as a fundamental part of clinical care and some regard 'gut feeling' or 'intuition' as an important part of this. However, realising that this inner knowledge, aided by evidence and education, is part of critical thinking may help nurses to recognise what they do as credible in a very scientific world. Furthermore, the practice of critical thinking should be encouraged to provide excellent care and improve patient well-being (Coutts, 2014).

REFLECTION

- Take a few minutes to think of a patient you have seen during a nursing visit.
- What helped you to make the right decisions for this patient's care?
- Did you learn anything about how the consultation went and has it made you think about how you would act next time?

4.4 Working Within One's Sphere of Knowledge

There are other considerations for a nurse working alone. Duty of care in nursing is an obligation to act towards patients in a certain way, following set standards both professionally and legally (Duncan, 2019). As registered professionals, community nurses are judged against the Nursing and Midwifery Council (NMC) (2018) Code of Conduct and are expected to act in a way that if tested against a body of professional opinion in situations where it is 'reasonably foreseeable' that the practitioner might cause harm through actions or omissions (Duncan, 2019). The nurse entering a patient's home to undertake an assessment or intervention needs to consider the patient's condition and the risk that condition might present to the person.

Patients who are seen in a community setting often present with conditions with increased risk factors such as long-term pain that can lead to falls (Cai et al., 2021), as well as other comorbidities that can be present in aging. There is an aim that nurses should provide competent care and clinical decision-making that safeguards a patient and leads to positive outcomes (Perez et al., 2014). This brings us back to the earlier discussions in this chapter regarding levels of autonomy and the need to ensure the nurse possesses a level of understanding of a patient's medical history and how this may affect any clinical treatments offered by the nurse. There will be times when a community nurse is required to ask for help from a district nurse, a more senior nurse or from another healthcare professional with a different set of skills and knowledge. Recognising limitations of knowledge is necessary to prevent unnecessary risk to patient care and is part of the NMC (2018) Code of Conduct.

REFLECTION

- Think of a time when you had to call another professional for advice on patient care.
- Did it provide the right outcome for the patient?
- If anything, what would have helped further for your patient?

4.5 Significant Developments in Nursing Autonomy

Although not available to all community nurses, the development of prescribing in nursing has led to a substantial increase in nursing autonomy. Following a change to legislation to enable nurses to prescribe, it was community nursing that was seen to lead the way (Rodden, 2001), prescribing is now a core component of many district nursing programmes and has led to greater autonomy of practice for many nurses working in a community setting.

Since the initial introduction of nurse prescribing, there have been further developments which have included independent prescribing and widening prescribing to some allied healthcare professionals. There is evidence in the literature that there is both patient and clinician satisfaction with nurse prescribing. Moreover, when nurses develop confidence in prescribing practice, it leads to greater autonomy and better patient outcomes (Chater et al., 2019).

4.6 Work-Based Pressures

There are always potential added pressures on nursing teams based on financial challenges, staffing levels, demands of workload and patient complexity (The King's Fund, 2022). This may present risks in practice, leading to safety being neglected at times of team pressure or requiring nurses and their team leaders to highlight increased risks to operational managers within an organisation (Duncan, 2019).

Some patients are seen in their own homes with little information and without knowing who else may be in their home. Therefore there is a need to always assess the risks when entering a patient's home and to mitigate or manage these risks. This might even include seeking guidance from a senior colleague or manager. To do this, there is a need to ensure adequate training for community nurses by employers to ensure they can manage this complex skill (Duncan, 2019). Nurses also have responsibilities for their own safety at work and it is important that community nurses understand that they should not undertake work that is not safe.

4.7 Recognising Safety in the Patient's Home

Community nursing could be described as a series of brief interventions either as single episodes of care or over multiple interactions with an individual patient. Because of the brief nature of interventions, there is a need for the community nurse to develop skills of self-efficacy and decision-making in order to provide the necessary nursing care to a person whom they may only see once (Chan et al., 2013).

Safe working environments are a cornerstone of nursing practice with community nurses facing unique challenges and dangers of working outside the safety of ward-based care (Flaubert et al., 2021). To enable good clinical care, that is delivered in a safe and effective setting, the nurse needs to understand 'what is safety' and to consider the circumstances they are working in. It is not just a personal consideration, but that of those around them and those who might enter the working environment. As a nurse providing essential care, it is crucial to promote and work in a safe and secure environment for the nurse, their patient and any carer or family member.

Challenges related to patient safety in the home are wide-ranging and include fragmentation of care, household hazards, ill-prepared family caregivers, limited training and regulation of home care workers, along with inadequate communication among patients, caregivers and providers. What is needed is to reevaluate decision-making around 'the right place, and right time'.

4.8 Managing Risks and Risk Assessment at Work

Prior to any clinical intervention, there is a need for the community nurse to have comprehensive assessment skills in identifying and recognising hazards and potential dangers (Table 4.1) (Tella et al., 2020).

Recognising and acting on safety as a community nurse are essential to protect both the nurse and the individual they serve. The nurse must always prioritise personal safety (RCN, 2022). By recognising potential risks, implementing preventative measures and promptly addressing any concerns that arise, community nurses can contribute to a safer environment for both themselves and their patients. Remember that specific safety considerations vary based on individual patient needs and their home environment.

Community nurses carry out a huge range of vital work with patients every day. For each home visit, it is important for a community nurse to carry out a dynamic risk assessment (RCN, 2023). Doing so allows the nurse to quickly assess a situation and take the necessary steps to remain safe. If it is the first time visiting the patient, the nurse must ensure that they have all the necessary information regarding the patient. Increasingly, technologies such as lone working apps that will log the location of the nurse, are being used as a safe tool for the protection of community staff. The Code (NMC, 2018) requires each nurse to balance risks in relation to the people they care for with their own safety. The nurse must consider other ways of delivering safe care and they may need to refuse to provide care because it is not safe to do so. The Employment Rights Act (1996) provides protection against detriment or dismissal if the nurse refuses to provide care because they believe there is a serious and imminent danger that they could not reasonably be expected to avoid.

TABLE 4.1 ■ **Points to Consider**

• Is the door locked behind you?
• Are you aware of any cognitive concerns of your patient?
• Are there any medical conditions that may increase the risk of accidents or injury to you or your patient?
• Do your colleagues know where you are?
• Is there adequate lighting?
• Do you have proper access to hand washing facilities?

CASE STUDY 4.1

Ola Yemi is a community nurse who has been in post for 4 years. It is a dark and wet afternoon when she visits Mary at her home to follow up on a previous wound. Mary lives on the fifth floor of a block of flats and Ola Yemi must take a lift to the front door. At some point during the consultation, Mary's son who has come to visit starts asking questions about why his mum's wound is not healing. Ola Yemi explains that the healing process can take a few weeks. Mary's son then starts to become confrontational saying that it is the nurse's fault that the wound is not improving.

Ola Yemi starts to feel unsafe and threatened.

Points to consider:

- Could Ola Yemi make a quick exit?
- Do her colleagues know where she is?
- Does she have a lone working device?
- Could she contact someone senior for support?

4.9 Duty of Care

Duty of care is a legal responsibility to provide care to a reasonable standard and to keep patients safe. Each employer has a primary duty of care and must do what is reasonably practicable to ensure the health and safety of their workers and others at the workplace, such as patients (HSE, 1974). All staff should expect to work within organisations which enable individuals to deliver safe and appropriate care in accordance with regulatory and professional standards.

Staff have a duty of care to:

- Take reasonable care for their own health and safety
- Be aware of different country laws and standards
- Take reasonable care that they do not adversely affect the health and safety of others
- Work according to health and safety instructions and co-operate with the employer's policies and procedures.

4.10 Conclusion

Community nursing has long been associated with lone working and a level of autonomy that is different from that seen in hospital-based care. This chapter has explained autonomy as a skill and considered how critical thinking helps with the development of community nursing practice. As development is cumulative and knowledge is gained through education and experience, it is important for nurses to work within their scope of practice and always adhere to the NMC code of practice. With increasing demands in clinical practice, the community nurse needs to ensure they recognise risks and manage these personally and through organisational policy. This is particularly important as many patients are seen briefly and therefore self-assurance and a high level of decision-making are often necessary.

References

Bate, L., Hutchinson, A., Underhill, J., & Maskrey, N. (2012). How clinical decisions are made. *British Journal of Clinical Pharmacology*, 74(4), 614–620.

Cai, Y., Leveille, S. G., Shi, L., Chen, P., & You, T. (2021). Chronic pain and risk of injurious falls in community dwelling older adults. *The Gerontological Society of America*, *76*, 9.

Chan, B. C., Jayasinghe, U. W., Christi, B., Laws, R. A., Orr, N., Williams, A., et al. (2013). The impact of a team based intervention on the lifestyle risk factor management practices of community nursing SNAP trial. *Biomedical Chromatography*, *13*, 54.

Chater, A. M., Williams, J., & Courtenay, M. (2019). The prescribing needs of community practitioner nurse prescribers: A qualitative investigation using the theoretical domains framework and COM-B. *Journal of Advanced Nursing*, *75*, 11.

Coutts, B. (2014). The complex decision making needed in significant event analysis. *Primary Healthcare*, *24*(2), 26–30.

Duncan, M. (2019). Employers' duty of care to district nursing team members: Health and safety concerns with lone domiciliary visits. *British Journal of Community Nursing*, *24*, 8.

Flaubert, J. L., Le Menestrel, S., & Williams, D. R. (2021). *The future of nursing 2020–2030: Charting a path to achieve health equity*. National Academies Press (US).

Health and Safety at Work etc. Act 1974, Section 2.

Majid, S., Foo, S., Luyt, B., Zhang, X., Theng, Y., Chang, Y., et al. (2011). Adopting evidence-based practice in clinical decision making: Nurses' perceptions, knowledge, and barriers. *Journal of Medical Library Association*, *99*(3), 229–236.

Nursing and Midwifery Council. (2018). *The code: Professional standards of practice and behaviour for nurses, midwives and nursing associates*. https://www.google.co.uk/url?sa=t&rct=j&q=&esrc=s&source=web&cd=&ved=2ahUKEwiunc3vkoaHAxW2Z0EAHdBHBbgQjBB6BAglEAE&url=https%3A%2F%2Fwww.nmc.org.uk%2Fstandards%2Fcode%2Fread-the-code-online%2F&usg=AOvVaw2Qw1LPcFHDMKKtfgMWWJPB&opi=89978449.

Oshodi, T., Bruneau, B., Crockett, R., Kinchington, F., Nayar, S., & West, E. (2019). Registered nurses' perceptions and experiences of autonomy: A descriptive phenomenological study. *BMC Nursing*, *18*, 51. https://doi.org/10.1186/s12912-019-0378-3. [Accessed 26 June 2023].

Perez, E. Z., Canut, M. T. L., Pegueroles, A. F., Llobet, M. P., Arroyo, C. M., & Merino, J. R. (2014). Critical thinking in nursing: Scoping review of the literature. *International Journal of Nursing Practice*, *21*.

Pursio, K., Kankkunen, P., Sanner-Stier-Stiehr, E., & Kvist, T. (2021). Professional autonomy in nursing: An integrative review. *Journal of Nursing Management*, *29*, 1565–1577.

Rodden, C. (2001). Nurse prescribing: Views on autonomy and independence. *British Journal of Community Nursing*, *6*, 7.

Royal College of Nursing. (2022). *Prioritising personal safety*. [Accessed 10 July 2023].

Royal College of Nursing. (2023). *Prioritising personal safety. Advice guides*. Royal College of Nursing. https://www.rcn.org.uk/Get-Help/RCN-advice/prioritising-personal-safety. [Accessed 13 September 2023].

Rutter, L., & Brown, K. (2013). Critical thinking at the bedside: Providing safe passage to patients. *Medsurg Nursing*, 22(2), 85–94.

Tella, S., Vaismoradi, M., Logan, P., Khakurel, J., & Vizcaya-Moreno, F. (2020). Nurses' adherence to patient safety principles: A systematic review. *International Journal of Environmental Research in Public Health*, *17*(6), 2028.

The Kings Fund (2022). The NHS Staff Survey, what do the results tell us. https://www.kingsfund.org.uk/insight-and-analysis/blogs/nhs-staff-survey-2022-results. (Accessed 01 July 2024).

Wolf, L. (2012). An integrated, ethically driven environmental model of clinical decision making in emergency settings. *International Journal of Nursing Practice*, 24(1), 49–53.

CHAPTER 5

Infection Prevention and Control in the Community

Helen Bosley ■ Gabbie Parham

LEARNING OUTCOMES

After reading this chapter you should be able to:

- Understand the fundamentals of infection control practice in the community
- Appreciate how to implement the principles of infection control in different environments in a person's own home
- Identify where to access appropriate and evidence-based information to facilitate best practice

5.1 Introduction

The incidence and prevalence of healthcare-associated infection (HCAI), especially those caused by antimicrobial-resistant microorganisms, have increased over recent years and are a serious concern for patient health and safety (Guest et al., 2020). HCAIs are defined as infections that were not present prior to a patient entering that care setting (World Health Organization (WHO), 2018). These infections can develop from contact with a health or social care setting or as a direct result of healthcare treatment (National Institute for Health and Care Excellence (NICE), 2017a).

It is estimated that HCAIs are the most common adverse event to occur, regardless of resources, in any healthcare system (WHO, 2011). The impact for patients who acquire HCAIs may include increased hospital stays, complex treatments (extended antibiotic treatments), ability to work (finance), possible complications to existing underlying long-term health comorbidities and ultimately death (WHO, 2011). A recent review of the annual National Health Service (NHS) costs and outcomes attributable to HCAIs has estimated there were 834,000 HCAIs, associated with 28,500 patient deaths, resulting in costs to the NHS of £2.7 billion (Guest et al., 2020).

5.2 Background

The majority of healthcare interventions occur in the community (Royal College of Nursing (RCN) and Queens Nursing Institute (QNI), 2019), and maintaining and delivering patient care within the home and the community remain a priority for the NHS. Providing good infection prevention and control (IPC) practice is a keystone for the delivery of safe patient care and reduces the risks of HCAIs developing. It is important to acknowledge that the existing HCAI data are based predominantly within the hospital settings. Community cases of mandatory reportable infections such as bloodstream infections or *Clostridioides difficile* infections are reported, however, this is not comprehensive for all potential HCAIs. This means the community prevalence of potentially infectious pathogenic (virus, bacteria or fungi) and multidrug-resistant microorganisms is unknown.

REFLECTION

- Why might people on the District Nursing caseload be more susceptible to infection?

The ability of the body to respond to infection declines progressively with age (Weltevrede et al., 2016), and this means older people on the District Nursing caseload will be more susceptible to the risk of infection. This patient group is also more likely to be living with long-term medical conditions and comorbidities including cardiovascular disease, diabetes, renal disease and respiratory disease such as chronic obstructive pulmonary disease (COPD). They may also be undergoing treatments or taking medications that affect their immune system, such as chemotherapy for cancer or disease modifying drugs (DMDs) for autoimmune conditions.

REFLECTION

- What are the ways that microorganisms could be transmitted in District Nursing practice?

Microorganisms can be transferred in several ways. These include via blood and other body fluids, secretions or excretions, nonintact skin or mucous membranes, any equipment or items that could have become contaminated, and the environment itself if it is not effectively cleaned and maintained appropriately (Otter et al., 2013). However, primary transmission is usually related to poor hand hygiene and inadequate decontamination of equipment/environment (Lee et al., 2020). This results in clinical staff acting as potential vectors for microorganism transmission.

In order to ensure patient safety and protect patients from potential life-threatening infections, correct application of IPC practices is vital (RCN, 2017) and additional resources to support IPC practice are available for staff to access (Loveday et al., 2014; NICE, 2017a; RCN, 2017). However, it is important to acknowledge that there are multiple challenges to delivering good IPC care within the patient's environment.

REFLECTION

- What types of environment is District Nursing care delivered in?
- What might be the challenges to delivering good IPC care in a patient's own home?

Some District Nursing care may be delivered in clinic settings or care homes, which should comply with legislative infection control environmental standards. Care homes offer shared living space and residents will be living close to each other. The risk of HCAIs is increased by a cohorted vulnerable, largely older population, often with existing comorbidities with lowered immunity, and sharing the same environment (Cousins, 2014).

5.3 Infection Prevention and Control in District Nursing Practice

5.3.1 STANDARD PRECAUTIONS

To manage the risk posed by the transmission of potentially pathogenic microorganisms, there are basic or standard infection prevention and control (IPC) precautions that can

TABLE 5.1 ■ **10 Elements of Standard Precautions**

1.	Patient placement
2.	Hand hygiene
3.	Respiratory and cough hygiene
4.	Personal protective equipment
5.	Safe management of the care environment
6.	Safe management of care equipment
7.	Safe management of healthcare linen
8.	Safe management of blood and body fluids
9.	Safe disposal of waste (including sharps)
10.	Occupational safety/managing prevention of exposure (including sharps)

(From National Infection Prevention Control Manual (NIPCM) (NHS England. (2022a). National Infection Prevention and Control Manual (NIPCM) for England. London. Retrieved from https://www.england.nhs.uk/national-infection-prevention-and-control-manual-nipcm-for-england/.)

be used. These are applicable to all care settings and should be always practiced. Possible sources of microorganisms (infection) include blood and body fluids (blood-borne viruses), contact with a contaminated environment or item of equipment and contact with unclean hands (staff). There are 10 elements of standard precautions (Table 5.1).

These precautions can be utilised based on a patient risk assessment and may not be applicable in some environments.

ACTIVITY

- Name five sources of infection transmission that are commonly experienced in District Nursing practice.

Some examples of standard precautions within a community setting are provided in Table 5.2.

5.3.2 HAND HYGIENE

Effective hand hygiene is vital in reducing the risk of HCAIs and guidance on the five moments of hand hygiene (WHO, 2009) have identified the key moments hands must be cleaned (see Fig. 5.1).

These are:

1. Before touching a patient
2. Before clean/aseptic procedures
3. After body fluid exposure/risk
4. After touching a patient
5. After touching patient surroundings

Hand washing with soap and water is required where there has been skin contact with organic material (e.g., body fluids). However, sinks, hand towels and soap will be of variable hygiene standards depending on the home. Therefore it is important to ensure that community nurses, if possible, carry their own portable hand hygiene bags, containing

TABLE 5.2 **Examples of Standard-Based Precautions**

Transmission via	Examples of District Nursing Care Where Transmission Could Occur	IPC Measures to Avoid Transmission Based on Standard and Transmission-Based Precautions (NHS England, 2022a)
Blood	Venous blood samples Intravenous lines Open wounds that are bleeding Capillary blood sampling (e.g. glucose)	Hand hygiene PPE (personal protective equipment) ANTT (aseptic nontouch technique) Safer sharps
Urine	Catheterisation—indwelling and intermittent Incontinence	Hand hygiene PPE ANTT Good continence assessment, treatment and, if required, appropriate products to manage intractable incontinence
Faeces	Bowel care Incontinence	Hand hygiene PPE Good continence assessment, treatment and, if required, appropriate products to manage intractable incontinence
Wounds	Pressure ulcers Leg ulcers Surgical wounds Lacerations Burns	Hand hygiene PPE ANTT
Mucous membranes	Eye care (e.g. eye drops) Vaginal pessary insertion	Hand hygiene PPE ANTT
Equipment	Glucometers Doppler equipment Dressings Catheters	Hand hygiene PPE ANTT Decontamination of equipment Correct storage of sterile appliances Ensuring sterile appliances are in date
Environment	Pets Personal care issues Household cleanliness issues Lack of laundry facilities Poorly managed incontinence	Hand hygiene PPE Working in partnership with the person Giving advice, support and onward signposting/referrals as needed for additional support with personal care, household functioning

IPC, Infection prevention and control.

liquid soap, paper towels, hand cream and alcohol gel. If the community nurse does not carry a hand hygiene bag, then as a minimum, they must ensure they carry alcohol gel dispensers which can be easily used and are readily available. If physical hand washing is required, washing up liquid and kitchen paper towels can be used, and hands cleaned with alcohol gel afterwards. However, it is better to carry a hand hygiene bag as some detergents, such as washing up liquid, are drying to the skin and may cause dermatitis (Angelova-Fischer et al., 2014).

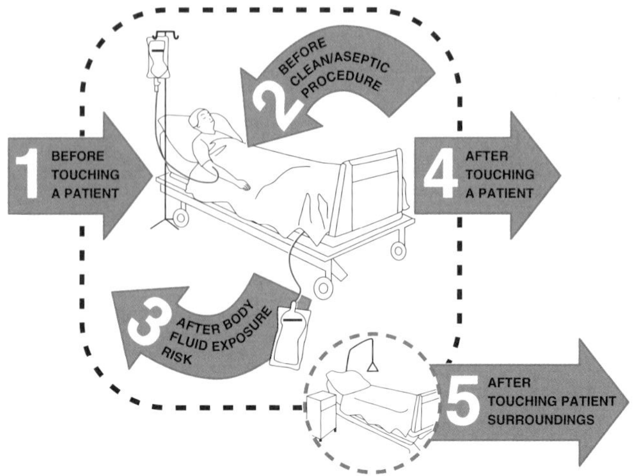

Fig. 5.1 Five moments for hand hygiene. (From World Health Organization: About SAVE Lives: Clean Your Hands: 5 moments for hand hygiene, 2017, https://www.who.int/multi-media/details/your-5-moments-for-hand-hygiene-poster.)

Fingernails may also be a source of microorganism transmission (NICE, 2017a); therefore when delivering clinical care, staff should:

- Be bare below the elbows, including no jewellery or watches (except one plain ring)
- Have short clean nails
- Have no false or painted nails

Hand hygiene audits should be performed regularly, according to the employing organisation's audit schedule, to check hand hygiene techniques are effective. Portable 'light boxes' are available that can be transported to community nursing bases for this purpose.

5.3.3 PERSONAL PROTECTIVE EQUIPMENT

The NHS accounts for around 5% of carbon emissions in England (NHS England, 2022c). In 2020, the NHS became the world's first health service to commit to reaching carbon net zero, in response to the profound and growing threat to health posed by climate change (for more information: www.england.nhs.uk/greenernhs/). Effective IPC for patients staff and the environmental impact needs to be balanced, and unnecessary use of personal protective equipment (PPE) is harmful to patients, healthcare staff, the environment and has a financial impact.

PPE is used to prevent transmission of potentially pathogenic microorganisms and should always be available to community nurses in their stock bags. PPE consists of disposable gloves, plastic aprons, facemasks and eye protection (shield or goggles). The decisions as to what PPE to use is based on assessment, and standard or transmission-based precautions need to be followed (NHS England, 2022a).

The RCN has a risk assessment toolkit around COVID-19 which guides employers and staff in identifying the appropriate use of PPE through assessment of the infection risks involved in procedures and environments. The RCN also runs a Glove Awareness Week annually to encourage appropriate glove use by raising awareness of sustainability factors and the importance of good skin health. Inappropriate use of gloves can increase the risk of dermatitis and an RCN survey published in 2020 showed that 93% of nurses had reported at least one symptom of hand dermatitis in the previous year.

Gloves need to be worn when the nurse is in contact with blood or body fluids, non-intact skin, mucous membranes and harmful drugs or chemicals, changing them for different procedures with the same patient and between patients. The changing of PPE equipment (particularly gloves) is defined by the nursing care being given, in relation to the aseptic nontouch technique (ANTT) principles.

In a standard situation, when providing hands-on nursing care, a plastic apron will largely prevent body fluids from contaminating clothing, and disposable gloves will prevent body fluids from contaminating hands.

In the event of transmissible infection outbreaks or pandemics, facemasks and eye protection may be needed in addition to protect both patients and nurses. National guidance should be followed and communicated clearly in these circumstances.

REFLECTION

- Think about your use of sterile gloves. Are you only using them when necessary? Are there circumstances where you could safely not wear gloves instead?

5.3.4 WASTE MANAGEMENT

Greener NHS principles also come into consideration when thinking about healthcare waste. Preventing waste in the first instance is key and disposal into correct waste streams thereafter is important (NHS England, 2022b).

When patients are treated at home by a community nurse, any waste produced as a result is considered as healthcare waste. If the waste is nonhazardous, it is acceptable for the waste to be disposed of with household waste (landfill). This is usually the case with noninfectious used dressings, urinary catheters and continence pads when they originate from a noninfectious person. When assessing whether the healthcare waste should be classed as infectious or not, consideration must be given to the medical history of the patient and any clinical signs and symptoms indicating a potential infectious risk, at the time the waste is generated (NHS England, 2022b).

Healthcare waste should be treated and disposed of as infectious if it has come from a patient with a known infection, from someone being treated for infection, or from contact with a patient with a transmissible disease (NHS England, 2022b).

If the waste is infectious then it is deemed hazardous. In this case, the community nurse should make sure that there is somewhere in the patient's home where the waste can be stored without harming residents and is not accessible to pets or pests. The householder's permission is required and waste should be double bagged ready for disposal. Liquid offensive waste such as urine, liquid faeces and vomit needs to be disposed of into the house sewer via the toilet if not infectious and must not be placed into landfill (unless it has been absorbed into a cloth or gelling agent first) (RCN, 2014).

If the patient is aware of the risks and has consented to store waste, then the community nurse should set up a clinical waste collection with the local authority. Orange hazardous waste bags will be used for this. However, some council areas may not provide a hazardous waste collection service. If this is the case, the community nurse should remove the waste from the home and the nurse should have received training of safe waste management. An approved waste storage container must be used to transport it to an appropriate clinical waste disposal site.

Training is required for all community nurses to handle even small quantities of waste to ensure they understand the segregation of waste and their role in supporting effective waste management.

ACTIVITY

- Read your employer's healthcare waste management policy and find out your local arrangements around healthcare hazardous waste generated in people's own homes and relevant training for staff.

Sharps waste management has further standards in order to prevent sharps injuries (NHS England, 2022b). With the use of invasive devices, there is an increased risk of sharps injuries, which can occur from a contaminated sharp and offer the potential risk of blood-borne virus transmission. In 2010, EU Directive 2010/32/EU was adopted by NHS employers, and legislation came into force in 2013 around the transition to safety engineered versions of syringes, needles, IV cannulas, blood collection systems and blood lancets to reduce needlestick injuries (more information can be found on the NHS Supply Chain website—https://www.supplychain.nhs.uk/programmes/safer-sharps). In addition to using safer sharps devices, to minimise the risks of needlestick injuries, a few key points should be followed (Health and Safety Executive (HSE), 2010):

- Do not overfill the sharps box
- Ensure prompt sharps bin disposal
- Use the temporary closing mechanisms on the sharps box
- Cover any cuts or abrasions with waterproof plasters
- Always use safer sharps devices when using needles/sharps
- Always have a sharps container available when using needles/sharps

Depending on the frequency of sharps use and the environment, it may be suitable to leave a sharps container at the patient's home. If a sharps box is left at the home, it is important to risk assess the situation in relation to vulnerable members of the household including children and pets and put appropriate mitigations into place (e.g., up high in a cupboard, with temporary closing mechanism activated). District Nursing staff should also carry a portable sharps box, in case they need to use it (carried safely, with the temporary closing mechanism activated).

5.4 Decontamination of Equipment

Decontamination is a combination of processes including cleaning, disinfection and sterilisation, which removes or destroys microorganisms, which in sufficient quantities can cause infection (Medicines and Healthcare Products Regulatory Agency, 2021).

The levels of decontamination are:

- Cleaning: the physical removal of microorganisms and organic matter on which they thrive
- Disinfection: the reduction of the number of viable microorganisms on a product to a level previously specified as appropriate for its intended further handling or use

- Sterilisation: the process used to render an object free from viable microorganisms including viruses and bacterial spores

In a community setting, the most common decontamination practice is cleaning followed by disinfection, using disinfection wipes.

All nurses need to make sure that they apply the principles of decontamination to the environment and the equipment they are using (RCN, 2017). Equipment can be patient specific, it might be carried by community nurses and used on more than one patient, and it may be stored in car boots and at district nurse bases. All of this needs to be decontaminated before and after use on each patient. Some medical devices used and carried by community nurses are susceptible to fluid ingress (e.g. syringe drivers, glucometers, electronic thermometers) and can be damaged by using standard disinfection wipes. In this case, 70% alcohol wipes should be used instead. The employer should advise on what is required. It is important to keep records of decontamination of the equipment that the individual nurse holds, and the team holds and stores in their bases.

Medical devices and consumables must be stored in a clean, designated area to avoid environmental contamination. When transporting equipment in community nurses' vehicles, a designated receptacle for transporting medical equipment and consumables should be used, that is cleanable.

5.4.1 UNIFORMS

The use of uniforms in District Nursing practice may vary between organisations. However, it is good practice to:

- Wear freshly laundered for every shift
- Change workwear if it becomes visibly contaminated during the shift
- Protect uniform from contamination by body fluids with a new disposable apron for any patient visit where there is a body fluids splash risk

(NHS England, 2020)

REFLECTION

- What types of District Nursing care might pose a risk of infection?
- What infections might be seen most commonly in relation to District Nursing practice?

5.4.2 WOUND MANAGEMENT AND INFECTION

Infection is defined as an '*invasion of the body by a harmful organism or infectious agent such as a virus, parasite, bacterium or fungus*' (NHS England, 2022a). A potential risk of infection in District Nursing practice is when caring for patients with wounds, where breaches in the normal skin barrier can lead to infection. Wound care accounts for a large proportion of care provided by district Nursing services, so preventing wound infection and recognising the signs of wound bed colonisation and infections are essential skills for the community nurse (Rutter, 2018).

The wound bed can become contaminated (bacteria are not multiplying or causing issues), colonised (bacteria are multiplying but not causing damage to wound tissues) and infected (bacteria have multiplied to the extent that wound healing is disrupted and there is further tissue damage). If this progresses, surrounding soft tissue can become infected and systemic infection occur (International Wound Infection Institute (IWII), 2016). It is important to recognise and treat colonisations and infections in wounds promptly to prevent delayed healing, deterioration of the wound and more serious local or systemic infections such as cellulitis or sepsis, with complications such as amputation and death (Rutter, 2018).

Prevention of infection is the first step. Correct ANTT must be applied when undertaking wound care, as this prevents the transmission of microorganisms. However, within a community setting, which is an uncontrolled environment, this can be a challenge (Boniface et al., 2016). The working environment may be cluttered, with little room to apply a sterile field (no stainless-steel dressings trolley) and possible pets on the loose! A flexible approach to the delivery of care, with a dynamic risk assessment regarding kneeling, bending and accessing the patient, is needed (Terry et al., 2015). Nurses will need a degree of creativity and flexibility and should work in partnership with patients and families to ensure a safe environment and to minimise infection risks. Practical solutions need to be utilised, including securing pets in another room, identifying a suitable table or chair to base the sterile field for wound care and sourcing a suitable bowl lined with a disposable bag, to wash ulcerated legs, for example.

Some patients are more at risk of an infection, for example, those with conditions that impact their immune or circulatory systems, those on certain medications and those where their lifestyle means more risk. Additionally, the classical signs of infection may not be present in those who are immunocompromised or have a dark skin tone.

If wound bed infection is suspected, then an assessment should be undertaken, which should include evaluation of the patient, the tissues around the wound and the wound itself for the signs and symptoms of wound infection. Acute (e.g., surgical, traumatic wounds or burns) wounds may present with signs and symptoms of localised infection, such as discolouration, erythema, heat, swelling, purulent exudate, with pain/tenderness reported by the patient. Other symptoms may include pyrexia (5–7 days postsurgery), delayed/stalled healing, abscess and malodour (Sandoz, 2022).

In chronic wounds, which are wounds persisting for more than 6 weeks (Jirawitchalert et al., 2022) (e.g., leg ulcers, pressure ulcers), localised infection may present as:

- New, increased or altered pain
- Delayed/stalled healing
- Periwound oedema
- Discolouration of wound bed
- Friable/bleeding granulation tissue
- Green/white/brown exudates
- Increased or altered/purulent exudate
- Malodour
- Pocketing/bridging of wound bed
- Cellulitis

Sending a wound bed swab to microbiology is only indicated when there are clinical symptoms of infection and an intention to treat with systemic antibiotics (Nagel et al., 2023). Wound colonisation and wound infection can be treated with a topical antimicrobial dressing as first line (Wounds UK, 2017). Treatment with systemic antibiotics should be reserved for localised soft tissue or systemic infections (Edwards-Jones, 2020).

5.4.3 INVASIVE DEVICES AND PROCEDURES

Care in the community is becoming more diverse, and more advanced treatments are now being routinely delivered. This means an increase in the use of invasive devices. An invasive device is a device which breaches the normal body defences either by accessing the body through breaks in the skin or via a body opening (Sepsis Alliance, 2022). This provides an opening for microorganisms to access the body.

Some common invasive devices managed in community nursing are:

- Intravenous lines (IV)—including peripheral, central lines and peripheral inserted central catheters (PICC)
- Urinary catheters—including long-term, intermittent and nephrostomies
- Tracheostomy tubes
- Gastrostomy tubes
- Butterfly needles for subcutaneous infusions
- Venepuncture equipment
- Needles for injections

Invasive devices should be avoided where possible. There should always be a management plan with review dates to ensure the continuing requirement of the device if it is indwelling. The risks of infection should be discussed with the patient as part of the joint decision-making process when considering any indwelling invasive device. However, often such devices are essential to patient care and so IPC principles including competent application of the ANTT is vital. To minimise risks from infection, a few key points should be followed:

- Staff must be appropriately trained in ANTT to insert and manage the device.
- The entry sites for the devices must be monitored for signs of infection and irritation and appropriate action taken—patients and carers should be educated about signs and symptoms to look out for and what to do to escalate if they detect any concerns.
- The rationale, date of insertion, review dates and date of removal of indwelling invasive devices should be clearly documented.

It is important to inform and empower patients, family and carers about good basic IPC practices (Higginson, 2018). It has been identified that a patient's risk of developing an infection is closely linked to their knowledge and understanding of their illness (Dowding et al., 2020).

Patients and carers may need to monitor and provide self-care of some indwelling invasive devices (i.e., an indwelling urinary catheter). In these cases, there should be education for them, which includes an emphasis on infection prevention. This education should be both verbal and written so there is guidance to refer back to in the home.

5.4.4 ENVIRONMENTAL CLEANLINESS AND HYGIENE ISSUES

The environment has the potential to increase the risk of HCAIs (Knox et al., 2016). Whilst hospitals and care homes have clear standards for environmental cleanliness (Department of Health and Social Care, 2022; NHS England, 2021), there are no such standards in a person's home.

Nurses are guests in the patient's home and must treat the patient and their home with respect and sensitivity. This can present a challenge to nurses delivering care as patients' homes will be variable in terms of their hygiene standards, and if there is an unclean environment, this will increase the risk of microorganism transmission (De Veer et al., 2022).

However, there may be some homes that present significant infection risks to the patient. This can include the presence of infestations of pests such as bedbugs and fleas, the presence of pets and their excrement or food that is going mouldy. Any concerns of this nature should be sensitively highlighted with the patient, and support and onward referrals offered, whilst remaining respectful of their home, life choices and lifestyle.

Equally in cases where the contamination of the environment is deemed high risk for health, other agencies, such as local council and environmental health agencies may need to be informed and asked to provide support to the patient (NHS England, 2022a).

There may even be a public duty to report environmental health issues that supersedes the wishes or consent of the patient to do so. Do take advice from a professional nursing union, safeguarding team and local environmental health experts if concerned and ensure there is communication and support for the patient throughout this process, as far as possible.

5.5 Keeping Your IPC Practice Up to Date and Evidence Based

5.5.1 STAFF EDUCATION

In order to provide safe IPC care, staff need to complete comprehensive training. In the Health and Social Care Act (2012) (criterion 6), it states 'education and training must be made available to all staff'. This education should explain the principles of IPC practices and include assessing risks from new and existing infectious diseases. This knowledge should be utilised and incorporated when assessing patients, equipment and the environment.

5.5.2 ACCESSING RESOURCES

Make use of local library services. Most Trusts and all universities will have a library service, including advice and support about accessing information and journals and some librarians will complete literature reviews.

It is a good idea to get involved in networking. There will always be new community nurses who are keen to share ideas and resources. Networking also creates support, facilitates creative ideas and increases opportunities for shared learning. There are also national organisations which offer additional resources and training opportunities, e.g., QNI and RCN.

5.6 Conclusion

People receiving care from the District Nursing service may be more susceptible to infections due to their general health, age or treatments which reduce the efficacy of their immune system. There can also be significant challenges to the delivery of safe IPC care within home environments. Therefore it is vitally important that District nurses undertake dynamic risk assessments in relation to IPC risks and adapt standard precautions to each individual patient and environment, using a creative, flexible and pragmatic approach.

It is important to ensure patients and carers are educated and empowered to minimise infection risk associated with their condition, treatment, including their hand, personal and environmental hygiene.

Education and care planning around infection risk must be carried out sensitively, in partnership and negotiation with patients and carers, whilst respecting their home and their lifestyle choices, and considering their mental capacity and ability to make decisions around self-care.

References

Angelova-Fischer, I., Dapic, I., Hoek, A. K., Jakasa, I., Fischer, T., Zillikens, D., & Kezic, S. (2014). Skin barrier integrity and natural moisturising factor levels after cumulative dermal exposure to alkaline agents in atopic dermatitis. *Acta Dermato-Venereologica*, *94*, 640–644.

Boniface, G., Ghosh, S., & Robinson, L. (2016). District nurses' experiences of musculoskeletal wellbeing: A qualitative study. *British Journal of Community Nursing*, *21*(7), 350–355. https://www.magonlinelibrary.com/doi/epub/10.12968/bjcn.2016.21.7.350.

Cousins, G. (2014). Role of environmental cleanliness and decontamination in care homes. *Nursing Standard*, *30*(19), 9. https://doi.org/10.7748/ns.30.19.39.s42

Department of Health and Social Care. (2022). *Health and Social Care Act 2012: code of practice on the prevention and control of infections*. London. Available: https://www.legislation.gov.uk/ukpga/2012/7/section/7/enacted.

De Veer, A. J. E., De Groot, K., & Verkaik, R. (2022). Home care for patients with dirty homes: a qualitative study of the problems experienced by nurses and possible solutions. *BMC Health Services Research*, *22*, 592. https://doi.org/10.1186/s12913-022-07988-2.

Dowding, D., McDonald, M. V., & Shang, J. (2020). Implications of a US study on infection prevention and control in community settings in the UK. *British Journal of Community Nursing*, *25*(12), 578–583. https://doi.org/10.12968/bjcn.2020.25.12.578

Edwards-Jones, V. (2020). Antimicrobial stewardship in wound care. *British Journal of Nursing*, *29*(15). https://doi.org/10.12968/bjon.2020.29.15.s10

Guest, J. F., Keating, T., Gould, D., & Wigglesworth, N. (2020). Modelling the annual NHS costs and outcomes attributable to healthcare-associated infections in England. *BMJ Open*, *10*, 1–11. https://doi.org/10.1136/bmjopen-2019-033367

Health and Safety Executive. (2010). *EU Directive to prevent injuries and infections to healthcare workers from sharp objects such as needle sticks*. Available: https://www.hse.gov.uk/healthservices/needlesticks/eu-directive.htm.

Higginson, R. (2018). Infection control in the community. *British Journal of Community Nursing*, *23*(12), 590–595. https://doi.org/10.12968/bjcn.2018.23.12.590

International Wound Infection Institute (IWII). (2016). *Wound infection in clinical practice*. Wounds International. https://woundinfection-institute.com/wp-content/uploads/2021/06/IWII-Consensus_Final-2017.pdf

Knox, J., Sullivan, S. B., Urena, J., Miller, M., Vavagiakis, P., Shi, Q., & Lowy, F. D. (2016). Association of environmental contamination in the home with the risk for recurrent community-associated, methicillin-resistant *Staphylococcus aureus* infection. *JAMA Internal Medicine*, *176*(6), 807–815 PubMed: 27159126.

Lee, M. H., Lee, G. A., Lee, S. H., & Park, Y. H. (2020). A systematic review on the causes of the transmission and control measures of outbreaks in long-term care facilities: Back to basics of infection control. *PLoS One*, *15*(3): Article e0229911. https://doi.org/10.1371/journal.pone.0229911. PMID: 32155208; PMCID: PMC7064182.

Jirawitchalert, S., Mitaim, S., Chen, C. Y., & Patikarnmonthon, N. (2022). Cotton cellulose-derived hydrogel and electrospun fiber as alternative material for wound dressing application. *International Journal Biomaterials*: Article 2502658.

Loveday, H. P., Wilson, J. A., Pratt, R. J., Golsorkhi, M., Tingle, A., Bak, A., … Wilcox, M. (2014). Epic 3: National evidence-based guidelines for preventing healthcare-associated infections in NHS hospitals in England. *Journal of Hospital Infection*, *86*(Suppl. 1), S1–S70. https://doi.org/10.1016/S0195-6701(13)60012-2. In press.

Medicines and Healthcare Products Regulatory Agency. (2021). *Managing medical devices. Guidance for health and social care organisations*. London: Government. https://assets.publishing.service.gov.uk/media/6089dc938fa8f51b91f3d82f/Managing_medical_devices.pdf.

Nagle, S. M., Stevens, K. A., & Wilbraham, S. C. (2023). Wound assessment. In *StatPearls [Internet]*. Treasure Island (FL): StatPearls Publishing. PMID: 29489199.

National Institute for Health and Care Excellence. (2017a). *Healthcare-associated infections: Prevention and control in primary and community care, Clinical guideline [CG139]*. London.

National Institute for Health and Care Excellence. (2017b). *Intravenous fluid therapy in adults in hospital, Clinical guideline [CG174]*. London.

NHS England. (2020). *Uniforms and workwear: guidance for NHS employers. Coronavirus: uniforms and workwear: guidance for NHS employers*. england.nhs.uk.

NHS England. (2021). *National standards of healthcare cleanliness*. London. Available: https://www.england.nhs.uk/wp-content/uploads/2021/04/B0271-national-standards-of-healthcare-cleanliness-2021.pdf.

NHS England. (2022a). *National Infection Prevention and Control Manual (NIPCM) for England*. London. Available: https://www.england.nhs.uk/national-infection-prevention-and-control-manual-nipcm-for-england/.

NHS England. (2022b). *Health technical memorandum 07-01: Safe and sustainable management of healthcarewaste*.Available:https://www.england.nhs.uk/wp-content/uploads/2021/05/B2159iii-health-technical-memorandum-07-01.pdf.

NHS England. (2022c). *Greener NHS. National ambition*. Available: https://www.england.nhs.uk/greenernhs/national-ambition/.

Otter, J. A., Yezli, S., Salkeld, J. A. G., & French, G. (2013). Evidence that contaminated surfaces contribute to the transmission of hospital pathogens and an overview of strategies to address contaminated surfaces in hospital settings. *American Journal of Infection Control*, *41*(5 Suppl). https://doi.org/10.1016/j.ajic.2012.12.004. In press.

Royal College of Nursing. (2014). *The management of waste from health, social and personal care*. London: Royal College of Nursing.

Royal College of Nursing. (2017). *Essential practice for infection prevention and control*. Royal College of Nursing. Available at: https://www.rcn.org.uk/Professional-Development/publications/pub-005940.

Royal College of Nursing and Queens Institutes. (2019). Outstanding models of district nursing. A joint project identifying what makes an outstanding district nursing service. Available: https://qni.org.uk/wp-content/uploads/2019/05/Oustanding-Models-of-District-Nursing-Report-web.pdf.

Rutter, L. (2018). Identifying and managing wound infection in the community. *British Journal Community Nursing*, *23*(Suppl 3), S6–S14. https://doi.org/10.12968/bjcn.2018.23.Sup3.S6. PMID: 29493306.

Sandoz, H. (2022). An overview of the prevention and management of wound infection. *Nursing Standard*, *37*(10), 75–82. https://doi.org/10.7748/ns.2022.e11889. In press

Sepsis Alliance. (2022). *Invasive devices. Sepsis alliance. The King's Fund. Healthcare-associated infections: Stemming the rise of superbug*. Invasive Devices | Sepsis Alliance (p. 2008). USA: Sepsis Alliance. In press.

Terry, D., Lê, Q., Nguyen, U., & Hoang, H. (2015). Workplace health and safety issues among community nurses: A study regarding the impact on providing care to rural consumers. *BMJ Open*, *5*(8), e008306. https://doi.org/10.1136/bmjopen-2015-008306. In press.

Weltevrede, M., Eilers, R., de Melker, H. E., & van Baarle, D. (2016). Cytomegalovirus persistence and T cell immunosenescence in people aged fifty and older: a systematic review. *Experimental Gerontology*, *77*, 87–95.

World Health Organization. (2009). *WHO guidelines on hand hygiene in healthcare*. World Health Organization. pesquisa.bvsalud.org.

World Health Organization. (2011). *Report* on the burden of endemic health care-associated infection worldwide. *World Health Organization*. Available: https://www.who.int/publications-detail-redirect/report-on-the-burden-of-endemic-health-care-associated-infection-worldwide.

World Health Organization. (2018). *A brief synopsis on patient safety 2010*. Available: http://www.euro.who.int/__data/assets/pdf_file/0015/111507/E93833.pdf?ua=1.

Wounds UK. (2017). *Best practice statement: Making day-to-day management of biofilm simple*. Wounds UK, London.

CHAPTER 6

Promoting Equity in Community Nursing

Vanessa Heaslip | Jonathan Parker | Kirsty Marshall

LEARNING OUTCOMES

After reading this chapter you should be able to:

- Recognise how some groups of people have poorer health outcomes as well as some of the factors inhibiting their access to care in the community
- Have a critical awareness of international and national policies pertaining to promoting equity and equality
- Develop professional practice and services that are inclusive, fair and respectful
- Have an awareness of the importance of multiagency working including working with nonstatutory partners

6.1 Introduction

The following chapter introduces how some people experience worse health outcomes and how they also experience poorer access to care. The chapter will provide definitions of key terms such as equity, equality, intersectionality and wider social determinates as well as a short overview of current international and national policy. It will explore the role of all nurses who work in community settings, particularly district nursing services, and examine how they can develop professional practice that is respectful, person centred, fair and inclusive. Lastly, it will consider how nurses can work in an integrated way across health and social care to promote health and well-being for those individuals, groups and communities who experience social exclusion and inequalities.

6.2 International Policy

The Sustainable Development Goals (SDGs) were published by the United Nations (UN) in 2015 in order to promote health, well-being and economic security for all. However, it is worth considering the degree to which these influence professional practice (see Reflection: Community Nurses and the SDGs).

REFLECTION: Community Nurses and the SDGs

Access and read about the UN Sustainable Developments Goals—https://sdgs.un.org/goals

Consider the following SDGs:

- No poverty (SDG 1)
- Zero hunger (SDG 2)
- Good health and well-being (SDG 3)
- Gender equality (SDG 5)
- Clean water and sanitation (SDG 6)
- Reduced inequalities (SDG 10)

Draw two columns on a page and, for each SDG, write a list of activities you currently do in your role as a community nurse that address this SDG.

In the previous reflection, very few activities identified may have been aligned to the UN SDGs. However, it could be argued that nurses are fundamental to meeting the SDGs yet the degree to which nurses feel connected to and empowered by them is questionable. A scoping review by Fields et al. (2021) noted that many individual nurses feel disconnected from the SDGs and struggle to relate these to their clinical role. In order to consider how community nurses can more meaningfully interact with the SDGs, an examination of the issues related to why some people have poorer health and access to care as well as key terminology is required.

6.3 Definitions of Equity and Equality

Within the UK, the predominate focus within policy is promoting equality and reducing inequalities. Although the terms 'equity' and 'inequity' are sometimes, albeit erroneously, used interchangeably, Heaslip et al. (2022b) argue there is a nuanced difference (Table 6.1).

Essentially, equality is about treating people the same way, providing the same services for all, and this is the foundation on which the NHS is based. However, remember the

TABLE 6.1 **Key Terms**

Health inequalities	Differences that exist between groups in health service access, health status and outcomes
Health equity	Achieving equity requires the provision of different attention to groups adversely affected so equality in access, status and outcomes can be achieved
Health inequities	Underpinned by social justice, health inequities refer to the unjust or unfair differences in health access, status and outcomes that exist between groups of people
Health disparities	Absolute and relative differences in health status and outcomes between groups. It is used to provide evidence of health inequities. For instance, differences in access to determinants of health and health services and quality of healthcare

(From Wilson, D., Heaslip, V., & Jackson, D. (2018). Improving equity and cultural responsiveness with marginalised communities: Understanding competing worldviews. *Journal of Clinical Nursing, 27*(19-20), 3810–3819. https://doi.org/10.1111/jocn.14546.)

adage, *'there is nothing more unequal than the equal treatment of unequal people'*. Consider the case in Case Study 6.1.

CASE STUDY 6.1

Alice	Alice is a 78-year-old female Romany Gypsy, who lives in a caravan on a council-maintained site. Alice has leg ulcers which the district nursing team are dressing 3 times a week. She has been referred to the hospital for a vascular assessment and has received a letter about an appointment in 6 weeks.
Meela	Meela is a 76-year-old female who lives in a bungalow with her husband; she also has leg ulcers managed by the district nursing team 3 times a week. She has also been referred to the hospital for a vascular assessment and has received a letter about an appointment in 6 weeks.

Looking at this case study, it could be argued that both Alice and Meela are being treated equally. Both have a letter for an appointment in 6 weeks, and so it could be perceived that this is fair treatment. However, consider, for example, that Alice may be unable to read and write, which is common in some Gypsy, Roma, Travellers (Office for National Statistics, 2022) and, therefore to promote equitable treatment, there should be another way to manage her appointment. If the appointment communication to Alice is written (via a letter), and she cannot read, then it is likely she will miss her appointment and probably be judged as 'nonconcordant' with treatment by the community nurses and the general practitioner (GP). Within this chapter, both equity and equality will be used: equity to highlight the systemic barriers that people face, and equality as this is the term used in the majority of UK policies.

To promote equitable treatment, nurses need to have a sound understanding of some of the challenges faced by individuals, groups and communities that may require a different approach.

6.4 Health Outcomes

Many different individuals and groups have poorer health outcomes, for example, Gypsy, Roma, Travellers (Heaslip et al., 2019b); people living with a disability (Ijezie et al., 2023) or mental health issue (Heaslip et al., 2019a); the global majority[1] or people from racialised communities (Public Health England, 2020); and people who are homeless (Heaslip et al., 2022a). In addition, belonging to a socially excluded group (Fig. 6.1) is also associated with poorer health outcomes (Marmot et al., 2010, 2020).

DEFINITION

The term 'global majority' refers to Black, African, Asian and Brown people, people of dual heritage, those native to the global south (Welsh Government, 2023).

A systematic review identified that socially excluded men's mortality rate was almost 8 times higher whilst socially excluded women's mortality rate was almost 12 times

[1]Term global majority refers to Black, African, Asian and Brown people, people of dual heritage, those native to the global south (Welsh Government, 2023).

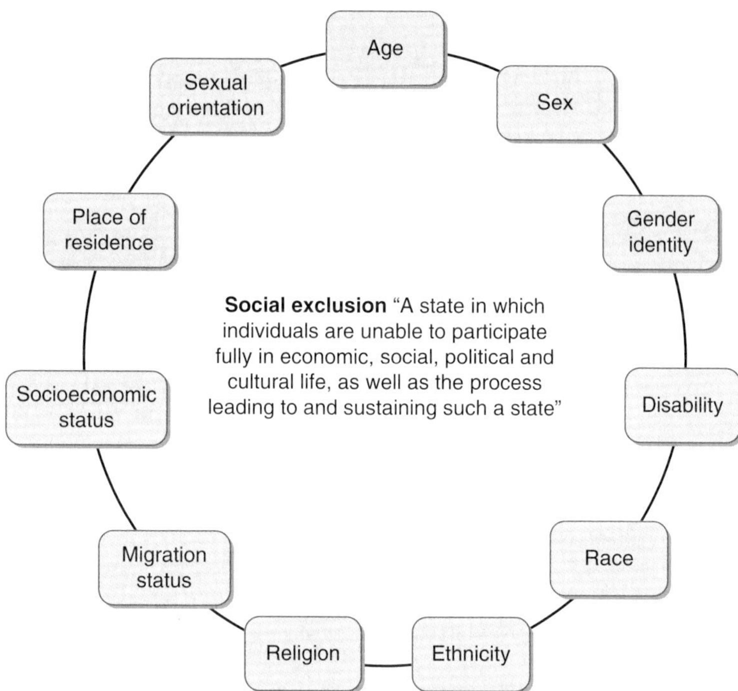

Fig. 6.1 Social exclusion. (From United Nations. (2016). Leaving no one behind: Equality and non-discrimination at the heart of sustainable development. Accessed 31 July 2023 from https://www.un.org/esa/socdev/rwss/2016/chapter1.pdf)

higher than those who belong to socially included groups, whilst deaths from cardiovascular disease, respiratory disease, cancer and asthma were also significantly increased in women (Aldridge et al., 2017). Social exclusion is, as Sacker et al. (2017) state, a multidimensional process that prevents people from engaging in mainstream society or gaining access to services that are meant to be universal. It is intersectional, meaning there are many diverse drivers of social exclusion, including educational attainment, unemployment and economic precarity, homelessness, lack of support and transport unavailability (Meer, 2014; Romero, 2017). These affect people across a range of dimensions and represent some of the structural barriers to engagement in appropriate health and social care (Parker, 2021a).

In addition to the groups mentioned earlier, the impact of poverty must be considered. Poverty is the single largest determinate of health as poorer people have shorter lives and greater health and well-being challenges (World Health Organization (WHO), 2021). Poverty is often considered broadly in terms of lower–middle-income countries, however, poverty within differentials within a single country, and higher-income countries, cannot be ignored. For example, in the UK, someone living in a deprived area of England is more likely to die 8½ years younger than someone living in a more affluent area (Office for National Statistics, 2021). They will also experience more ill health and reduced well-being compared to their wealthier counterparts. Marmot et al. (2010) argue there is a social gradient of health, that is, the lower an individual's social position

TABLE 6.2 **Core20PLUS5**

Core 20	The most deprived 20% of the national population identified by Index of Multiple Deprivation
PLUS	This includes population groups: • ethnic minority communities • inclusion health (people experiencing homelessness, drug and alcohol dependence, vulnerable migrants, Gypsy, Roma, Travellers, sex workers, people in the justice system, victims of modern slavery and other socially excluded groups) • people with a learning disability and autism • deprived coastal communities • people with multimorbidities • people in protected characteristic groups The Plus group also notes that consideration also needs to be taken for young carers, looked after children/care leavers and those in contact with the justice system
5	The 5 refers to five clinical areas of focus including: • Asthma • Diabetes • Epilepsy • Oral health • Mental health These five areas are designated for integrated care boards and integrated care partnerships to ensure system change and to improve care for children and young people

(From NHS England. (2021). *Core20PLUS5 – An approach to reducing health inequalities for children and young people.* NHS England. Retrieved 7 September 2023 from https://www.england.nhs.uk/about/equality/equality-hub/national-healthcare-inequalities-improvement-programme/core20plus5/core20plus5-cyp/.)

in society, the worse their health experience/outcomes, and conversely, the higher their social position, the better their health (Parker, 2023). In 2020, 10 years after his initial report, Marmot undertook a subsequent review in the UK (Marmot et al., 2020) examining any progress made during the preceding 10 years. Rather than identifying improvements in health inequalities, he found that the opposite was true, that there was a widening of health inequalities in England, most notably for women. It is important to note that many of the socially excluded groups identified earlier will also be living in poverty which can compound their heath inequity, for example inability to attend hospital appointments because you cannot afford to pay for the transport to attend, or lack of food or secure housing.

The COVID-19 pandemic had a disproportionate impact on some of the most disadvantaged groups in society, and the repercussions of this are still being felt as the gap in levels of well-being between low and high incomes has increased by 50% (Bambra et al., 2021; Parker, 2021b, 2023; WHO, 2023). These health disparities are often exacerbated by health and social care services, which are not designed to support people with multiple and intersecting health issues. These fragmented services do not link support mechanisms together, resulting in people falling between gaps of services (Marshall, 2023).

There is an increasing recognition, nationally, of the health impact of social exclusion, and to begin to address this, the Core20PLUS5 framework (NHS England, 2021) was introduced. This framework (see Table 6.2) aims to reduce health inequalities at both national and systems level.

Considering the groups identified in the Core20PLUS5 framework, it is easy to see why community nurses are ideally placed to recognise the impact health inequalities have on the people they work with and to enable them to access health and social care service (Marshall, 2023). However, many nurses do not always have the skills and knowledge to support individuals and their families with complex health and social care issues.

REFLECTION: How Well Do You Know Your Local Community and Services?

Consider the local community in which you work and ask yourself:

- How many of the Core20PLUS5 groups do you have within your service; how are they identified? Initially, you may think they are categories on GP records, but are they? For example, Gypsy, Roma, Traveller groups are often not identified in the NHS Data Dictionary ethnicity category codes (GOV UK, Undated), so are they recorded in your systems?
- How aware are you of the local community support services offered in your local community, how people can access them—consider:
  - Community fridges
  - Soup kitchens/meals for vulnerable families
  - Night shelters
  - Food banks
  - Half-way houses to supported or community living
  - Faith groups and support
  - Pop-up clinics
  - Clothes banks
  - Youth groups
  - Walking groups
- In your assessments of people, do you consider these wider aspects and how you share information in an inclusive way, considering that some people may have difficulty reading or have lack of internet access?

As nurses are the main care coordinators who work across the health and social care interface, they are pivotal in helping people to access the services they need (Royal College of Nursing, 2016). However, research by Wain (2020) identified multiple perceptions of professionals regarding what it meant for them to work in integrated ways. Case Study 6.2 captures good practice within integrated care delivery and how services can support people who may otherwise be excluded.

CASE STUDY 6.2

An example of integrated working in more inclusive ways is the leg ulcer service offered by Manchester Local Care Organisation. It was recognised that people who are homeless were underserved in terms of wound assessment and management, as many of the individuals struggled to make or keep appointments due to the challenges of living in the streets. In response to this, a nurse-led service run by community nurses was set up which offers a drop-in clinic for people who are homeless. People do not require an appointment to attend, they simply can turn up to three different clinics held at local GP practices (3 days a week) to have their wound assessed and treated. As the clinics are run in GP practice, the GPs are also on hand which has benefits; for example, if the nurses identify an infection, leading to a one-stop service. This service is very successful, seeing on average 10–20 patients a week who would otherwise struggle to access care. The benefits of this community-based nurse led service are that the nurses are able to build a rapport with the clients who in turn feel they are treated with respect and dignity.

For more information about this service, see https://www.manchesterlco.org/services/north-manchester-community-services/leg-ulcer-service/#1679485858520-678f40dd-2576.

6.5 Conclusion

This chapter has examined how some people and groups have worse health outcomes and how they also experience poorer access to care. It has explored how this is influenced by wider societal processes as well as examining the role of community nurses in promoting health access for all. It then presented some national and international policies linked to health equity and explored how community nurses have a vital role in helping people access care.

Finally, draw up a personal action plan (Reflection: Personal Action Plan).

REFLECTION: Personal Action Plan

Review the activities presented in this chapter and develop an action plan which you shall work on over the next 6 months to help you further develop your knowledge and skills as an inclusive community nurse. Separate your plan into immediate learning and development needs, medium-term ones and longer-term needs. Once you have done this, add to each point in your action plan, what you need to achieve, what resources you need to do so, and how you aim to complete the action plan. Check this over the next 6 months and add and adjust as necessary. It is your choice how to develop this, but you may wish to follow something like the following example. You could colour or shade each point when achieved:

Action	*Short-Term Needs*	*Medium-Term Needs*	*Long-Term Needs*
1.			
2.			
3.			
4.			

References

Aldridge, R. W., Story, A., Hwang, S. W., Nordentoft, M., Luchenski, S. A., Hartwell, G., et al. (2017). Morbidity and mortality in homeless individuals, prisoners, sex workers, and individuals with substance use disorders in high-income countries: A systematic review and meta-analysis. *Lancet*, *391*, 241–250. https://doi.org/10.1016/S0140-6736(17)31869-X

Bambra, C., Lynch, J., & Smith, K. E. (2021). *The unequal pandemic: COVID-19 and health inequalities*. Bristol: Policy Press.

Fields, L., Perkiss, S., Dean, B. A., & Moroney, T. (2021). Nursing and the sustainable development goals: A scoping review. *Journal of Nursing Scholarship*, *53*(5), 568–577.

GOV UK. (Undated). Ethnicity classifications. Available from https://www.ethnicity-facts-figures.service.gov.uk/. (Accessed 1 July 2024).

Heaslip, V., Green, S., Simkhada, B., Dogan, H., & Richer, S. (2022a). How do people who are homeless find out about local health and social care services: A mixed method study. *International Journal of Environmental Research and Public Health*, *19*, 46. https://doi.org/10.3390/ijerph19010046

Heaslip, V., Thompson, R., Tauringana, M., Holland, S., & Glendening, N. (2022b). Health inequity in the UK: Exploring health inequality and inequity. *Practice Nursing*, *33*(2), 84–87.

Heaslip, V., Vahdaninia, M., Hind, M., Darvill, T., Staelens, Y., O'Donoghue, D., et al. (2019a). Locating oneself in the past to influence the present: Impacts of Neolithic landscapes on mental health well-being. *Health and Place*, *62*. Article 102273. https://doi.org/10.1016/j.healthplace.2019.102273

Heaslip, V., Wilson, D., & Jackson, D. (2019b). Gypsy roma travellers: An indigenous population? *Public Health*, *176*, 43–49. https://doi.org/10.1016/j.puhe.2019.02.020

Ijezie, O. A., Healy, J., Davies, P., Balaguer-Ballester, E., & Heaslip, V. (2023). Quality of life in adults with down syndrome: A mixed methods systematic review. *PLoS ONE, 18*(5): Article e0280014. https://doi.org/10.1371/journal.pone.0280014

Marmot, M., Allen, J., Boyce, T., Goldblatt, P., & Morrison, J. (2010). *Fair society, healthy lives.* London: Institute of Health Equity. Available at https://www.instituteofhealthequity.org/resources-reports/fair-society-healthy-lives-the-marmot-review. [Accessed 28 July 2023].

Marmot, M., Allen, J., Boyce, T., Goldblatt, P., & Morrison, J. (2020). *Health equity in England: The marmot review 10 years on.* The Health Foundation. Available from https://www.health.org.uk/publications/reports/the-marmot-review-10-years-on?gad_source=1&gclid=EAIaIQobChMI342rurOFhwMVn5hQBh1YBgBXEAAYASAAEgIZe_D_BwE. (Accessed 28 July 2023).

Marshall, K. (2023). Chapter – 5. What is integrated care and why is it different. In K. Marshall, H. Bamber, R. Garbutt, & Easton, C. (Eds.), *Demystifying integrated care: A handbook for practice.* Elsevier.

Meer, N. (2014). *Key concepts in race and ethnicity.* London: SAGE.

NHS England. (2021). *Core20PLUS5 – an approach to reducing health inequalities for children and young people.* NHS England. Available from: https://www.england.nhs.uk/about/equality/equality-hub/national-healthcare-inequalities-improvement-programme/core20plus5/core-20plus5-cyp/. (Accessed 7 September 2023).

Office for National Statistics. (2021). *Health state life expectancies by national deprivation deciles, England: 2017 to 2019. Office for national statistics.* Available from https://www.ons.gov.uk/peoplepopulationandcommunity/healthandsocialcare/healthinequalities/bulletins/healthstatelifeexpectanciesbyindexofmultipledeprivationimd/latest. [Accessed 28 July 2023].

Office for National Statistics. (2022). *Gypsies' and travellers' lived experiences, education and employment, England and Wales: 2022.* Office for National Statistics. Available at https://www.ons.gov.uk/peoplepopulationandcommunity/educationandchildcare/bulletins/gypsiesandtravellerslivedexperienceseducationandemploymentenglandandwales/2022. [Accessed 5 September 2023].

Parker, J. (2021a). *Social work practice: Assessment, planning, intervention and review.* London: SAGE.

Parker, J. (2021b). Structural discrimination and abuse: COVID-19 and people in care homes in England and Wales. *The Journal of Adult Protection, 23*(3), 169–180. https://doi.org/10.1108/JAP-12-2020-0050

Parker, J. (2023). *Analysing the history of British social welfare: Compassion, coercion and beyond.* Bristol: Policy Press.

Public Health England. (2020). *Beyond the data: Understanding the impact of COVID-19 on BAME groups.* Available from https://assets.publishing.service.gov.uk/government/uploads/system/uploads/attachment_data/file/892376/COVID_stakeholder_engagement_synthesis_beyond_the_data.pdf. (Accessed 7 September 2023).

Romero, M. (2017). *Introducing intersectionality.* Cambridge: Polity Press.

Royal College of Nursing. (2016). *The nursing role in integrated care models; Reflecting on the United States' experience.* London: Royal College of Nursing.

Sacker, A., Ross, A., MacLeod, C. A., Netuveli, G, & Windle, W (2017). Health and social exclusion in older age: Evidence from Understanding Society, the UK household longitudinal study. *Journal of Epidemiology and Community Health, 71*(7), 681–690.

United Nations. (2015). *Resolution adopted by the general assembly on 25 september 2015.* Available from https://sdgs.un.org/2030agenda. [Accessed 28 July 2023].

United Nations. (2016). *Leaving no one behind: Equality and non-discrimination at the heart of sustainable development.* Available from https://www.un.org/esa/socdev/rwss/2016/chapter1.pdf. [Accessed 31 July 2023].

Wain, L. (2020). Does integrated health and care in the community deliver its vision? A workforce perspective. *Journal of Integrated Care*, *29*(2), 170–184. https://doi.org/10.1108/JICA-10-2020-0061

Welsh Government. (2023). *Welsh language race and ethnicity terminology*. Available from: https://www.gov.wales/sites/default/files/publications/2023-05/welsh-language-race-and-ethnicity-terminology.pdf. [Accessed 29 September 2023].

Wilson, D., Heaslip, V., & Jackson, D. (2018). Improving equity and cultural responsiveness with marginalised communities: Understanding competing worldviews. *Journal of Clinical Nursing*, *27*(19-20), 3810–3819. https://doi.org/10.1111/jocn.14546

World Health Organization. (2021). *Poverty and social determinates. Social determinants of health*. Available at https://www.who.int/health-topics/social-determinants-of-health#tab=tab_3. (Accessed 28 July 2023).

World Health Organisation. (2023). *Transforming the health and social equity landscape; Promoting socially just and inclusive growth to improve resilience, solidarity and peace*. Available from https://www.who.int/europe/publications/i/item/WHO-EURO-2023-7761-47529-69924. [Accessed 28 July 2023].

CHAPTER 7

Intersecting Pathways: Exploring Population Health, Public Health and Health Promotion

Michelle McBride   Katie Romanillos

LEARNING OUTCOMES

After reading this chapter you should be able to:

- Understand the differences between population health, public health and health promotion
- Explain the role of the community nurse within population health, public health and health promotion
- Understand the relevance of behaviour change models and how to apply them to practice
- Recognise how public health and sustainability are closely intertwined concepts

7.1 Population Health, Public Health and Health Promotion

Community nursing can be delivered across different settings and reach out to communities that may be otherwise invisible and unsupported. District nurses and their community teams work closely with general practitioners (GPs) and other specialists with a focus on patients and families and offer support to patients to manage their own long-term conditions and therefore are best placed to promote health and prevent further complications (Queens' Nursing Institute (QNI), 2019). Community nurses often have privileged access to patients in their homes, can build a level of trust (Khumalo & Brown, 2022) and have tacit knowledge about local populations (Duncan, 2019). However, the role they play within population health and public health domains can be less clear and not always documented with clarity. The definitions of these terms can sometimes be misunderstood.

DEFINITIONS

Population health management (PHM): PHM is a data-based approach to identify the current and future health risks of a local population. This may join up information about health behaviours and status, clinical care access, use and quality of available services and social determinants of health (Duncan, 2019). These are often referred to as the four pillars of a population Health System (King's Fund, 2018). See Fig. 7.1.

Public health: Public health is an overall term that covers aspects of disease prevention and health promotion, and is about supporting people to stay well and helps to improve the health of the population through protection, prevention and promotion (RCN, 2024).

Health promotion: Health promotion is about improving the health status of individuals and the population as a whole, which is essentially a process of enabling people to increase control over, and to improve, their health (Evans et al., 2017).

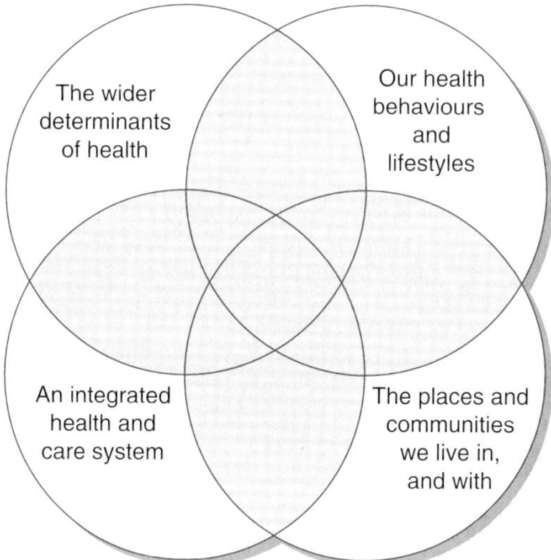

Fig. 7.1 A vision for population health: towards a healthier future. (The King's Fund. (2018). A Vision for population health: Towards a Healthier Future. https://www.kingsfund.org.uk/insight-and-analysis/reports/vision-population-health)

7.2 Population Health and Community Nursing

REFLECTION

- How are community nursing teams involved in PHM in your area?
- Are you aware of any training or education material available that relates to population health?

In general, population health addresses four groups of society: firstly those who are generally well and who could maintain this status using health interventions, for example, screening programmes for hypertension, and secondly those that have been identified as being at risk of developing long-term conditions (Duncan, 2019). These areas might be the focus of primary care interventions. The latter two focus on those that already have long-term conditions and could benefit from support to delay progression and those who have complex needs and require a high level of individualised coordinated care. This group of individuals may find themselves on the caseloads of community nurses and this is not a new concept for these teams (Khumalo & Brown, 2022). It has been well documented that community nurses play a strategic role in the delivery of the NHS Long Term Plan and yet sometimes terminology can be difficult to understand, and there is a lack of awareness around frameworks. However, community nurses often cite a lack of time, permission and resources to be proactive within PHM and access to training is often limited (Khumalo & Brown, 2022). Therefore for community nurses to be confident in delivering PHM, they require additional education materials. Moreover, they should be involved in the planning of these services and have their voices heard, as they will already be aware of the impact of lifestyle choices on the risk of developing preventable illnesses and have an awareness of deprivation issues (Duncan, 2019).

For PHM to be successful, there needs to be joined-up thinking and information about local health, social care and well-being needs, which is a fundamental building block for integrated care systems (NHS England, 2024).

7.3 Public Health in Community Nursing

Community nurses play a valuable role in minimising the impact of illness, promoting health and helping individuals to function well in any environment (RCN, 2024). All nurses and midwives have a role in improving public health:

- Public health is everyone's responsibility and should be a fundamental part of all nursing roles.
- Nursing skills are rightly valued as being able to provide meaningful public health interventions across all health and social care settings as part of holistic patient centred care (RCN, 2016).

The public health element of the community nurse's role is decreasing due to other pressures (QNI and RCN, 2019), yet there is an awareness that promoting health and preventing ill health are key standards of proficiency for preregistration and post registration nursing education in the UK (Donaghy et al., 2022; NMC, 2022). Therefore there is a disparity between what is addressed in the curriculum for preregistration nurses and what might be observed in practice. Much of what nurses do will fall under the heading of public health but is often not recognised as such; they are involved in disease prevention through immunisation and sometimes even screening (Evans et al., 2017) or perhaps engage in cold weather or heatwave campaigns to ensure the safety and well-being of vulnerable individuals or wider concepts such as antibiotic stewardship or disease surveillance. Whatever the context, community nurses are in an optimum position to support people to stay well. It is also important to remember that the circumstances within which people live their lives have a great influence on their health and they may not always be able to control the determinants that limit their choices in relation to health behaviours and that social isolation and lack of family support often contribute to the struggle (Wild & McGrath, 2018).

7.4 Health Promotion in Community Nursing

An emphasis on promoting good health is not a new concept and has been around since the 1970s (Pronk et al., 2021). However, over time it has become apparent that for individuals to 'own' their health and to make a sustainable change, not only do they need education, but they also need support to act on this knowledge (Wild & McGrath, 2018). As seen in Fig. 7.2, Tannahill's (2009) model of health promotion combines health protection, prevention and health education as key elements of health promotion. Community nursing teams will deliver elements of all of these but not always be aware of how their practice aligns with the local healthcare priorities.

REFLECTION

Consider the following:

- Which elements of your current role would be considered either health protection, prevention or promotion?
- What public health campaigns are currently delivered in your own local trust?

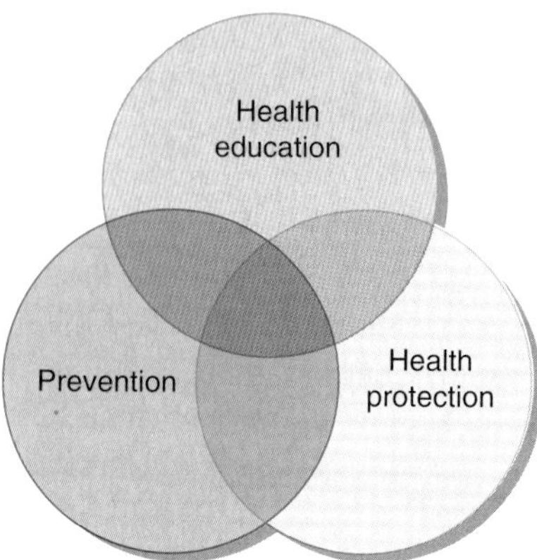

Fig. 7.2 Tannahill model of health promotion (2009). (From Tannahill, A. (2009). Health promotion: the Tannahill model revisited. *Public Health, 123*(5), 396–399, https://doi.org/10.1016/j.puhe.2008.05.021.)

Within community nursing, many of the activities that are performed and care provided to patients will include those that could be considered health promotion. This could involve:

- Immunisations
- Health check and disease monitoring for diabetes and or/heart disease which could involve blood tests, blood pressure (BP) monitoring and body mass index (BMI) monitoring
- Smoking cessation
- Dietary advice
- Oral hygiene (promotion and advice)
- Obesity management—particularly in vulnerable groups such as clients with a learning disability (LD)
- Identifying those with depression and promoting well-being (Public Health England (PHE), 2016).

One of the previously mentioned areas of patient care is that of promoting oral hygiene. This is often overlooked within the community setting and careful consideration should be made as the patient is often at risk if this is neglected (Palmer, 2023). It has also been noted that oral hygiene issues often affect the poorer, marginalised and vulnerable groups in society. If this group of people also have an inability to maintain good oral care, they would quite likely be on the community nursing caseload (Palmer, 2023). See Box 7.1 for further information.

There is a clear role for community nurses in promoting the oral health of those patients that they may already visit at home or within residential care. This may involve performing accurate oral assessments, training care home staff and highlighting those individuals who may have limited dexterity or capacity and may require assistance or aids. It might also involve the care of dentures and the appropriate use of toothpaste or mouthwashes (NICE, 2022; Palmer, 2023).

Low quality of life and chronic health conditions can often be linked back to poor oral health, and meeting the needs of the patient who lives in their own home may often prove challenging (Palmer, 2023). As the Chief Medical Officer (2023) stated, poor oral health can be a result of a poor diet or actually contribute to poor nutritional intake. As Stark et al. (2022) noted, it is not yet clear how community nurses can deliver effective oral health

BOX 7.1 ■ NICE (2022) Improving Oral Health for Adults in Care Homes

Patients often have higher risk of poor oral health due to:

- Long-term condition such as Parkinson's disease, arthritis and dementia
- Multiple medications can reduce saliva in the mouth
- Older people often now keep their own teeth, leading to complex dental needs over time.

education for this group of patients but support when appropriate with daily oral care, training and supporting informal carers, identifying those at risk and overseeing the need for dentist referrals will all contribute to effective health promotion in this area.

7.5 Behaviour Change in Community Nursing

When promoting health in nursing, there is often a change or modification in lifestyle choices that is required in order to make a sustainable difference in health. Behaviour change approaches are unlikely to be effective unless the impact of the environment in which they live in, is taken into account (Wills, 2023). To enable people to make a change, approaches need to be client-centred and focus on promoting and maintaining a person's independence in the decisions they make about their health (Wills, 2023). Information alone is not sufficient for behaviour change; often, attitudes and values need to be taken into consideration. An individual will decide whether they wish to change their own behaviour by evaluating the change's feasibility and its benefits weighed against its costs as illustrated in the Health Belief Model (Fig. 7.3). As community nurses have a unique relationship with their patients and insight into the environment in which they live and the lifestyle choices they make, they are often in the best position to facilitate behaviour change.

CASE STUDY 7.1 Part 1

Gagandeep is a 75-year-old male who has been smoking tobacco for 50 years of his life. He finds that it helps him relax and admits that he is possibly addicted. He also says that there is no point in giving up as he is old and it will not make any difference to his health or life expectancy.

Five years ago, Gagandeep was diagnosed with type 2 diabetes which he thought he was managing quite well. Last month, he attended his GP with a wound on his right foot, which was exuding fluid, which the GP informed him was an infected ulcer. Now his mobility has become so poor, he is having to receive community nurse visits to receive wound care.

He has realised that he has never really understood his diabetes and is now getting concerned that smoking might be one of the causes of his painful wound.

REFLECTION

If this person was a patient who you were going to visit today, consider how you might contribute positively to their behaviour change (giving up smoking) using the Health Belief Model.

- What are their perceptions of his condition?
- Do they understand the severity of the disease?
- What cues or prompts might help them to change his behaviour?
- What might they perceive as the benefits of giving up smoking?
- What might be the barriers to giving up smoking?
- What is the likelihood of this person giving up smoking at this point?

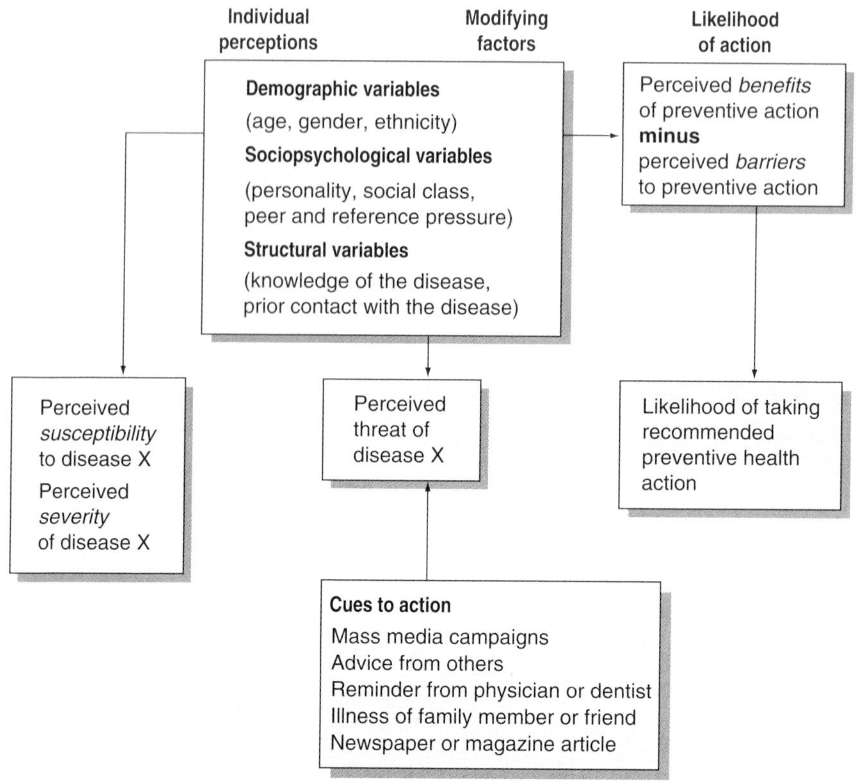

Fig. 7.3 The Health Belief Model. (From Becker, M. H. (Ed.). (1974). *The Health Belief Model and personal health behaviour*. Thorofare, NJ: Slack.)

In order to facilitate any behaviour change in patients, they need to be ready for it, which is often context driven and relates to outcomes but will involve multiple internal and external factors (Wild & McGrath, 2018). Community nurses who are working with patients who could be making a change in their behaviour need to consistently assess motivation and how confident the individual might be alongside any perceived threats (Wild & McGrath, 2018). It should also be noted that an individual's choice can be affected by both automatic and reflective aspects of their decision-making (PHE, 2016).

Many health professionals are aware of the Prochaska and DiClemente's (1984) stage of change model, where the premise is that before any change can take place, a person needs to believe there's an advantage to changing (see Fig. 7.4). For this to work, they also need to be willing to put an effort into making this happen and then they have the control over deciding what this might look like and how they do it (RCN, 2024).

It is also important to ensure that any interventions support self-efficacy to ensure a sense of optimism and self-belief and support patients understanding that they can shape their future. Bandura (1997) identified four major influences on the generation of self-efficacy which are still referred to in current practice:

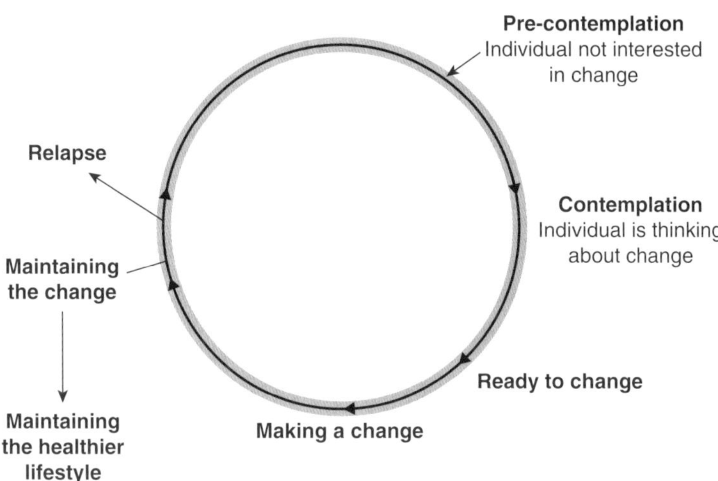

Fig. 7.4 The stages of change model. (Adapted from Prochaska, J. O., & DiClemente, C. (1984). *The transtheoretical approach: crossing traditional foundations of change* (1st ed.). Homewood, IL: Dow Jones-Irwin.)

1. **Mastery experience (performance outcomes):** this relates to a person's previous experiences in behaviour change and can include both successes and failures.
2. **Vicarious experience:** seeing other people make successful changes in behaviour can often provide exposure to techniques or strategies that could work.
3. **Verbal persuasion/social persuasion:** in order to promote self-efficacy, it is important to give consistent encouragement and to truly believe that an individual can change their behaviour.
4. **Perceptions of somatic/affective states (physiological feedback):** it is important to gauge how physically and emotionally ready an individual might be to make the change to their behaviour. It is important to understand how their current behaviour has an impact on their physical health and mood and feelings.

To be effective in supporting individuals in making these changes, it is important to try and see the situation from their point of view, encourage a realistic first step, build on their existing strengths, use small measurements to track their progress so that they can see the benefit of changing, respect their decisions, be open to honest discussions regarding support mechanisms and explore the potential of relapse.

7.6 Making Every Contact Count in Community Nursing

Making Every Contact Count (MECC) is an approach to behaviour change that enables the opportunistic delivery of healthy lifestyle interventions and facilitates conversations with individuals about their health (PHE, 2016). It also maximises the opportunities during routine health and care interactions for a brief discussion on health and well-being. With this in mind, it is useful to consider how visits from community nurses can provide opportunities to address unhealthy behaviours and be the catalysts for change.

CASE STUDY 7.1 Part 2

Gagandeep has been reading some information online that his daughter has found for him, which links poorly controlled diabetes and smoking with lower limb wounds that are slow to heal, and he is worried.

A course of antibiotics and analgesia have reduced the pain and exudate, but Gagandeep is constantly aware of the presence of the wound and is embarrassed.

He is still receiving weekly visits for wound care.

REFLECTION

- You are making a routine visit for wound management to Gagandeep's home. Considering the Prochaska and DiClemente's (1984) stage of change model and Bandura's (1997) influences on self-efficacy, how could you plan to address giving up smoking and support him to make this behavioural change? What skills might you need to achieve this?

7.7 Environmentally Sustainable Care in Community Nursing to Linking Sustainability to Public Health in Community Nursing

Community nurses provide complex care throughout the life course, maintaining population health and well-being, managing long-term conditions, palliative care, supporting rapid discharges, hospital avoidance and acuity care at home (Nursing and Midwifery Council (NMC), 2022; QNI, 2019). Much of this work already aligns with the principles in lower carbon care, in particular keeping people healthy, providing care in the right place, at the right time and at home. This work also points to the vital leadership and advocacy roles that District Nurses hold and the importance of interdisciplinary collaboration. Taken together, this high-quality care benefits patients and families whilst contributing to carbon reduction.

7.8 Climate Change and Health

Changes to the climate and the environment are having an impact on people's mental and physical health and exacerbating health inequalities, as outlined in the Lancet Countdown on health and climate change and by the World Health Organisation (The Lancet, 2023; WHO, 2024).

Climate change is a health crisis; it is a public health emergency and a patient safety issue. Climate change refers to long-term changes in temperature and weather patterns (United Nations, 2023). These changes are mostly driven by human activity, due to the burning of fossil fuels releasing greenhouse gas emissions, such as carbon, into the planet's atmosphere (United Nations, 2023). The impacts of climate change on health include heat-related illness and death during periods of extreme heat, asthma and cardiovascular disease linked to air pollution, mental health impacts linked to severe weather events and increases in vector-borne diseases (National Center for Environmental Health, 2022). Likewise, climate change is impacting on how we can deliver health and care services (NHS England, 2022). As nurses working in the community, work can be disrupted by severe weather and flooding, and working in buildings/homes during extremes of heat can place staff under additional physical and mental pressure.

Health systems are a significant source of greenhouse gas emissions and clinical activity through the delivery of care contributes to these emissions (Department of Health and Social Care (DH), 2021). The UK health and care system accounts for nearly 5% of the UK's total carbon emissions (Council of Deans of Health (CODH), 2023). In October 2020, the NHS in England became the world's first health service to commit to reaching carbon net zero (NHS England, 2022) and now all four United Kingdom (UK) Health Services have made similar commitments (DH, 2021).

Broadly speaking as a society, we can act to mitigate and adapt to climate change. Mitigation involves reducing greenhouse gas emissions (IPCC, 2018) to abate the impact of climate change worldwide. To reduce and prevent emissions of greenhouse gases into the environment by tackling the source of these emissions for example, can be done by changing the way in which we travel (European Environment Agency, 2024). Climate change adaptation refers to the adjustments needed in response to changes to our planet's climate (Department for Environment, Food and Rural Affairs (DEFRA), 2023), p. 13) and can include safeguarding water quality and investing in schemes to reduce flood risks and coastal erosion (DEFRA, 2023). It is imperative that healthcare professionals recognise, act and evaluate the management of risks posed by climate change to protect population health (Stanford, 2022) and prioritise reducing the emissions associated with health and social care. Prioritising action on climate change brings opportunities for improvements in public and societal health, reducing the demand on health and care services in the long-term (Fig. 7.5) (NHS England, 2022).

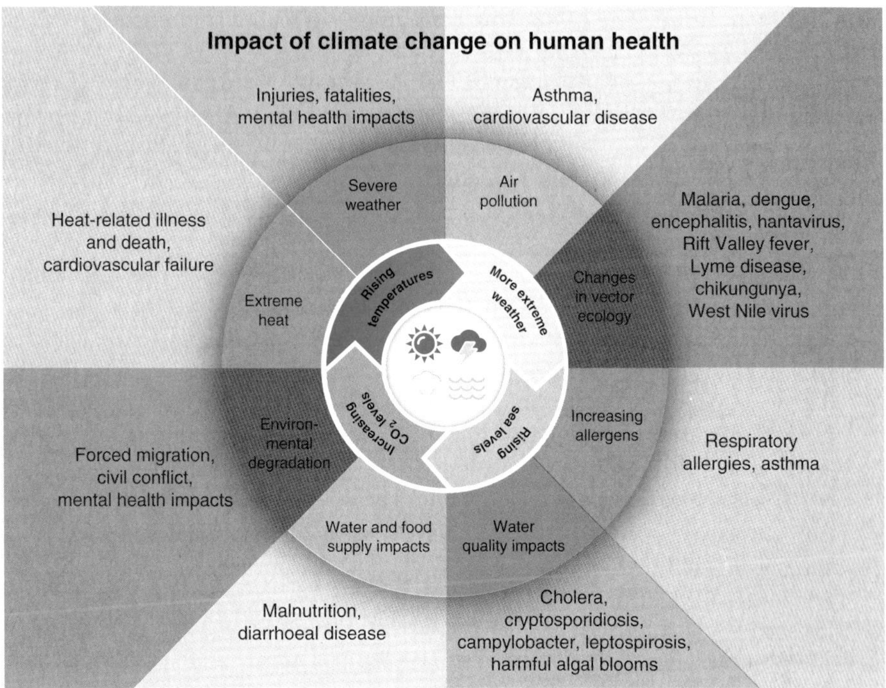

Fig. 7.5 Significant climate change impacts (rising temperatures, more extreme weather, rising sea levels, and increasing carbon dioxide levels), their effect on exposures and the subsequent health outcomes that can result from these changes in exposures. (From National Center for Environmental Health. https://www.cdc.gov/nceh/.)

As one of the most trusted professions, and a profession with arguably the most reach across and within communities, nurses have a central role to play in addressing climate change through leadership and scholarship, by advocating for the communities they serve and providing more environmentally sustainable care. Nursing colleagues from across the world recognise the need for urgent, coordinated action to tackle climate change both in terms of its causes and impacts. The nursing role in addressing climate change is recognised internationally (International Council of Nurses (ICN), 2023) and reflected the Chief Nursing Officer (CNO) for England's vision for nurses, midwives and nursing associates, which includes a focus area on 'protecting our planet' (Devereux, 2023), which will ultimately benefit the health of our environment and our population.

7.9 Lower Carbon Care

Achieving net zero means there is an equal balance of emissions being released into and removed from the atmosphere (IPCC, 2018). This requires human action to reduce the emissions we produce through our activity. The NHS is responsible for approximately 4% of the UK's total carbon footprint, with 40% of emissions from the public sector (The Health Foundation, 2023). On 1 July 2022, the NHS became the first health system to embed net zero into legislation, through the Health and Care Act 2022. To achieve carbon net zero, robust responses to climate change need to minimise emissions of care delivery through new duties on NHS England, all trusts, foundation trusts and integrated care boards to contribute towards statutory guidance in emissions and environmental targets (NHS England, 2022).

The principles of lower carbon care delivery have evolved over the past few years as awareness has grown on the escalating risks of climate change. All bring unique opportunities to improve the health and care of our patients/public in an efficient way (The Health Foundation, 2023) whilst also reducing carbon emissions.

These principles include (CODH, 2023; National Collaborating Centre for Mental Health, 2023):

- Clinical leadership, systems and workforce: leadership to support sustainable healthcare, training and education, time to get involved.
- Keeping people healthy: improving population health, reduce need for care, reducing health inequalities, primary and secondary prevention.
- Right care, right place, right time: efficiency, reducing inefficient and inappropriate care, using evidence-based practice, includes Getting It Right First Time (GIRFT) methodology (NHS England, 2023b).
- Low carbon treatment and care settings: using lower carbon alternatives, looking to the principles of circular economy and resource stewardship (Circular Economy Introduction, 2023).

In addition, recent work from the CODH proposes the inclusion of adaptation and resilience, whereby actions may not contribute to reducing carbon however, they may be necessary to support a resilient health system (CODH, 2023). These principles can be used to guide actions and care delivery in community settings and act as a structure to help identify and make visible the contribution of community nurses to delivering lower carbon environmentally sustainable care.

7.10 Community Nurses and Environmentally Sustainable Care

Over the last few years, colleagues within the Queen's Nursing Institute have been addressing issues of environmental sustainability and climate change through changes to their practice, for example, as outlined here: https://qni.org.uk/individual-actions-for-a-greener-planet/. Through a range of actions, including but not limited to using e-bikes or electric cars, recycling products, working with procurement colleagues to use the most appropriate products, implementing the 'Gloves off' campaign (RCN, 2023), considering prescribing practices to reduce overprescribing and promoting the use of evidence-based clinical practice, colleagues are reducing different sources of carbon that make up the NHS carbon footprint plus (see Fig. 7.6). Thus addressing environmental sustainability is not new for community nurses.

7.11 Examples in Focus: High-Quality Care in the Community

An example of how nurses are shaping and implementing new models of high-quality care that also align with principles of lower carbon care has its root in the Buurtzorg Model, which was first developed in the Netherlands as a nurse-led model of holistic

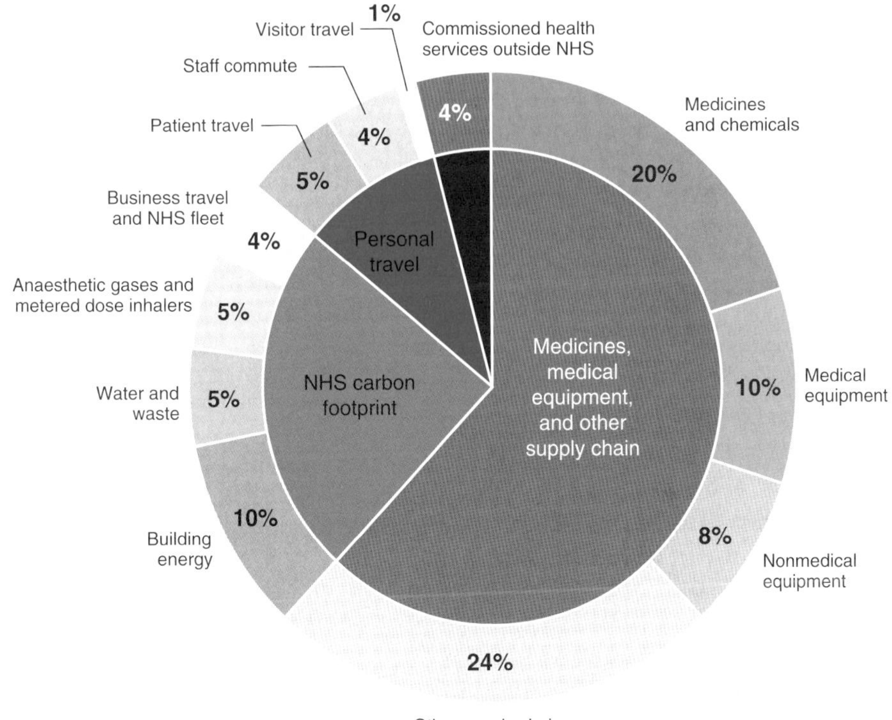

Fig. 7.6 Sources of carbon emissions by proportion of NHS Carbon Footprint Plus. (From NHS England 2021 – Delivering a 'Net Zero' National Health Service. https://www.england.nhs.uk/greenernhs/a-net-zero-nhs/.)

BOX 7.2 ■ Tips to Deliver Environmentally Sustainable Care

Nursing practice can be both high quality and low carbon and there are a range of actions that can be taken at an individual, team and service level:

- As a starting point, there is a need for each community nurse to understand climate change and the health impacts on the communities they serve.
- Then, there is a requirement to recognise what is already being done that aligns with the principles of lower carbon care.
- In addition, community nurses can also make a conscious effort to visibly support achieving net zero, for example, actions linked to good clinical practice and that focus on preventing ill health through measures including promoting healthy, sustainable diets, promoting active travel and environmentally friendly social prescribing for mental and physical health, all of which supports environmentally sustainable care and contributes to building healthier communities (QNI, 2022).
- Further ideas such as reducing polypharmacy, using green inhalers and reducing waste can also make a difference. For example, prescribing accounts for over 60% of the average general practice's carbon footprint. Additional actions include reducing unnecessary patient and staff travel and engaging with the voluntary sector in promoting community awareness and education (from QNI, 2022).

homecare that supports, empowers and encourages independent living and fosters the notion of 'humanity over bureaucracy' (Iriss, 2020). This model of care is known as 'a whole systems healing'; it is seen as a way of cultivating and improving the health and well-being of individuals and communities through sustaining economic, environmental and social structures (Kreitzer et al., 2015).

Neighbourhood models of care allow more time with patients, understanding what matters most and addressing health issues which are most important to the patient, in the end, providing a holistic and personalised package of nursing care which could help avoid hospital admissions and keep patients healthy and at home (Oxtoby, 2021). Keeping people healthy and reducing hospital admissions are important components to lower carbon care. Community nurses are in an ideal position to lead on and provide environmentally sustainable care (Box 7.2) and deliver on current recommendations set out in national policy (NHS England, 2019, 2022).

7.12 Conclusion

Community nurses have an important role to play within promoting health and well-being. Although sometimes limited by knowledge and resources, community nursing teams can inform population health strategies and become implicit in its delivery. Public health is everyone's responsibility and community nurses are in an optimum position to deliver this, however, this is often not transparent and goes unrecognised. Health promotion encompasses health education, prevention and protection, and community nurses already engage in activities within these areas. In order to make a sustainable impact on negative health behaviour choices, it is vital that community nurses understand what influences the choices that individuals make and that health education on its own is insufficient without appreciating the values and beliefs that underpin the motivation to succeed. It is also essential to recognise how important it is for individuals to have self-efficacy and a sense of self belief if they are going to make sustainable changes. In addition, community nurses are also ideally placed to contribute towards environmentally sustainable care. They are already making a meaningful impact for the health of the planet and the communities they serve. Working more sustainably is not about stopping or reducing needed resources; it is about the effective stewardship of resources and the provision of high-quality patient and community care. Community nurses are clinical leaders providing unique clinical decision-making to support equity and personalised care that works in the context for that patient improving population health. Community nurses can provide unique insights and solutions for alternative ways of working to improve planetary and population health.

References

Becker, M. H. (Ed.). (1974). *The Health Belief Model and personal health behaviour*. Thorofare, New Jersey: Slack.

Bandura, A. (1977). Self-efficacy: Towards a unifying theory of behaviour change. *Psychological Review*, *84*, 191–215.

Chief Medical Officer's annual report 2023 health in an ageing society. https://assets.publishing.service.gov.uk/media/6674096b64e554df3bd0dbc6/chief-medical-officers-annual-report-2023-web-accessible.pdf.

Circular Economy Introduction. (2023). *What is a circular economy?* Available at: https://www.ellenmacarthurfoundation.org/topics/circular-economy-introduction/overview. [Accessed 22 January 2024].

Council of Deans of Health. (2023). *Education for sustainable healthcare within UK pre-registration curricula for allied health professions*. Council of Deans of Health. Available at: https://www.councilofdeans.org.uk/wp-content/uploads/2023/12/ES-curricula-guidance-CoDH-version_SM-final-no-links.pdf. [Accessed 22 January 2024].

Department for Environment, Food and Rural Affairs (DEFRA). (2023). *The Third National Adaptation Programme (NAP3) and the Fourth Strategy for Climate Adaptation reporting*. Available at: https://assets.publishing.service.gov.uk/media/64ba74102059dc00125d27a7/The_Third_National_Adaptation_Programme.pdf. [Accessed 22 January 2024].

Department of Health and Social Care. (2021). *UK health services make landmark pledge to achieve net zero*. Available at: https://www.gov.uk/government/news/uk-health-services-make-landmark-pledge-to-achieve-net-zero. [Accessed 22 January 2024].

Devereux, E. (2023). *New 7Ps for nursing unveiled as part of CNO strategy*. Nursing Times. Available at: https://www.nursingtimes.net/news/leadership-news/new-7ps-for-nursing-unveiled-as-part-of-cno-strategy-16-11-2023/. [Accessed 22 January 2024].

Donaghy, P. H., Greenhalgh, C., Griffiths, P., & Verma, A. (2022). Preregistration adult nursing. Programmes and promotion of a population health agenda: An investigation. *British Journal of Community Nursing*, *27*(1), 40–44.

Duncan, M. (2019). Population health management and its relevance to community nurses. *British Journal of Community Nursing*, *24*(12), 595–599.

European Environment Agency. (2024). *What is the difference between adaptation and mitigation?* European Environment Agency. Available at: https://www.eea.europa.eu/help/faq/what-is-the-difference-between#:~:text=In%20essence%2C%20adaptation%20can%20be,(GHG)%20into%20the%20atmosphere. [Accessed 22 January 2024].

Evans, D., Coutsaftiki, D., & Fathers, C. P. (2017). *Health promotion and public health for nursing students*. Exeter: Sage.

International Council of Nurses. (2023). *ICN's key messages on climate change and health echoed in COP28's climate and health declaration*. ICN. Available at: https://www.icn.ch/news/icns-key-messages-climate-change-and-health-echoed-cop28s-climate-and-health-declaration. [Accessed 22 January 2024].

IPCC. (2018). Annex I: Glossary. Matthews, J.B.R. (ed.). In V. Masson-Delmotte, P. Zhai, H.-O. Pörtner, D. Roberts, J. Skea, P. R. Shukla, et al. (Eds.), *Global warming of 1.5°C. An IPCC special report on the impacts of global warming of 1.5°C above pre-industrial levels and related global greenhouse gas emission pathways, in the context of strengthening the global response to the threat of climate change, sustainable development, and efforts to eradicate poverty* (pp. 541–562). Cambridge, UK and New York, NY, USA: Cambridge University Press. https://doi.org/10.1017/9781009157940.008. [Accessed 22 January 2024].

Iriss. (2020). *The Buurtzorg model.* https://www.iriss.org.uk/sites/default/files/2020-03/iriss_on.the_buurtzorg_model.pdf.

Khumalo, M., & Brown, N. (2022). The role of the community nurse in population health management. *British Journal of Community Nursing*, *27*(6), 302–304.

King's Fund. (2018). *A vision for population health: Towards a healthier future*. Available at: https://www.kingsfund.org.uk/insight-and-analysis/reports/vision-population-health OR https://assets.kingsfund.org.uk/f/256914/x/25fa862dd5/vision_for_population_health_2018.pdf.

Kreitzer, M. J., Monsen, K. A., Nandram, S., & Blok, J. D. (2015). Buurtzorg Nederland: A global model of social innovation, change, and whole-systems healing. *Global Advances in Health and Medicine*, *1*(4), 40–44. Available at: https://journals.sagepub.com/doi/pdf/10.7453/gahmj.2014.030.

National Center for Environmental Health. (2022). *Climate effects on health*. Centers for Disease Control and Prevention. Available at: https://www.cdc.gov/climateandhealth/effects/default.htm. [Accessed 22 January 2024].

National Collaborating Centre for Mental Health. (2023). *Delivering greener, more sustainable and net zero mental health care: Guidance and recommendations*. London: National Collaborating Centre for Mental Health. Available at: https://www.rcpsych.ac.uk/docs/default-source/improving-care/nccmh/net-zero-mhc/delivering-greener--more-sustainable-and-net-zero-mental-health-care---guidance-and-recommendations.pdf?sfvrsn=c119e9d4_3. [Accessed 22 January 2024].

NHS England. (2019). *NHS long term plan*. Available at: https://www.longtermplan.nhs.uk/. [Accessed 3 May 2023].

NHS England. (2022). *Delivering a 'net zero' National Health Service*. NHS England. Available at: https://www.england.nhs.uk/greenernhs/wp-content/uploads/sites/51/2022/07/B1728-delivering-a-net-zero-nhs-july-2022.pdf. [Accessed 22 January 2024].

NHS England. (2023a). *Integrated care systems*. NHS England. Available at: https://www.england.nhs.uk/integratedcare/.

NHS England. (2023b). *Getting It Right First Time (GIRFT)*. NHS England. Available at: https://gettingitrightfirsttime.co.uk/. [Accessed 22 January 2024].

NHS England. (2024). *Population health management*. Available at: https://www.england.nhs.uk/integratedcare/phm/.

NICE. (2022). *Improving oral health for adults in care homes*. Available at: https://www.nice.org.uk/about/nice-communities/social-care/quick-guides/improving-oral-health-for-adults-in-care-homes.

NMC. (2022). *Standards of proficiency for community nursing specialist practice qualifications.* London: Nursing & Midwifery Council. Available at: https://www.nmc.org.uk/globalassets/sitedocuments/standards/post-reg-standards/nmc_standards_of_proficiency_for_community_nursing_spqs.pdf. [Accessed 11 June 2023].

Nursing and Midwifery Council. (2022). *Standards of proficiency for community nursing specialist practice qualifications.* NMC.

Oxtoby, K. (2021). *Can the Buurtzorg model of nursing transform the NHS? Independent Nurse.* Available at: https://www.independentnurse.co.uk/content/news/can-the-buurtzorg-model-of-nursing-transform-the-nhs/.

Palmer, S. J. (2023). Oral healthcare in the community. *British Journal of Community Nursing, 28*(5), 244–246.

Prochaska, J. O., & DiClemente, C. (1984). *The transtheoretical approach: Crossing traditional foundations of change.* Harnewood: Don Jones/Irwin.

Pronk, N. P., Kleinman, D. V., Goekler, S. F., Ochiai, E., Blakey, C., & Brewer, K. H. (2021). Promoting health and well-being in Healthy People 2030. *Journal of Public Health Management and Practice, 27*(6), S242–S248.

Public Health England. (2016). *Making Every Contact Count (MECC): Consensus statement.* PHE.

QNI. (2019). *District nursing today. The view of district nurse team leaders in the UK.* QNI. Available at: https://qni.org.uk/wp-content/uploads/2019/11/District-Nursing-Today-The-View-of-DN-Team-Leaders-in-the-UK.pdf.

QNI and Royal College of Nursing. (2019). *Outstanding models of district nursing. A joint project identifying what makes an outstanding district nursing service.* Available at: https://www.qni.org.uk/wp-content/uploads/2019/05/Oustanding-Models-of-District-Nursing-Report-web.pdf.

QNI. (2022). *Climate change. Actions community nurses can take.* https://qni.org.uk/climate-change-actions-community-nurses-can-take/.

Royal College of Nursing (RCN). (2016). *Nurses 4 Public Health Promote, Prevent and Protect. The value and contribution of nursing to public health in the UK: Final report.* Available at: https://www.rcn.org.uk/Professional-Development/publications/pub-005497.

Royal College of Nursing (RCN). (2023). *Glove awareness.* Available at: https://www.rcn.org.uk/Get-Involved/Campaign-with-us/Glove-awareness. [Accessed 22 January 2024].

Royal College of Nursing (RCN). (2024). *Public health: Improving the public's health is at the heart of health and social care across the UK.* Available at: https://www.rcn.org.uk/clinical-topics/Public-health#:~:text=Public%20health%20refers%20to%20all,the%20population%20as%20a%20whole.

Stanford, V. (2022). *Climate change adaptation: A guide for health and care professionals.* Centre for Sustainable Healthcare. Available at: https://sustainablehealthcare.org.uk/blog/climate-change-adaptation. [Accessed 22 January 2024].

Stark, P., McKenna, G., Wilson, C. B., Tsakos, G., Brocklehurst, P., Lappin, C., … Mitchell, B. (2022). Interventions supporting community nurses in the provision of oral healthcare to people living at home: A scoping review. *BMC Nursing, 21*, 269.

Tannahill, A. (2009). Health promotion: The Tannahill model revisited. *Public Health, 123*, 396–399.

The Health Foundation. (2023). *Net zero care: What will it take?* The Health Foundation. Available at: https://www.health.org.uk/publications/long-reads/net-zero-care-what-will-it-take#:~:text=The%20NHS%20in%20England%20has,estates%2C%20energy%20and%20supply%20chains. [Accessed 22 January 2024].

The Lancet. (2023). The Lancet countdown on health and climate change. *The Lancet*. Available at: https://www.thelancet.com/countdown-health-climate. [Accessed 22 January 2024].

United Nations. (2023). *What is climate change? United Nations*. Available at: https://www.un.org/en/climatechange/what-is-climate-change. [Accessed 22 January 2024].

Wild, K., & McGrath, M. (2018). *Public health and health promotion for nurses at a glance*. USA: Wiley & Sons.

Wills, J. (2023). *Foundations for health promotion* (5th ed.). Scotland: Elsevier.

World Health Organisation. (2024). *Climate and health are inextricably linked*. WHO. Available at: https://climahealth.info/understand/chapter-1/. [Accessed 22 January 2024].

CHAPTER 8

Clinical Assessment

Sandra Dilks

LEARNING OUTCOMES

After reading this chapter you should be able to:

- Describe and discuss the role of holistic assessments in district nursing
- Explain how patients are empowered to be part of the assessment pathway
- Discuss effective verbal and nonverbal communication as part of the assessment process
- Understand mental capacity assessment in the community

8.1 Introduction

Assessment is a fundamental aspect of the district nursing process and ensures the district nurse gathers all the information required to provide a clear structure with which to plan, implement and evaluate episodes of care. High-quality care that is focused on addressing the patient's needs requires a holistic assessment to take into account the patient's physical, psychological, social and spiritual well-being (Queen's Nursing Institute, 2015a).

8.2 Background

As people are living longer with more long-term and often complex health conditions and care needs, the district nurse as an autonomous practitioner is required to adopt an evidence-based approach to provide the framework with which to base decision-making and developing a plan of care (Queen's Nursing Institute, 2015b). A key element of this approach is a holistic assessment, the purpose of which is to gain a complete picture of the patient, their health needs and their perspectives and concerns as the foundations of providing individualised care. As a vital component, the assessment process is a fundamental skill of all nursing disciplines, however, district nurses are seen as specialists when assessing patients within their own homes (Horner, 2022). The principles of assessment are outlined in Fig. 8.1.

In 1958 a research associate, Ida Jean Orlando, described a nursing process based on her own research known as The Deliberate Nursing Process, which continues to influence nursing practice today. The foundation of this approach is to apply critical thinking, be patient centred, evidence based and using nursing intuition when following five sequential steps as shown in Fig. 8.2.

The assessment is the first stage in any nursing process and requires the district nurse to gather data systematically and continuously: to sort and analyse the data using

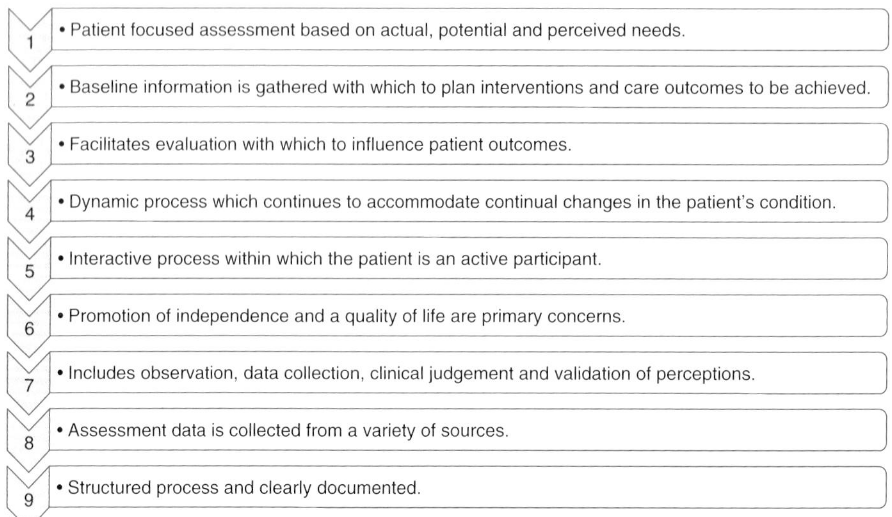

Fig. 8.1 Principles of assessment. Adapted from Lister, S., Hofland, J., & Grafton, H. (2020). *The Royal Marsden manual of clinical nursing procedures; professional edition* (10th ed.). Chichester: Wiley Blackwell.

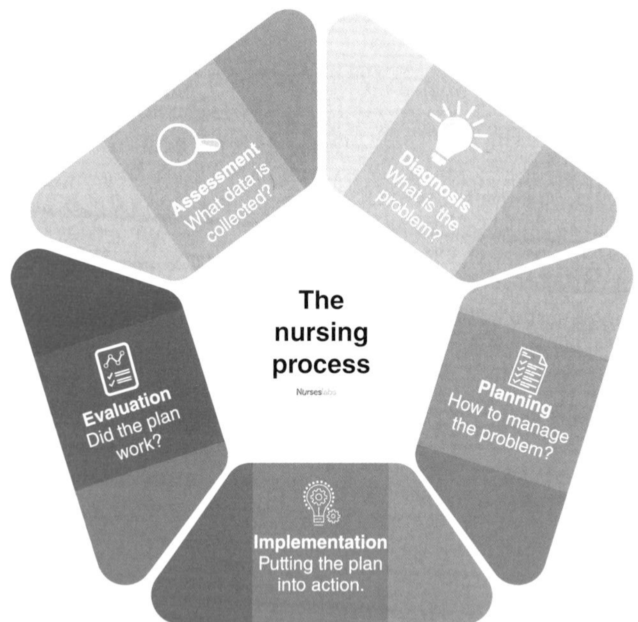

Fig. 8.2 The nursing process. (From Wayne, G. (2022). The nursing process: a comprehensive guide. Nurseslabs. https://nurseslabs.com/nursing-process/.)

evidence-based tools to organise the information gained to form an overview of the patient's concerns, symptoms and overall health (Mayo, 2017). The district nurse then interprets the data into information with which to inform the decision-making process and to devise a care plan and any ongoing decisions. Finally, this is documented and communicated with the patient, family or carers and potential other services, identifying any normal or abnormal findings which may impact on acute, urgent, long-term or life-limiting conditions (Carrier & Newbury, 2016).

Information and data gathered will include the collection of objective data by obtaining baseline observations such as blood pressure, respiratory rate and temperature but will also include subjective data such as the effects on daily living and pain levels, which will require the use of appropriate nursing assessment tools such as appropriate pain and dyspnoea scales (Lister et al., 2020).

Through an accurate and comprehensive gathering of information, the district nurse is then able to prioritise the care required, without which delayed or incomplete assessments can result in adverse consequences for patients. As evidenced in numerous reports which have highlighted failings in the National Health Service (NHS), poor and inadequate care results in poor patient experience, increased risk of infection and complications due to undetected deterioration (Cho et al., 2015; Kalisch et al., 2012; Keogh, 2013). Therefore an inadequate assessment can have a negative impact on patient safety and must be seen as a dialogue between the district nurse and the patient where they can discuss the individual needs of the patient in order to promote their health and well-being, empowerment and shared decision-making.

8.3 Holistic Assessment

Conducting an accurate assessment will aid the district nurse to identify the presenting and any continuing healthcare needs (Ajibade, 2021). The structure of the assessment will include reviewing any existing health records, identifying any potential presenting complaints, gathering a comprehensive patient history and performing a physical examination (Wilson and Giddens, 2022). However, most importantly, the earlier the initial history taking, and physical examination is completed, the higher the likelihood any potential life-limiting conditions can be recognised and stabilised ensuring better patient outcomes.

To ensure the district nurse provides high-quality care that is focused and patient centred and meets the patients' individual needs requires a holistic approach to the assessment and avoiding becoming solely focused on a particular condition or task at hand (Kwame & Petrucka, 2021). This is achieved by the district nurse engaging with the patient and including family and carers where necessary and acknowledging that the patient may have multiple problems or conditions for which they will have their own opinions or preferences. Intrinsic factors such as mental health, values and beliefs and previous experiences will often not only manifest in physical conditions but will affect patient concordance with healthcare treatment and advice (World Health Organization, 2022).

Through a holistic approach, the district nurse will ensure that the aspects of physical, psychological, spiritual, social and cultural care are all included, assessing and seeing the patient as a whole rather than a diagnosis or a series of tasks to complete. Therefore essentially holistic care requires the patient to be shown respect, treated in a nonjudgemental manner and seen as an individual instead of a medical condition. The principles which underpin holistic care are emulated in the 'house of care', a model which has been universally adopted across the NHS to ensure patients are at the heart of the delivery of care (Coulter et al., 2013) (Fig. 8.3).

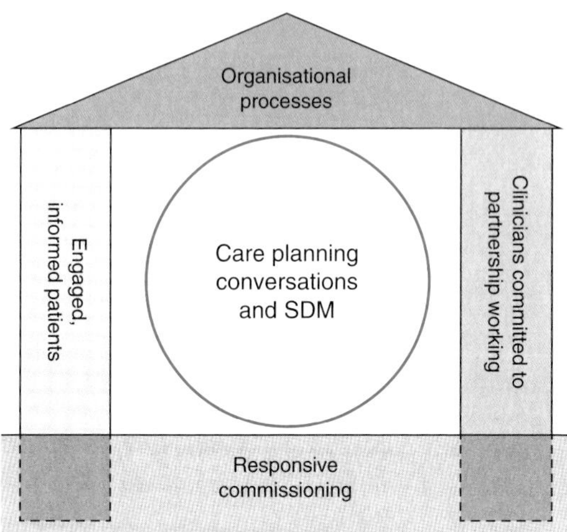

Fig. 8.3 House of care. *SDM,* Shared decision-making. (Adapted from Coulter, A., Roberts, S., & Dixon, A. (2013). Delivering better services for people with long term conditions: building the house of care. Retrieved 7 September 2023 from https://www.kingsfund.org.uk/sites/default/files/field/field_publication_file/delivering-better-services-for-people-with-long-term-conditions.pdf.)

8.4 Initial Impression

The initial relationship with a patient depends on the first encounter where with limited information, the initial few minutes of a conversation and rapid automatic judgments, a first impression will be formed which will influence the establishment of a therapeutic relationship. Research suggests that it takes just a few seconds or a quick glance to form an opinion based on appearance, body language, mannerisms and demeanour (South Palomares & Young, 2017). These first impressions are formed each time we meet someone new and are often impossible to reverse setting the tone of the relationship moving forward.

During this initial impression, the district nurse will begin the assessment by gathering clues to identify any issues with communication, mobility and assessing the home environment. At the same time, the patient will form an initial impression of professionalism and develop a preconceived level of care anticipated that may have significant implications and influence continued interactions and concordance.

8.5 Developing a Rapport

An expected outcome from the initial meeting is the establishment of a nurse–patient rapport which is essential to an effective relationship (Molina-Mula & Gallo Estrada, 2020). As a foundation for trust and parallel with respect and empathy, a good rapport will have positive outcomes on the patient experience and satisfaction and overall concordance with treatment. Therefore developing a rapport and establishing a therapeutic relationship which is harmonious and patient centred are crucial for shared decision-making and the quality of care provided (Butt, 2021).

8.6 Privacy and Dignity

For most of the district nurse workload, assessments will most likely be conducted within the patient's own home. Regardless of which, it continues to be important for the district nurse to have an awareness of the surrounding environment and aim for a private, unoccupied room that is free from distractions. The patient should be physically comfortable during the assessment and where possible seated or positioned to suit their preferences during the initial stages. The principles of privacy and dignity remain relevant even in the patient's own home as they are less likely to be open and honest with personal and potentially sensitive information if they are in discomfort or fearful of being overheard or interrupted (Maybin et al., 2016). Conducting a physical examination in the patient's home can be challenging, as the environment will have a significant impact and therefore it is essential to continue to maintain privacy and dignity. Therefore the patient should be positioned as comfortably as possible, in a suitable position but also so that the minimum number of positional moves is required.

8.7 History Taking

The importance of gathering a comprehensive patient history should not be underestimated, with research suggesting that the information required for a diagnosis can be identified from a patient's history alone in 70%–90% of cases (Fitzgerald, 2012), thus indicating that history taking alone is the single most important aspect of the holistic process and is crucial to guide and direct care.

Many newly qualified district nurses or those new to the assessment process may follow a recognised consultation model such as Neighbour's (1987) 'The Inner Consultation' (Fig. 8.4) or Kurtz and Silverman's (1996) 'Calgary–Cambridge Guide' (Fig. 8.5). However, over time and through experience, it is essential nurses develop their own framework,

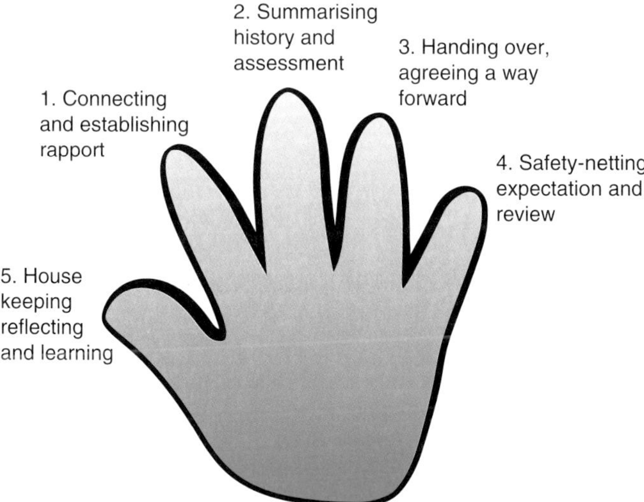

Fig. 8.4 Inner consultation. (Adapted from Neighbour, R. (1987). *The inner consultation*. London: Springer.)

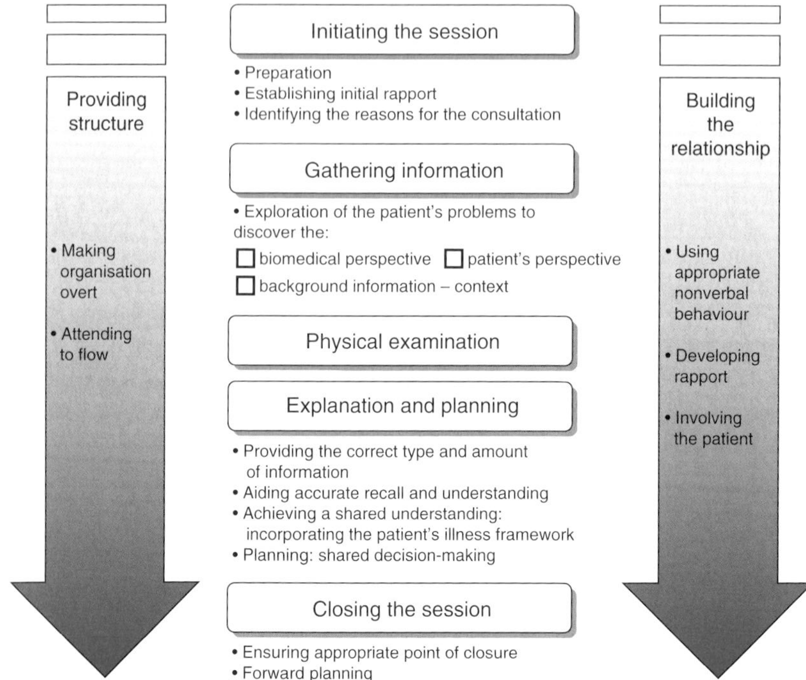

Fig. 8.5 Calgary–Cambridge guide. (Adapted from Kurtz, S., & Silverman, J. (1996). The Calgary–Cambridge referenced observation guides: an aid to defining the curriculum and organizing the teaching in communication training programmes. *Medical Education, 30*, 83–89.)

taking elements from the existing models and building on them, so that they avoid relying on them as a set of rules rather than an aid to the overall consultation.

A comprehensive history taking assessment should cover both general and focused components with which to gather the patient's story (Bickley et al., 2021). There are several approaches to history taking with the main principles of using a framework to gather the information required in a sequential order and to listen to the patient's responses. The primary aim of gathering a history is to develop an understanding of the patient's state of health, secondary to which is to determine if there is any further potential harm that can be negated. The process should be structured to enable the district nurse to gain a clear picture of the patient's presenting and existing complaints by gathering the data and information in order to reach a potential diagnosis and develop a treatment plan.

The components of history taking adapted from The Royal Marsden Manual of Clinical Nursing Procedures (Lister et al., 2020) are summarised in Table 8.1.

8.8 Differential Diagnosis

Taking time to gather a comprehensive history will allow the district nurse time to ask open-ended questions and actively listen to the patient's perspective, ultimately ensuring

TABLE 8.1 ■ **Comprehensive History**

Identifying Data	Name, Date of Birth, Gender
Presenting complaint	Opening gambit. 'How can I help you today?' Clear chronological order history of symptoms. Avoiding interruptions to patient explanation. Documenting in patient's own words, 'difficulty in breathing'
I.C.E.	Ascertain the patient's ideas, concerns and expectations from the consultation
History of presenting complaint	Gather information using a prompt such as a mnemonic to ask questions regarding symptoms: 'OLD CARTS': **O**nset, **L**ocation, **D**uration, **C**haracteristics, **A**ssociated Symptoms/**A**ggravated factors, **R**adiation/**R**evealing factors and **T**iming/In**T**ensity
System enquiry	Gathering additional information, either general such as unintentional weight loss/altered appetite or system specific such as for a head injury to include headache, dizziness. Consider pertinent positives and pertinent negatives such as chest pain, associated nausea/dizziness, shortness of breath, radiation
Past medical history	Gather information using a prompt such as a mnemonic to ask if the patient has any past or existing medical conditions: 'JAMTHREADS': **J**aundice, **A**naemic, **Myocardial** infarction, **T**uberculosis, **H**ypertension, **R**heumatic fever, **E**pilepsy, **A**sthma, **D**iabetes, **S**troke
Medication history	What medication is the patient taking? Gather a full list including dose, frequency and route, whether they are taking any over-the-counter (OTC) herbal or recreational remedies
Allergy history	Check for an adverse drug reaction (ADR) to determine if a known side effect or a true allergy
Family history	To ascertain relevant patient/sibling/grandparent history. Can adopt the same new mnemonic 'JAMTHREADS'
Social history	Gather information regarding: • Occupation as this may include exposure to industrial risk factors • Social—family, married, children, dependants, etc. • Infectious disease—recent foreign travel • Contacts—recent exposure next to • Dependents • Social service/safeguarding
Lifestyle/risk factors	Gather information regarding: • Smoking history (pack years)—packs smoked per day × years smoked • Alcohol consumption—units/week; alcohol-free days—current and past • Exercise • Diet • Salt

they can begin to formulate a list of potential conditions which indicate the cause of symptoms (Henly, 2016). Although occasionally it is possible to arrive at a single diagnosis, most district nurses will identify one of two primary diagnoses whilst additionally identifying a list of potential alternatives. The history can present clues to the potential cause and aid the district nurse to continuously refine the list of potential diagnoses. This continuous systematic process is known as differential diagnoses and requires the district nurse to understand the aetiology of disease and will continue throughout the consultation as they discover new information with which to evaluate the pertinent positives and negatives from the patient history, undertake a physical examination and review any further investigations. At the same time, the district nurse will be confirming or refuting differentials until reaching the final diagnosis.

8.9 Physical Examination

A physical examination is a systematic assessment of one or several body systems depending on the indications and nature of the presenting complaint guided by the gathering of the patient's history (Dover et al., 2023). Whilst it has been identified that a comprehensive history will provide between 70% and 90% of the potential diagnosis, it is further suggested that the physical examination and any further investigations will only add a further 10% to the information gained. By this stage in the health assessment process, the physical examination should essentially provide the confirmation of the primary diagnosis. However, the physical examination remains paramount as it can provide confirmation evidence such as visible discolouration, bruising or rashes or identify areas of tenderness which may be too subtle for x-rays and scans. When conducting an appropriate physical examination, it will not only offer confirmation of a primary diagnosis but can also avoid the need for nonessential investigations.

During the initial impression stage, the district nurse should have been identifying general observations from the patient such as levels of consciousness, distress, pain or laboured breathing and these observations will have extended to the environment to include safety hazards, lighting and medical equipment (Dover et al., 2023). Prior to conducting any physical contact during the examination, the district nurse should adhere to the standard universal precautions applied by infection control standards including hand washing and donning any required personal protective equipment.

The district nurse will evaluate further objective data findings by adopting the approach of inspection, palpation, percussion and auscultation which should be seen as a continuum to the information gathered from the history. The sequence of inspection, palpation, percussion and auscultation relies on the district nurse's knowledge of normal anatomy and common presentation patterns in order to identify abnormal findings associated with the potential differentials.

8.10 Appropriate Investigations

Undertaking a comprehensive holistic history and an appropriate physical examination can provide more information than conducting investigations and tests and assist the district nurse to refine the diagnostic process avoiding unnecessary investigations (Balogh et al., 2015). Although medical science has seen rapid advancements in technology, it is important to consider the patient and the limitations of excessive and unnecessary tests. Investigations can often be time consuming and expensive for both the patient and the wider NHS (NHS England, 2019). The process of waiting for an investigation and yielding results can cause the patient unwanted stress and can produce incidental findings that cannot be ignored. Therefore the district nurse should consider the implications of further investigations which often result in a greater cost to the patient.

8.11 Diagnosis and Continuous Assessment

The information gathered from the history and the physical examination is crucial for the diagnostic and decision-making stage of the process (Nichol et al., 2022). On the balance of probability, the components of the assessment will enable the district nurse to reach a final diagnosis which is often from pattern recognition. Although acknowledging the element of uncertainty, the district nurse will anticipate potential future healthcare needs and long-term prognosis by reviewing and reevaluating the history and physical examination, as and when required through continuous assessment.

8.12 Patient Empowerment

The term 'patient empowerment' generally refers to having independent control over one's own health and being actively involved in decisions regarding the care received by working in partnership with healthcare providers, rather than being passive recipients of care (NHS England, 2017).

Patient empowerment is not a new phenomenon, although it repeatedly has renewed significance and has become increasingly popular within nursing. Historically, the clinician or healthcare service provider made the decisions regarding the care required and there was little or no emphasis on patient choice. The transfer of care from such a paternalistic approach towards one of patient empowerment has now been linked to improved health outcomes, patient satisfaction and greater compliance and improves the financial sustainability of the NHS (NHS England, 2017).

The NHS Long Term Plan (NHS England, 2019) has more recently set out to endorse and increase the support available to enable patients to have more control over their own health and for care to become increasingly individualised depending on their needs. The aim of this approach is to ensure the patient becomes the key driver in their healthcare needs and is now recognised as a core value for delivering high-quality patient-centred care, placing a strong emphasis on patient participation in the assessment and clinical decision-making process.

The district nurse can play a pivotal role in promoting patient empowerment by encouraging and enabling them to share their views and opinions, thus demonstrating they are valued and can take ownership of the decisions regarding their own health. Treating the patient as an individual, recognising the impact of the symptoms or condition and respecting their views and preferences empowers the patient in the assessment process (Fig. 8.6).

When conducting a holistic assessment, patient control, choice and empowerment rebalance the power during the consultation and can be of particular importance with informed decision-making. The basis of active patient empowerment begins during the consultation process, where the formation of a partnership frequently occurs whilst establishing a rapport and a one-to-one relationship at the history gathering stage. Therefore by empowering the patient whilst eliciting detailed and accurate information and obtaining consent for examination and investigations can reveal the nature, extent and context of the symptoms or condition.

Furthermore, as the NHS continues to evolve, and patients have greater access to medical information, this in turn can enhance patient empowerment through their increased knowledge and expectations enabling them to become partners in healthcare

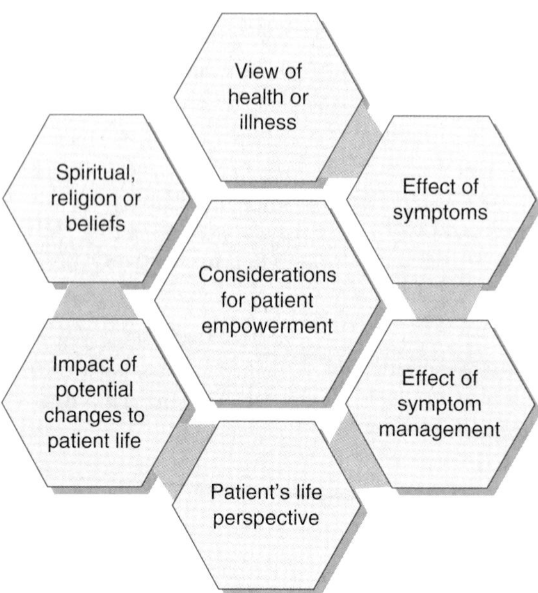

Fig. 8.6 Considerations for patient empowerment during the history gathering stage of the assessment process.

decisions. Their contribution to healthcare is then not only reflected in taking ownership of their own health decisions but can also increase their participation in health promotion and move towards a more consumer-led healthcare service as they make informed decisions regarding resources within the healthcare system (NHS England, 2017).

8.13 Effective Communication

Communication is a two-way process which is multidimensional and can be simultaneously simple and complex in nature. In its simple format communication is the exchange of information however, this exchange can be complex as a result of a variety of modes and impacted by intentional or unintentional behaviours.

Within a multicultural society, there will be a significant proportion of the population who will not have English as their first language (Squires, 2018), thus creating a barrier between the district nurse and the patient due to the absence of a common language. Whilst care should not be compromised as a result, the language barrier can affect nursing practice unless the cultural divide is bridged (Lee, 2021). A readily available option would be to use family or friends to translate; unfortunately, doing so can create shortcomings in key information being inaccurately communicated or misunderstood (Squires, 2018). Therefore professional interpreters offer a valuable service of translation that will assist to ensure that care can be delivered which considers specific cultural phrasing (Rimmer, 2020).

Whilst the spoken word is recognised as verbal communication in the age of technology, this is often extended to modes of written communication such as emails and text

BOX 8.1 ■ Communicating Effectively

Section 7 of the NMC Code (2018)

You communicate effectively, keeping clear and accurate records and sharing skills, knowledge and experience where appropriate.

To achieve this:

7.1 use terms that people in your care, colleagues and the public can understand.

7.2 take reasonable steps to meet people's language and communication needs, providing, wherever possible, assistance to those who need help to communicate their own or other people's needs.

7.3 use a range of verbal and nonverbal communication methods and consider cultural sensitivities, to better understand and respond to people's personal and health needs.

7.4 check people's understanding from time to time to keep misunderstanding or mistakes to a minimum.

7.5 be able to communicate clearly and effectively in English.

(Adapted from Nursing and Midwifery Council (2018). The Code: Professional standards of practice and behaviour for nurses, midwives and nursing associates. London: Nursing and Midwifery Council.)

messaging. Communication does not occur in isolation with words as it also includes modes of nonverbal communication. Primarily nonverbal communication is the interplay of body language such as facial expressions, eye contact, appearance, stance and gestures. Each can convey a subtle message of empathy and are uniquely dependent on the individual and situation. However, as nonverbal communication can be more compelling than words, to be an effective communicator, the district nurse must have an awareness of all communication channels to prevent any negative influences.

The ability to communicate effectively is the most important skill a district nurse can possess (Afriyie, 2020). The experience of healthcare and overall patient satisfaction is principally determined by the extent of the provider's communications skills. A failure or inability to demonstrate an array of effective communication skills can negatively impact patient care. McDonald (2016) estimated that poor communication skills cost the NHS over £1 billion per year, leading to poor compliance with treatment regimes, repeated visits to clinics and disputes leading to litigation.

Compassion in Practice (Department of Health (DH), 2012) identified communication as a central component of its vision and values for healthcare professionals and this is further reflected within the Nursing and Midwifery Council (2018) The Code: Professional standards of practice and behaviour for nurses, midwives and nursing associates, as identified in Box 8.1.

As the foundation to a positive patient–nurse relationship, effective communication is pivotal within the assessment process not only for gaining trust and building a rapport but also for obtaining of a detailed and accurate history, gaining consent to examination and investigations, discussing a diagnosis and the management of a treatment plan which overall improves patient outcomes.

The district nurse requires a wide range of skills for communication to be effective, including empathy for the delivery of care to be patient centred; this level of understanding is key to the provision of high-quality care which is compassionate. Fig. 8.7 demonstrates the range of skills required.

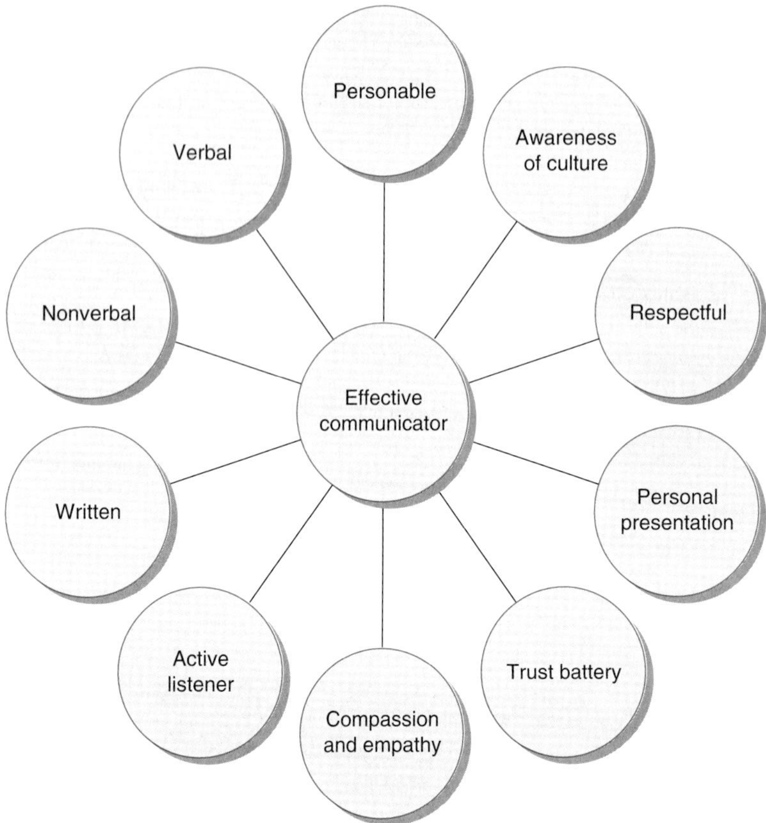

Fig. 8.7 Skills of an effective communicator.

8.14 Mental Capacity

Whilst caring for patients in their own homes and in the community, district nurses often face assessing acute complex care needs which are multifaceted affecting both physical and mental health. The correlation between health and well-being is a two-way relationship as physical health problems can significantly influence poor mental health and vice versa. This interrelationship between physical and mental health is an important consideration within any patient assessment as mental health is the largest determinant of disability within the UK (DH, 2011). Furthermore, the influence of mental health on how an individual patient thinks, feels and behaves in daily life affects their ability to deal with challenges within their own health and the building of relationships required to work in partnerships with healthcare professionals.

Each episode of care requires valid informed consent, and it must be assumed that all patients have the capacity to consent to care and treatment unless proven otherwise (Health Research Authority, 2021). Implemented in 2007 in England and Wales the Mental Capacity Act (MCA) 2005 is statutory legislation which is designed to improve the protection and empowerment of vulnerable adults who lack or have lost the capacity

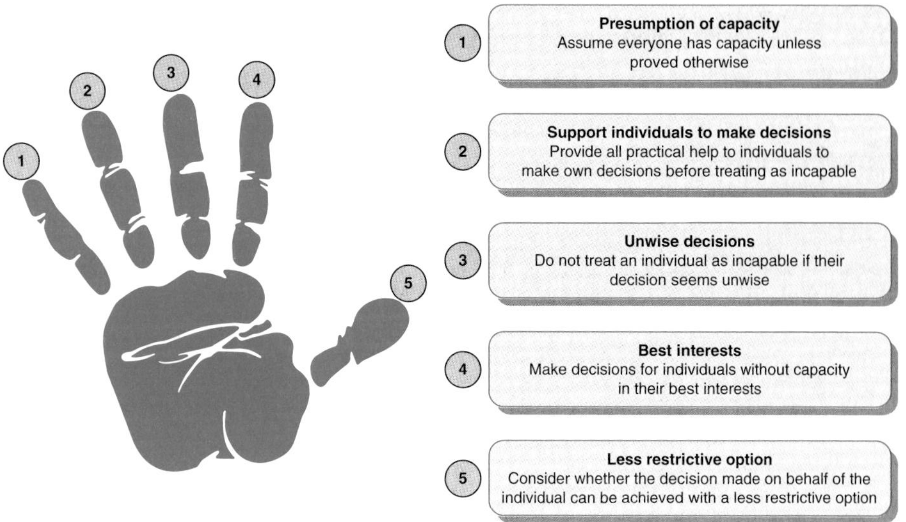

Fig. 8.8 Five principles of the Mental Capacity Act, 2005.

to make decisions about their care and treatment (HM Government, 2005). Those within Scotland operate under the Adults with Incapacity Act 2000, whilst Northern Ireland operates under the Mental Capacity Act (Northern Ireland) 2016.

The five statutory principles which apply to assessing an individual's capacity can be found in Fig. 8.8.

Under the Mental Capacity Act, an individual lacks capacity if they are unable to make decisions due to an impairment or disturbance in the functioning of the brain or mind which is limiting their ability to understand and evaluate information which was provided and required at the time the decision needs to be made. Although some individuals may experience fluctuating periods of capacity, either due to an acute or chronic illness such as an infection or dementia, the Mental Capacity Act is clear that a diagnosis alone should not be used to determine mental capacity.

Unfortunately, in healthcare, decisions regarding care and treatment cannot always be postponed until a time when the individual has regained capacity. Therefore decisions can be made in their best interests if an assessment of mental capacity has been recorded and the decision can be justified. Where there is an element of doubt the district nurse should adopt the two-stage test for capacity as shown in Box 8.2.

8.15 Conclusion

A holistic and comprehensive history taking is the fundamental starting point for any health assessment, and accurately completing the process ensures the district nurse can prioritise the health care needs required. The process should be logical and ensure patient safety, dignity and privacy at all times even in the challenging environments of patients' own homes. As the aspect of physical examination requires the element of touch, it is important that the district nurse establishes an effective rapport and builds a good initial

BOX 8.2 ■ Two-Stage Capacity Test

Stage two—passed the test

To assess whether an individual lacks capacity to make a decision, the two-stage capacity test should be followed. The test is time and decision specific and must be repeated for each episode, consent is required.

1. Does the individual have an impairment or disturbance of the brain or mind, regardless if permanent or temporary?

If yes:

2. Is impairment or disturbance sufficient resulting in the individual's inability to make particular decision?

This is determined by ensuring all appropriate support and information has been provided to make the decision and that the individual cannot do at least one of the following:

- Understand the information
- Retain sufficient information long enough to make a decision
- Evaluate and weigh up the information for its advantages and disadvantages
- Communicate their decision.

When any of the above applies, it can be deemed that the individual lacks capacity to make the decision.

(Adapted from Department for Constitutional Affairs, (2007). *Mental Capacity Act 2005: Code of Practice*. London: Stationary Office.)

impression. The initial visit or consultation with a patient will require the information gathered from a full and comprehensive history and physical examination, whereas subsequent consultations will generally involve a review of the history and examination in order to modify any management or treatment plan.

References

Afriyie, D. (2020). Effective communication between nurses and patients: An evolutionary concept analysis. *British Journal of Community Nursing*, *25*(9), 438–445.

Ajibade, B. (2021). Assessing the patient's needs and planning effective care. *British Journal of Nursing*, *30*(20), 1166–1171.

Balogh, E., Miller, B., & Ball, J. (2015). *Improving diagnosis in health care*. Washington: The National Academic Press.

Bickley, L., Szilagyi, P., & Hoffman, R. (2021). *Bates' pocket guide to physical examination and history taking* (9th ed.). Philadelphia: Wolters Kluwer.

Butt, M. (2021). Approaches to building rapport with patients. *Clinical Medicine*, *21*(6), 662–663.

Carrier, J., & Newbury, G. (2016). Managing long-term conditions in primary and community care. *British Journal of Community Nursing*, *21*(10), 504–508.

Cho, S., Kim, Y., Yeon, K., You, S., & Lee, I. (2015). Effects of increasing nurse staffing on missed nursing care. *International Nursing Review*, *62*(2), 267–274.

Coulter, A., Roberts, S., & Dixon, A. (2013). Delivering better services for people with long term conditions: Building the house of care. Available at https://www.kingsfund.org.uk/insight-and-analysis/reports/better-services-people-long-term-conditions (Accessed on 7th September 2023).

Department for Constitutional Affairs. (2007). *Mental capacity act 2005: Code of practice. London: Stationary office.*

Department of Health. (2011). *No health without mental health: A cross-government mental health outcomes strategy for people of all ages*. London: Department of Health.

Department of Health. (2012). *Compassion in practice: Nursing, midwifery and care staff, our vision and strategy*. London: Stationary Office.

Dover, A., Innes, J., & Fairhurst, K. (2023). *Macleod's clinical examination* (15th ed.). Edinburgh: Elsevier.

Fitzgerald, F. (2012). History and physical examination: art and science. In M. Henderson, L. Tierney, & G. Smetana (Eds.), *The patient history: An evidence based approach to differential diagnosis* (2nd ed.) (pp. 3–4). New York: McGraw Hill Medical.

Health Research Authority. (2021). *Mental capacity act*. Available at https://www.hra.nhs.uk/planning-and-improving-research/policies-standards-legislation/mental-capacity-act/ (Accessed on 8th September 2023).

Henly, S. (2016). Health Communication Research for Nursing Science and Practice. *Nursing Research*, *65*(4), 257–258.

Horner, R. (2022). The role of the district nurse in screening and assessment for frailty. *British Journal of Community Nursing*, *27*(5), 226–230.

HM Government. (2005). *Mental capacity act, 2005*. London: The Stationary Office. Available at https://www.legislation.gov.uk/ukpga/2005/9/contents (Accessed on 28th April 2023).

Kalisch, B., Tschannen, D., & Lee, K. (2012). Missed nursing care, staffing and patient falls. *Journal of Nursing Care Quality*, *27*(1), 6–12.

Keogh, B. (2013). *Review into the quality of care and treatment provided by 14 hospital trusts in England: Overview report*. Available at https://www.basw.co.uk/system/files/resources/basw_85333-2_0.pdf (Accessed on 30th June 2023).

Kurtz, S., & Silverman, J. (1996). The Calgary–Cambridge Referenced Observation Guides: An aid to defining the curriculum and organizing the teaching in communication training programmes. *Medical Education*, *30*(2), 83–89.

Kwame, A., & Petrucka, P. (2021). A literature-based study of patient-centered care and communication in nurse–patient interactions: barriers, facilitators, and the way forward. *BMC Nursing*, *20*(1), 1–10.

Lee, M. (2021). Supporting patients whose first language is not English. *British Journal of Nursing*, *30*(4), 3–4.

Lister, S., Hofland, J., & Grafton, H. (2020). *The royal marsden manual of clinical nursing procedures; Professional edition* (10th ed.). Chichester: Wiley Blackwell.

Maybin, J., Charles, A., & Honeyman, M. (2016). *Understanding the quality in district nursing services: Learning from patients, carers and staff*. London: The Kings Fund.

Mayo, P. (2017). Undertaking an accurate and comprehensive assessment of the acutely ill adult. *Nursing Standard*, *32*(8), 53–61.

McDonald, A. (2016). *A long and winding road. Improving communication with patients in the NHS*. Available at: https://www.mariecurie.org.uk/globalassets/media/documents/policy/campaigns/the-long-and-winding-road.pdf (Accessed on 17th May 2023).

Molina-Mula, J., & Gallo-Estrada, J. (2020). Impact of nurse-patient relationship on quality of care and patient autonomy in decision-making. *International Journal of Environmental Research and Public Health*, *17*(3), 835–859.

Neighbour, R. (1987). *The Inner Consultation*. London: Springer.

NHS England. (2017). *Involving people in their own health and care: Statutory guidance for clinical commissioning groups and NHS England*. Available at: https://www.england.nhs.uk/publication/nhs-long-term-workforce-plan/ (Accessed on 16th May 2023).

NHS England. (2019). NHS long term plan. Available at https://www.england.nhs.uk/long-term-plan/ (Accessed on 16th May 2023).

Nichol, J., Sundjaja, J., & Nelson, G. (2022). *Medical history*. Available at https://www.ncbi.nlm.nih.gov/books/NBK534249/ (Accessed on 7th September 2023).

Nursing and Midwifery Council. (2018). *The Code: Professional standards of practice and behaviour for nurses, midwives and nursing associates*. London: Nursing and Midwifery Council.

Queen's Nursing Institute. (2015a). *The QNI/QNIS voluntary standards for district nurse education and practice*. Available at https://www.qni.org.uk/wp-content/uploads/2017/02/District_Nurse_Standards_WEB.pdf (Accessed on 16th May 2023).

Queen's Nursing Institute. (2015b). *The value of the district nurse specialist practitioner qualification: A report by the Queen's Nursing Institute*. Available at https://www.qni.org.uk/wp-content/uploads/2016/09/SPQDN_Report_WEB2.pdf (Accessed on 17th July 2023).

Rimmer, A. (2020). *Can patients use family members as non-professional interpreters in consultations?*. Available at: https://www-bmj-com.ezproxy.wlv.ac.uk/content/368/bmj.m447 (Accessed on 8th September 2023).

South Palomares, J., & Young, A. (2017). Facial first impressions of partner preference traits: Trustworthiness, status, and attractiveness. *Social Psychological and Personality Science*, *9*, 8. Available at https://doi.org/10.1177/1948550617732388 (Accessed on 2nd July 2023).

Squires, A. (2018). Strategies for overcoming language barriers in healthcare. *Nursing Management*, *49*(4), 20–27.

Wilson, S., & Giddens, J. (2022). *Health assessment for nursing practice* (7th ed.). Missouri: Elsevier.

World Health Organization. (2022). *Mental health*. Available at https://www.who.int/news-room/fact-sheets/detail/mental-health-strengthening-our-response (Accessed on 5th September 2023).

CHAPTER 9

Long-Term Conditions Management

Sue Brooks ■ Neesha Oozageer Gunowa ■ Michelle McBride

LEARNING OUTCOMES

After reading this chapter you should be able to:

- Define the complexities of living with a long-term condition
- Understand the concepts of self-care, empowerment and autonomy
- Identify the Individual needs of people with long-term conditions, who may need referral to members of the health and social care team

9.1 Introduction

Across the world, around 74% of deaths are caused by noncommunicable diseases (NCDs), also known as long-term conditions (LTCs), that cannot be cured but can be managed for optimum outcomes and to maximise diminishing healthcare resources (World Health Organisation (WHO), 2022a).

District nurses (DNs) and nurses working in the community regularly meet people living with LTCs, but there is variation across the UK regarding diagnostic processes and support received by those with ongoing physical and mental challenges (Watt et al., 2022). Further disparity can be found in the impact of the condition or conditions on the person receiving care. Indeed, some indicate little or no effect on daily life (Office for National Statistics, 2022; WHO, 2022b), but many are severely and frequently impacted, reducing their quality of life and that of those living with them. The burden of treatment cited by Rosbach and Andersen (2017) indicated that there are complex challenges and negative effects of living with multimorbidity. Different ways to address these varying needs include integration of care provision across medical, nursing and social services, one example being the Kaiser Permanente framework which emerged from the USA (The King's Fund, 2010a; Fig. 9.1).

There is no doubt that the number of people diagnosed with LTCs continues to rise in the UK (NHS England, 2018a) and around the world, partly due to many societies seeing increasing longevity but also experiencing the effects of health behaviour choices alongside environmental factors that are not yet fully understood (Public Health England, 2018; WHO, 2022b). Approximately 26 million people are living with at least one LTC in the UK (The Patients Association, 2023). The broad range of people requiring resources and support indicates how management approaches need to be varied. The emphasis on care being delivered in the community in preference to the hospital has impacted the workload and challenges for District nursing teams (The Queen's Nursing Institute (QNI), 2019), meaning that patients can be more unwell on their return to the community (Ashworth, 2020).

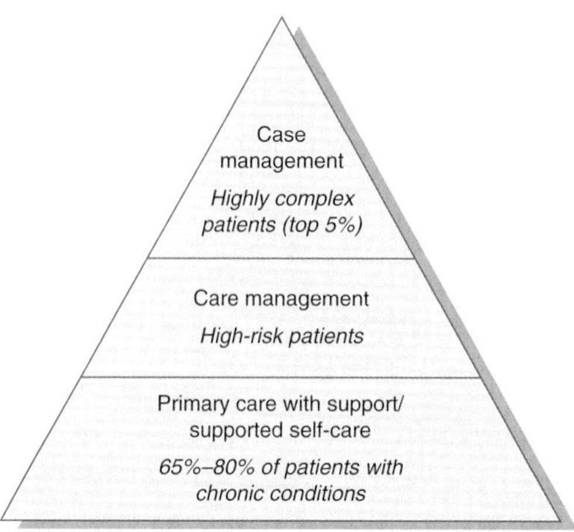

Fig. 9.1 Kaiser Permanente framework.

NHS England's (2017a) Five Year Forward View update cited the increasing complexity of the conditions being managed and the need to embrace technological advances, and this was reiterated in the National Health Service (NHS) Long Term Plan (NHS England, 2019) in its preventative approach and focus on tackling health inequalities and encouraging people to aim for more control over their own health. It is debatable whether these goals have been addressed when the NHS is experiencing its toughest period since its inception and the global pandemic of COVID-19 impacted and continues to impact the health and economics of all nations (Deakin, 2022).

A repeated thread in the narrative written about caring for people living with LTCs is the need for person-centredness and empowerment of individuals to maximise their abilities and resources for self-care and management (Owen et al., 2022). The voices of those experiencing life with one or more LTCs must be the focus of any management or planning of care if service users are to be treated compassionately, appropriately and in economically viable ways through the 21st century and beyond (NHS England, 2023a).

9.2 Support Planning for People With LTCs

Frameworks from the government and the NHS that aim to improve consulting such as the Year of Care (NHS England, 2017b) and the House of Care (Roberts & Dixon, 2013) focus on person-centred care planning and delivery with emphasis on autonomy and respect for peoples' wishes. The Year of Care initiative aimed to integrate services and began with local population analysis and consultation of stakeholders including people living with LTCs. But it could be argued that the outworking of these programmes could be compromised when set against audits or targets such as the Quality and Outcomes Framework (QOF) linked to payment in general practice (Forbes et al., 2017). Forbes's team conducted a systematic review of evidence and concluded that the use of QOF did not produce significantly improved outcomes for people living with

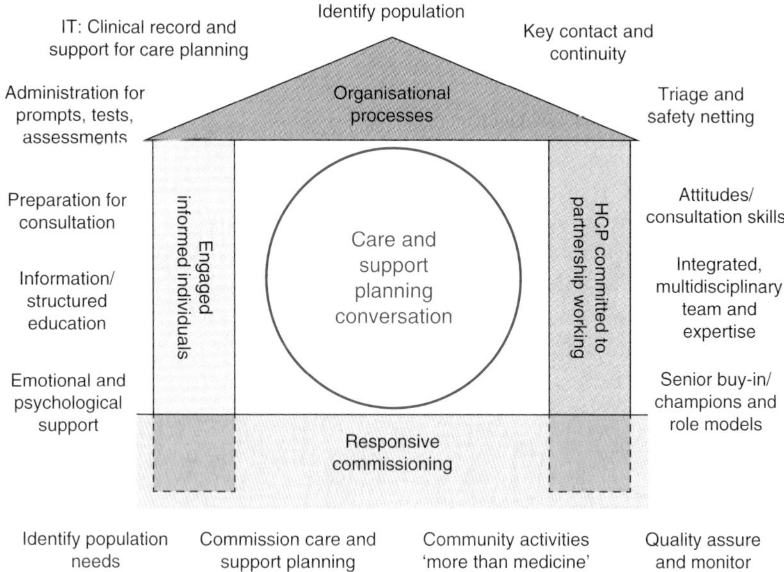

Fig. 9.2 Year of care. *HCP,* Healthcare professional. (From Dixon, A., and Roberts, S. (2013). Delivering better services for people with long-term conditions – building the House of Care. King's Fund. https://www.kingsfund.org.uk/insight-and-analysis/reports/better-services-people-long-term-conditions.) (Accessed 29 July 2024).

LTCs. However, there have been recent changes (NHS England, 2023b) to reduce the number of QOF indicators in favour of focusing on workforce wellbeing, and optimisation of demand and capacity management in general practice. The coproduction of health and social care plans for each person living with one or more LTC has become the bedrock of integrated teams, and despite many challenges including low staffing levels and financial constraints, the ethos of person-centred and supportive nursing, medical and social input continues to strive for improved outcomes and quality care (Crocker et al., 2020) (Fig. 9.2).

Remote consultations and evaluation of their effectiveness have emerged as a result of the COVID-19 pandemic. Face-to-face consultations remain the usual norm for DNs and community nurses but remote access via phone, video and email have transformed the possibilities for people to access care (The Health Foundation, 2021), assessments to be made of patients' needs, and for teams to communicate online (Williams, 2022). This brings challenges such as data protection, personal security and privacy if being overheard could cause issues with family and friends, and impact the veracity of history-taking, assessment strategies and treatment options (Neve et al., 2020). Despite the benefits of mobile working for contemporaneous and complex documentation by DNs and community nurses, there has been critique of the use of digital devices which include barriers such as poor connectivity in peoples' homes, potential limits to verbal or nonverbal cue acquisition, and the practical interventions required that cannot be addressed by telehealth (Williams, 2022). However, there has been positive feedback from people living with LTCs regarding access to resources for self-management and support (Castle-Clarke, 2018). Further research is needed in this area to inform best practice and avoid pitfalls of miscommunication.

9.3 Self-Care for People With LTCs

Wagner's (1998) chronic care model began to focus the healthcare community on the importance of system design to enhance self-management support, delivery options, decision support and clinical information systems. There was an emphasis on better health for people living with chronic illness but also on increasing economic productivity and job satisfaction for healthcare professionals (HCPs) (Davy et al., 2015). More than a decade ago, shared decision-making (SDM) was the growing focus of The King's Fund (2010b) and authors such as Barry and Edgman-Levitan (2012) cited how collaboration with people was needed that truly recognises and accepts:

- peoples' values,
- preferences
- and expert knowledge of their own condition(s).

This shift from a previously paternalistic approach where knowledge of medical and treatment options was kept in the domain of HCPs requires both respectful consulting and active sharing of relevant resources from the evidence-base of practice (Richards et al., 2015). Griffith and Tengnah (2013) argued that DNs are well placed both to provide understandable information and to respect and collaborate with their patients to ensure SDM occurs in practice. Indeed, the tenet of autonomy is threaded throughout the NHS Constitution (Department of Health and Social Care (DH), 2021), valuing each person as a unique individual with equal rights for respect and compassionate care when they require it.

Barriers to optimising self-care for people living with one or more LTCs fall into two main domains:

- **Lack of understanding or the outworking of the principle of SDM.** This may be based on pragmatic constraints of poor staffing levels limiting opportunities for skilled communication and transfer of information (Crocker et al., 2020) or possible resistance to relinquish control to people. Spiers et al. (2021) have consistently indicated how people wish to be involved in their care and make decisions based on their values and priorities at the time. Therefore, there is an educational imperative for DNs to gain and sustain their understanding of these principles, including the vital use of language that is inclusive, empathetic and based on respect (NHS England, 2018b). The 'Language Matters' guide was aimed at those working in diabetes care, but it can be argued that its tenets are applicable to all of us who seek to support those living with LTCs.
- **Lack of understanding or uptake of self-care by people who live with LTCs.** There are still difficulties with literacy and health literacy for some parts of the UK population (Public Health England, 2015) which may add to the barriers to self-management. Some cite a lack of motivation along with a paucity of time to self-manage, but life with one or more LTCs is a complex phenomenon and human nature does not always respond with logical decisions (Riegel et al., 2021).

Case Study to Consider Self-Management and Autonomy for Ms Bhatt

Ms Bhatt, who is 78 years old, had been diagnosed with bipolar disorder for many years. She lived alone and had an estranged son living close by. After a fall 5 weeks ago in a local supermarket, she had sustained a flap injury to the anterior border of her tibia which was not healing as she hoped. She required a DN visit to review and redress the wound.

During a consultation, it became clear that she had been dressing her wound at home using Manuka honey and lint pads from an old first-aid kit taped to her skin with Elastoplast. She also admitted to pain whenever she tried to change these.

- **What would you have said to Ms Bhatt? Have you experienced situations like this where people have tried self-care?**
- **What might have empowered her to use dressings that would maximise healing and reduce her pain?**

Improved accessibility and offering different approaches to support people through their conditions' trajectory are challenges for the healthcare system to tackle to embrace as many people as possible to maximise their ability to care for themselves and improve their outcomes such as quality or quantity of their lives (Davy et al., 2015). Poor mental health is often experienced concurrently with physical LTCs, and this can be a distinct barrier to self-management, especially when acknowledging difficult to manage issues such as social isolation and perceived or actual stigma experienced by people with mental health problems (Chief Medical Officer, 2023). National Institute of Health and Care Excellence (NICE) (2016) cites how the identification of people living with multimorbidity (more than two LTCs that can be physical or mental health conditions) is a key activity for stakeholders such as primary care to be able to offer appropriate support that aligns with peoples' aims for their quality of life.

Once identified, *encouragement and empowerment to share the decision-making* regarding their condition(s) are paramount to effective collaborative care. Some people require signposting to discover their own information, and some have already become experts prior to a consultation. *The Expert Patient Programme* (DH, 2013) was adopted in England from the USA in 2002 and has developed through various iterations to be run by private companies with some challenges to parity of coverage and access across the country. Some have cited that the programme does not necessarily engender closer collaboration between clinicians and those living with LTCs, nor reach those who need to be empowered and supported (Vadiee, 2012). Positive feedback is also evident, and the programmes continue to offer online and other resources for many living with LTCs (Office of the Regulator of Community Interest Companies and Department for Business, Innovation & Skills, 2013).

However, for others, motivation to look after themselves in whatever way they prefer can be difficult to find or maintain. This is documented in the literature with many attempts to discover what will help people find their own goals and methods of achieving them (NHS England, 2023c).

9.4 Motivational Interviewing

Motivational Interviewing (MI) was first identified by Rollnick and Miller (1995) as a tool for guiding rather than directing with many subsequent applications to areas of health and social care, including community nursing. The premise is to encourage 'change talk' with the person who wishes to alter something in their life using some or all of the acronym DARN-CAT (Miller & Rollnick, 2013):

- Desire
- Ability
- Reason
- Need
- Commitment
- Activation
- Taking steps

Frost et al.'s (2018) systematic review of studies examined the effectiveness of MI and concluded that short-term benefits can be found in changing health behaviour, but that high-quality research is needed to identify the components that are most useful and resilient.

REFLECTION

- Which *tools have you seen used in practice* that encourage empowerment and self-management and allow people to act autonomously?
- Which of the *principles are omitted or compromised* in your experience? Why?
- What *could you adopt* from some of the evidence discussed in this chapter?

9.5 Collaborative Working

Working within competency and scope is vital for patient safety, and this is certainly true for liaison and support of those living with one or more LTCs (Health and Care Professions Council (HCPC), 2016; Nursing and Midwifery Council (NMC), 2018). Silo working and lack of understanding regarding the skills and knowledge of different practitioners and multidisciplinary teams (MDTs) can result in poor or limited care being offered (Damarell et al., 2020). Indeed, a recurrent theme in patient complaints is poor communication between the various health and social care systems and practitioners (Spiers et al., 2021). Integrated health and social care teams aim to reduce these barriers that can be detrimental to people living with LTCs and there are initiatives to streamline data sharing and improve communication channels (NHS England, 2017b). Some primary care networks (PCNs) support direct referral by DNs so patients can access practitioners providing physiotherapy, oxygen therapy and various specialist services to support those with conditions such as dementia, Parkinson's disease and mental health problems. However, the authorisation for DNs to refer directly to streamline services is not standard across the country. The use of technology to provide frailty virtual wards with the MDT and wider virtual reviews at PCN level can enhance integrated care and improve communication for the benefit of patients and their families and investment in these systems, partly because of COVID-19, continues to develop (NHS England, 2023d). Hunter (2022) considers the benefits of virtual services but warns of capacity and staffing limitations that can hinder even the best of intended care provision.

People must receive regular health checks relevant to their condition to prevent avoidable complications and excess morbidity or, indeed, mortality. A recent report highlighted the stark effects of the COVID-19 pandemic when many were not able to access these checks, resulting in terrible consequences (Diabetes UK, 2023). And this is echoed across many other conditions where face-to-face investigations and monitoring were stopped and then severely limited for many months, for example, for those living with respiratory conditions such as asthma and COPD (NICE, 2020) and those being diagnosed with cancer (Maringe et al., 2021). The challenging task for the entire NHS to provide a system with enough capacity for screening and diagnostics as well as treatment is an ongoing battle.

9.6 Conclusion

The challenge to help people live with their LTCs in the best way they define is one that will always require an individual approach. This is aligned to our own personalities, experiences and the tools we adopt to use with those we consult with, but also directly informed by each person's proclivities and health beliefs. To successfully support people living with LTCs, systems need to place the person at the centre and healthcare professionals need to work collaboratively.

References

Ashworth, L. (2020). Challenges and opportunities: The role of the district nurse in influencing practice education. *British Journal of Community Nursing, 25*(8). Available at: https://www.britishjournalofcommunitynursing.com/content/professional/challenges-and-opportunities-the-role-of-the-district-nurse-in-influencing-practice-education.

Barry, M., & Edgman-Levitan, S. (2012). Shared decision-making: The pinnacle of patient-centred care. *New England Journal of Medicine, 366*, 780–781. Available at: https://www.nejm.org/doi/10.1056/NEJMp1109283?url_ver=Z39.88-2003&rfr_id=ori:rid:crossref.org&rfr_dat=cr_pub%20%200pubmed.

Castle-Clarke, S. (2018). *What will new technology mean for the NHS and its patients? (King's Fund, London).* Available at: https://www.kingsfund.org.uk/sites/default/files/2018-06/NHS_at_70_what_will_new_technology_mean_for_the_NHS_0.pdf.

Chief Medical Officer's annual report 2023 health in an ageing society. https://surreyac.sharepoint.com/sites/FHMSResearchThemes762/_layouts/15/viewer.aspx?sourcedoc={889f6ae1-7293-4309-95f6-fcce4eafa359}.

Crocker, H., Kelly, L., Harlock, J., Fitzpatrick, R., & Peters, M. (2020). Measuring the benefits of the integration of health and social care: qualitative interviews with professional stakeholders and patient representatives. *BMC Health Services Research, 20*, 515. Available at: https://doi.org/10.1186/s12913-020-05374-4.

Damarell, R. A., Morgan, D. D., & Tieman, J. J. (2020). General practitioner strategies for managing patients with multimorbidity: A systematic review and thematic synthesis of qualitative research. *BMC Primary Care, 21*, 131. Available at: https://bmcprimcare.biomedcentral.com/articles/10.1186/s12875-020-01197-8.

Davy, C., Bleasel, J., Liu, H., Tchan, M., Ponniah, S., & Brown, A. (2015). Effectiveness of chronic care models: Opportunities for improving healthcare practice and health outcomes: A systematic review. *BMC Health Services Research, 15*. Article number: 194 Available at: https://bmchealthservres.biomedcentral.com/articles/10.1186/s12913-015-0854-8.

Deakin, M. (2022). NHS workforce shortages and staff burnout are taking a toll. *British Medical Journal, 377*, 945. Available at: https://www.bmj.com/content/bmj/377/bmj.o945.full.pdf.

Department of Health and Social Care. (2013). *The Expert patients programme.* Available at: https://www.gov.uk/government/case-studies/the-expert-patients-programme.

Department of Health and Social Care. (2021). *The NHS constitution for England*. Available at: https://www.gov.uk/government/publications/the-nhs-constitution-for-england/the-nhs-constitution-for-england.

Diabetes UK. (2023). *Diabetes care: Is it fair enough*. Available at: https://www.diabetes.org.uk/about_us/news/too-many-people-diabetes-still-not-receiving-vital-care-our-new-report-shows.

Forbes, L., Marchand, C., Doran, T., & Peckham, S. (2017). The role of the quality and outcomes framework in the care of long-term conditions: A systematic review. *British Journal of General Practice*, *67*(664), 775–784. Available at: https://bjgp.org/content/bjgp/67/664/e775.full.pdf.

Frost, H., Campbell, P., Maxwell, M., O'Carroll, R. E., Dombrowski, S. U., Williams, B., et al. (2018). Effectiveness of motivational interviewing on adult behaviour change in health and social care settings: A systematic review of reviews. *PLOS ONE*, *10*, 1371. Available at: https://journals.plos.org/plosone/article?id=10.1371%2fjournal.pone.0204890.

Griffith, R., & Tengnah, C. (2013). Shared decision-making: Nurses must respect autonomy over paternalism. *British Journal of Community Nursing*, *18*(6). Available at: https://www.magonlinelibrary.com/doi/full/10.12968/bjcn.2013.18.6.303.

Health and Care Professions Council (HCPC). (2016). Standards of conduct, performance and ethics. Available at: https://www.hcpc-uk.org/standards/standards-of-conduct-performance-and-ethics/.

Hunter, W. (2022). Virtual wards: A bridge between hospitals and the community? *Nursing in Practice*. Available at: https://www.nursinginpractice.com/analysis/virtual-wards-a-bridge-between-hospitals-and-the-community/.

Maringe, C., Spicer, J., Morris, M., Purushotham, A., Nolte, E., Sullivan, R., ... Aggarwal, A. (2021). The impact of the COVID-19 pandemic on cancer deaths due to delays in diagnosis in England, UK: A national, population-based, modelling study. *The Lancet*, *21*(Issue 8), 1023–1034.

Miller, W., & Rollnick, S. (2013). *Motivational Interviewing: Helping people change* (3rd ed.). New York, NY: Guildford Press.

National Institute of Health and Care Excellence (NICE). (2016). *Multimorbidity: Clinical assessment and management*. Available at: https://www.nice.org.uk/guidance/ng56.

National Institute of Health and Care Excellence (NICE). (2020). *NICE impact respiratory conditions*. Available at: https://www.nice.org.uk/about/what-we-do/into-practice/measuring-the-use-of-nice-guidance/impact-of-our-guidance/nice-impact-respiratory-conditions.

Neve, G., Fyfe, M., Hayhoe, B., & Kumar, S. (2020). Digital health in primary care: Risks and recommendations. *British Journal of General Practice*, *70*(701), 609–610. Available at: https://bjgp.org/content/70/701/609.

NHS England. (2017a). *Next steps on the NHS five year forward view*. Available at: https://www.england.nhs.uk/wp-content/uploads/2017/03/NEXT-STEPS-ON-THE-NHS-FIVE-YEAR-FORWARD-VIEW.pdf.

NHS England. (2017b). *The long term conditions year of care commissioning programme. Implementation Handbook*. Available at: https://www.england.nhs.uk/wp-content/uploads/2017/02/ltc-yoc-handbook.pdf.

NHS England. (2018a). *Enhancing the quality of life for people living with long term conditions*. Available at: https://cpe.org.uk/wp-content/uploads/2018/02/Infographic-FINAL.pdf.

NHS England. (2018b). *Language matters: Language and diabetes*. Available at: https://www.england.nhs.uk/long-read/language-matters-language-and-diabetes/.

NHS England. (2019). *The NHS long term plan*. Available at: https://www.england.nhs.uk/wp-content/uploads/2022/07/nhs-long-term-plan-version-1.2.pdf.

NHS England. (2023a). *Our work on long term conditions*. Available at: https://www.england.nhs.uk/ourwork/clinical-policy/ltc/our-work-on-long-term-conditions/.

NHS England. (2023b). *Quality and outcomes framework guidance for 2023/24*. Available at: https://www.england.nhs.uk/publication/quality-and-outcomes-framework-guidance-for-2023-24/.

NHS England. (2023c). *Supported self-management: the evidence base*. Available at: https://www.england.nhs.uk/personalisedcare/supported-self-management/evidence/.

NHS England. (2023d). *Virtual wards*. Available at: https://www.england.nhs.uk/virtual-wards/.

Nursing and Midwifery Council (NMC). (2018). The Code. *Professional standards of practice and behaviour for nurses, midwives and nursing associates*. Available at: https://www.nmc.org.uk/standards/code/.

Office of the Regulator of Community Interest Companies and Department for Business, Innovation & skills. (2013). *Case study. The expert patients programme*. Available at: https://www.gov.uk/government/case-studies/the-expert-patients-programme.

Office for National Statistics. (2022). *UK health indicators 2019–2020*. Available at: https://www.ons.gov.uk/peoplepopulationandcommunity/healthandsocialcare/healthandlifeexpectancies/bulletins/ukhealthindicators/2019to2020.

Owen, N., Dew, L., Logan, S., Denegri, S., & Chappell, L. (2022). Research policy for people with multiple long term conditions. *Journal of Multimorbidity and Comorbidity*, *12*, 1–8. Available at: https://www.ncbi.nlm.nih.gov/pmc/articles/PMC9201348/pdf/10.1177_26335565221104407.pdf.

Public Health England. (2015). *Local action on health inequalities. Improving health literacy to reduce health inequalities*. Available at: https://assets.publishing.service.gov.uk/government/uploads/system/uploads/attachment_data/file/460709/4a_Health_Literacy-Full.pdf.

Public Health England. (2018). *Research and analysis. Chapter 3: trends in morbidity and risk factors*. Available at: https://www.gov.uk/government/publications/health-profile-for-england-2018/chapter-3-trends-in-morbidity-and-risk-factors.

Riegel, B., Dunbar, S., Fitzsimons, D., Freedland, K., Lee, C., Middleton, S., et al. (2021). Self-care research: Where are we now? Where are we going? *International Journal of Nursing Studies*, *116*: Article 103402.

Richards, T., Coulter, A., & Wicks, P. (2015). Time to deliver patient centred care. *British Medical Journal*, *350*, h530. Available at: https://www.bmj.com/content/350/bmj.h530.

Roberts, S., & Dixon, A. (2013). *The Kings Fund: Delivering better services for people with long term conditions*. Available at: https://www.kingsfund.org.uk/insight-and-analysis/reports/better-services-people-long-term-conditions.

Rollnick, S., & Miller, W. R. (1995). What is motivational interviewing? *Behavioural and Cognitive Psychotherapy*, *23*(4), 325–334.

Rosbach, M., & Andersen, J. S. (2017). Patient-experienced burden of treatment in patients with multimorbidity – a systematic review of qualitative data. *PloS One*, *12*(6): Article e0179916.

Spiers, G., Boulton, E., Corner, L., Craig, D., Parker, S., Todd, C., & Hanratty, B. (2021). What matters to people with multiple long-term conditions and their carers? *Postgraduate Medical Journal BMJ*, *0*, 1–6. Available at: https://pmj.bmj.com/content/early/2021/12/17/postgradmedj-2021-140825.

The Health Foundation. (2021). *How has the COVID-19 pandemic impacted primary care?*. Available at: https://www.health.org.uk/news-and-comment/charts-and-infographics/how-has-the-covid-19-pandemic-impacted-primary-care.

The King's Fund. (2010a). *Clinical and service integration: The route to improved outcomes*. Available at: https://www.kingsfund.org.uk/publications/clinical-and-service-integration.

The King's Fund. (2010b). *How to deliver high-quality, patient-centred, cost-effective care. Consensus solutions from the voluntary sector*. London: The King's Fund.

The Patients Association. (2023). *Long term conditions*. Available at: https://www.patients-association.org.uk/long-term-conditions.

The Queen's Nursing Institute. (2019). *District nursing today. The view of district nurse team leaders in the UK*. Available at: https://qni.org.uk/wp-content/uploads/2019/11/District-Nursing-Today-The-View-of-DN-Team-Leaders-in-the-UK.pdf.

Vadiee, M. (2012). The UK "Expert Patient Program" and self-care in chronic disease management: An analysis. *European Geriatric Medicine*, *3*(3), 201–205.

Wagner, E.H. (1998). Chronic disease management: What will it take to improve care for chronic illness? Effective Clinical Practice, 1, 2–4.

Watt, T., Raymond, A., & Rachet-Jacquet, L. (2022). *Quantifying health inequalities in England*. The Health Foundation REAL Centre. Available at: https://www.health.org.uk/news-and-comment/charts-and-infographics/quantifying-health-inequalities.

Williams, F. (2022). The use of digital devices by district nurses in their assessment of service users. *British Journal of Community Nursing*, *27*(7). Available at: https://www.magonlinelibrary.com/doi/full/10.12968/bjcn.2022.27.7.342.

World Health Organisation. (2022a). *Noncommunicable diseases. Key facts*. Available at: https://www.who.int/news-room/fact-sheets/detail/noncommunicable-diseases.

World Health Organization WHO. (2022b). *Ageing and health*. Available at: https://www.who.int/news-room/fact-sheets/detail/ageing-and-health.

CHAPTER 10

Physical Health in Community Nursing

Roseline Agyekum ■ Richard Green ■ Sue Green ■ Janine Lane ■ Ashley Luchmun ■ Caroline Nicholson ■ Samantha Wakefield ■ Caroline Knott ■ AnnMarie Whyte ■ Janine Lane ■ Paul McAleer ■ Ann Marie Devitt ■ Alison Child

LEARNING OUTCOMES

After reading this chapter you should be able to:

- Identify some of the more prevalent long-term conditions that are managed by community nursing teams
- Gain an awareness of where to access appropriate and evidence-based information to facilitate best practice
- Understand how to provide support for individuals and their families at home when care needs can be complex and when to refer on for advice

10.1 Introduction

The role of community nursing within the management of long-term conditions has been well established, and the care that these teams provide is integral to maintaining quality of life. The following chapter aims to provide an overview of some of the more prevalent long-term conditions that impact physical health and how to manage these using a safe, evidence-based approach. These include:

- Diabetes
- Heart Failure
- Chronic Kidney Disease
- Respiratory Disease
- Neurological conditions
- Fraility

There is also a focus on some of the more challenging aspects of providing care to individuals in their homes, which include wound care, continence management and the provision of nutritional support. It is widely accepted that all of these conditions may have a psychological, social and emotional impact on the individual and can lead to stigma and social isolation. These aspects are addressed in more detail in the next chapter.

10.2 Diabetes and Community Nursing

10.2.1 INTRODUCTION

Diabetes is currently one of the most common chronic diseases in the UK, affecting almost 5 million people (National Institute for Health and Care Excellence (NICE), 2022c). It occurs when the pancreas either does not produce enough insulin or cannot use its insulin effectively (World Health Organisation (WHO), 2023b) and results in high blood glucose levels. Insulin, a hormone produced by the pancreas to regulate blood sugar levels, acts as a key, opening the body's cells, allowing glucose entry where it can be used as energy (Diabetes UK, 2022a). As a result of an increasing prevalence in recent years, caring for someone living with the condition has become an integral aspect of all community nursing caseloads (Diabetes UK, 2021).

10.2.2 TYPES OF DIABETES

There are several classifications of diabetes. Box 10.1 outlines the most common types.

10.2.3 THE ROLE OF THE COMMUNITY NURSE AND DIABETES

10.2.3.1 Insulin Administration

Community nurses, often tasked with administrating injectable therapies for those unable to do so independently, need to consider many aspects of good injection technique to avoid suboptimal glycaemic control (Hicks & James, 2023). Insulin is administered subcutaneously into the upper arm, abdomen, upper thighs or buttocks. Regular rotation of injection sites is vital in avoiding the development of lipohypertrophy (Smith et al., 2017).

When administering insulin to patients, 5-mm safety needles are preferred to reduce the risk of needlestick injuries. All insulin pen needles should be used only once, primed

BOX 10.1 ■ Most Common Types of Diabetes

Type 1 diabetes, an autoimmune disease usually diagnosed in children and young adults, occurring when the immune system destroys the cells that produce insulin in the pancreas, leaving the body unable to produce any insulin. The only treatment available is insulin.

Type 2 diabetes, accounting for 90% of cases (Diabetes UK, 2021), is the most common type in the UK and occurs when the body either does not produce enough insulin or is unable to use that insulin effectively (insulin resistance). It is managed with lifestyle modifications, oral medications or insulin and is often associated with poor lifestyle choices.

Gestational diabetes, occurring in women with no earlier history of the condition, presents during pregnancy and usually resolves following childbirth. It requires careful monitoring and management to ensure the health of both the mother and the baby.

There are also other less common types of diabetes, such as steroid-induced diabetes, cystic fibrosis-related diabetes, latent autoimmune diabetes in adults (LADA) and maturity-onset diabetes of the young (MODY).

(From American Diabetes Association. (2021). Classification and diagnosis of diabetes: Standards of medical care in diabetes. *Diabetes Care, 44* (Supplement 1), S15–S33.)

BOX 10.2 ■ Safety Considerations for Insulin Administration

- Prescriptions should never be shortened to 'iu' or 'u', but always be written as 'units'.
- The timing of the injection should ensure it is appropriate concerning food intake.
- NEVER draw insulin out of a cartridge or disposable pen.
- Only use an INSULIN SYRINGE (measures in units) to draw up insulin.
- Use a safety needle if you are giving insulin to someone else.
- Never recap pen needles.
- Dispose of sharps safely, as per local guidelines

(From Diggle, J. (2022). How to minimise insulin errors. *Diabetes & Primary Care*, *24*, 181–182.)

before use, and safely disposed of in a sharps bin when finished (Forum for Injection Technique (FIT), 2016). Once in use, insulin pens can be stored for up to 4 weeks at room temperature, with spare insulin pens stored in a fridge door (NHS England, 2017b).

Insulin regimes can be very complex, and each insulin will have a different action profile and administration time concerning food intake; therefore, a sound knowledge of these action profiles is crucial in providing good diabetes care in the community (NHS England, 2019). As Bain et al. (2019) identified, adverse effects involving insulin are the most common medication errors worldwide (Box 10.2).

10.2.3.2 Glucose Monitoring

Understanding blood glucose monitoring and safely completing the procedure are an integral part of living with diabetes and an essential skill for all nurses (Delves-Yates, 2022). Nurses need a good understanding of blood glucose targets. It is important to remember that blood glucose targets need to be individualised and will vary according to age, frailty and risk of hypoglycaemia. While a glucose range of 4–7 mmol may be considered normal (NICE, 2015a), a target of 6–9 mmol for an elderly patient under the community nurse caseload may be more realistic (Leung et al., 2018).

While most patients on a community nurse caseload will use a traditional blood glucose meter, today, some may have access to continuous glucose monitoring. The continuous glucose monitor, a small sensor worn on the arm for 2 weeks, sends glucose readings to a mobile phone or reader and checks glucose levels without the need to prick a finger. Studies are already showing that continuous glucose monitors are beneficial tools for managing diabetes within the community setting (Gregory & Curtis, 2022).

10.2.4 HYPOGLYCAEMIA

Hypoglycaemia, a common side effect of insulin therapy, has considerable consequences in the elderly population living with diabetes, with recurrent episodes of hypoglycaemia increasing the risk of cardiovascular events and impairing cognitive function (Lacy et al., 2020; Standl et al., 2019). When faced with an episode of hypoglycaemia, the community nurse must have excellent knowledge of how to manage the situation.

10.2.4.1 Common Symptoms and Causes of Hypoglycaemia

According to the National Health Service (NHS) (2020), the patient may appear shaky, sweaty, dizzy, confused or anxious.

Hypoglycaemia occurs for many reasons, most commonly when a meal is missed or delayed. Medicine administration can also be a cause of hypoglycaemia; more medication than needed could be taken, especially if suffering from reduced appetite or impaired cognition, or taken/administered at an incorrect time. Alcohol intake can also be a cause of hypoglycaemia (NHS, 2020).

REFLECTION

Mohammed is a 75-year-old male who has been living with type 2 diabetes for 15 years. The community nurse visits once daily to give his insulin: *Abasaglar, 12 units* in the morning. His blood glucose was 3.5 mmol when checked before his insulin administration.

- Would you administer his insulin?
- Are there any other measures you would take to provide safe care?

10.2.4.2 Treating Hypoglycaemia

NICE (2022b) recommends the following quick and effective treatment of hypoglycaemia.

If the person is conscious and able to swallow:

- 15–20 g glucose orally, such as, 200 mL orange juice, 5–6 Jelly Babies or 5–6 dextrose tablets.
- Repeat blood glucose after 10–15 minutes; the fast-acting glucose treatment can be further given up to three times if needed.
- Once blood glucose is above 4 mmol, a long-acting carbohydrate snack must be eaten, for example, two biscuits, one slice of bread, a banana.

10.2.4.3 Caution

Chocolates and biscuits are not recommended to treat hypoglycaemia due to the high-fat content that delays glucose absorption.

If the person is unconscious, this is considered a medical emergency, and the following steps should be taken:

- Call 999/ambulance.
- Oral hypoglycaemia treatment should **not** be administered, due to the increased risk of choking or aspiration.
- Glucagon should be administered intramuscularly.
- If there is no response from glucagon, then intravenous 10% glucose should be administered.
- Once recovered and blood glucose levels have risen above 4 mmol, a long-acting carbohydrate-based snack should be provided as earlier.

The insulin should *not* be omitted if due, but the dose will require review by a doctor or Diabetes Specialist Nurse.

10.2.5 HYPERGLYCAEMIA

Hyperglycaemia is defined as a blood glucose level over 11 mmol (NICE, 2015b). People frequently feel similar symptoms to when they were initially diagnosed, the more common being frequent urination (polyuria), especially at night (nocturia), thirst (polydipsia), tiredness and lethargy, weight loss, thrush or other recurring bladder and skin infections (Diabetes UK, 2022b).

Hyperglycaemia can occur due to missing medications, stress, infections or merely eating more food than needed. The overtreating of a previous hypo can also lead to hyperglycaemia (Diabetes UK, 2022b).

When a person with diabetes is unwell and hyperglycaemic, the blood must be tested for ketones, although ketones can develop even at normal glucose levels during illness (Plewa et al., 2021). Ketones, a sign of diabetes ketoacidosis, are a waste product occurring when the body starts to break down body fat, instead of glucose, for energy, and are often accompanied by symptoms such as shortness of breath, nausea, and vomiting and sweet-smelling breath (American Diabetes Association, 2024).

10.2.6 DIABETES COMPLICATIONS

With poorly managed glycaemic control comes an increased risk of serious complications, including cardiovascular disease, kidney disease, nerve damage, eye problems and foot complications (see Box 10.3). However, effective management, including lifestyle changes, medication and regular monitoring, can reduce the risk (NICE, 2015b).

A significant diabetes-related complication for community nursing caseloads is diabetes foot ulcers, leading to more than 180 amputations weekly in the UK (Diabetes UK, 2023). With both neuropathic and ischaemic ulcerations, the pathway to deterioration can be swift if not recognised early and appropriate referral is made (Phillips et al., 2020).

BOX 10.3 ■ Complications of Diabetes

Macrovascular

- Cardiovascular disease
  - Stroke
  - Myocardial infarction
  - Peripheral vascular disease

Microvascular

- Diabetic kidney disease
- Retinopathy
- Peripheral neuropathy
- Autonomic neuropathy

Foot Problems

- Including ulceration and amputation

Metabolic

- Dyslipidaemia
- Diabetic ketoacidosis (DKA)
- Hyperosmolar hyperglycaemic state (HHS)

Psychosocial

- Anxiety
- Depression
- Diabetic distress

Reduced life expectancy

National Institute for Health and Care Excellence (NICE). (2015b). Diabetes (type 1 and type 2) in children and young people: diagnosis and management NICE guideline. Available at: https://www.nice.org.uk/guidance/ng18/resources/diabetes-type-1-and-type-2-in-children-and-young-people-diagnosis-and-management-pdf-1837278149317.

BOX 10.4 ■ The ACT NOW Acronym

A—Accident? Recent or history of an accident, injury or trauma?
C—Change: Is there any new swelling, redness or change of shape of the foot?
T—Temperature: Is there a change in temperature present? Either hot or cold. Could this be an infection or possible Charcot?
N—New pain? Is there pain present? Is it localised or generalised throughout the foot?
O—Oozing? Would colour is any exudate? Is there an odour?
W—Wound: Can you document the size, shape and position of the wound in the foot affected?

(From Phillips, A., Edmonds, M., Holmes, P., Robbie, J., Odiase, C. and Grumitt, J. (2020). ACT NOW in diabetes and foot assessments: an essential service. *Practice Nursing*, 31(12), pp. 516–519.)

Community nurses, often visiting frequently for diabetes or wound care, are ideally placed to change the long-term outcomes of these patients. The adoption of sound assessment tools, for example, the ACT NOW (Box 10.4) assessment tool, has demonstrated a significant reduction in the volume of diabetes-related amputations (Phillips et al., 2020) and is an excellent tool for recognising when urgent referral to specialist services is required.

10.2.7 CONCLUSION

Diabetes is a very common long-term condition and therefore community nurses recurrently encounter patients with this condition. It is important to understand how to store and administer insulin safely and to provide support for patients who wish to increase their independence. It is also essential to understand the causes of hypoglycaemia and hyperglycaemia and how to treat accordingly to minimise risks to patients. Poorly controlled diabetes can lead to several complications, and community nurses need a broad understanding of how to identify these and provide nursing care to prevent further deterioration.

10.3 Heart Failure

10.3.1 INTRODUCTION

According to the European Society for Cardiology (ESC; McDonagh et al., 2021), heart failure (HF) is not a single pathological diagnosis but rather a clinical syndrome that has typical symptoms of breathlessness, ankle swelling and fatigue. HF also presents with elevated jugular venous pressure, basal crepitations and peripheral oedema and can be caused by structural and/or functional abnormality (NICE, 2018c).

'Heart failure' is an alarming term and may cause anxiety to patients, but the term simply means a failure to effectively pump blood, and therefore oxygen, around the body. It can occur as an acute syndrome but is more commonly seen in the community as chronic heart failure (CHF). This is a common, progressive condition and occurs mainly in older adults. About 98% of people living with CHF will have another long-term condition (British Heart Foundation, 2020). Therefore community nurses will commonly visit, not necessarily because of this diagnosis, but due to comorbidities or frailty. As such, community nurses are well placed to monitor and support people with this condition in both physical and psychological care.

There is no cure for CHF, but medical management, device therapy and surgery are used to reduce and manage symptoms and mortality, with the primary goals being to improve prognosis, enhance quality of life, avoid recurrent hospital admissions and/or reduce the incidence of acute exacerbations (McDonagh et al., 2021). HF affects 1%–2% of the global population (Schwinger, 2021), however, the prevalence of CHF in the UK is 1 in 15 people between 75 and 84 and just over 1 in 7 in those over 85 years of age (NICE, 2023f), again highlighting the importance of good understanding for community nurses as this group of patients makes up a large proportion of their caseloads.

As Kumar and Clark (2020) suggest, there are numerous causes of HF including postmyocardial infarction, prolonged hypertension, cardiomyopathy—a weakness of the heart muscle which can be hereditary—infection, pregnancy or excess alcohol intake. There are other, less common causes including chemotherapy treatment.

According to NICE (2023f), patients with heart failure can experience a number of symptoms. One of these is shortness of breath which initially starts on exertion but may develop further at rest and is caused by an accumulation of fluid in the lungs; thus impairing effective gaseous exchange. Secondly, patients may experience increased tiredness and muscle fatigue due to the reduced oxygen levels in the muscles as a consequence of the heart struggling to pump oxygen around the body. Lastly, reduced pumping leads to accumulation of fluid in the tissues so patients might experience swelling in the lower limbs due to gravity and this may also be detected in the sacrum or abdomen. The latter is often a sign of worsening heart failure.

10.3.2 DIAGNOSIS

The diagnosis of CHF requires the presence of symptoms and/or signs of HF and objective evidence of cardiac dysfunction (ESC, 2021). The following tests may also be carried out (see algorithm in Fig. 10.1).

- Electrocardiogram (ECG)
- B-type natriuretic peptide (BNP) blood test
- Serum urea and electrolytes, creatinine, full blood count, liver and thyroid function tests
- Echocardiography
- Chest x-ray

HF is investigated using a BNP blood test; elevated levels suggest that the heart is failing. When BNP is above 400 ng/L, a referral should be made for specialist intervention and echocardiogram to confirm diagnosis (NICE, 2023f), and for urgent referral, levels should be above 2000 ng/L. HF with a reduced ejection fraction (HFrEF) is diagnosed with an ejection fraction (EF) less than 40%. Further diagnoses of HF with moderately reduced or preserved EF are now common.

DEFINITION

Ejection fraction:

- HF is classified by measurement of the left ventricular ejection fraction (LVEF). A reduced LVEF of 40% or less is HFrEF (HF with reduced EF). Just over half of people with HF have evidence of reduced LVEF on echocardiography (NICE, 2018a).
- People with an LVEF between 41% and 49% have a mildly reduced EF—HF with mildly reduced EF (HFmrEF).
- People who have symptoms of HF, cardiac structure or function abnormalities and/or raised levels of natriuretic peptides with a preserved LVEF of 50% or more have HF with preserved EF (HF-PEF).
- Nearly half of people with HF have preserved LVEF on echocardiography (NICE, 2018a).

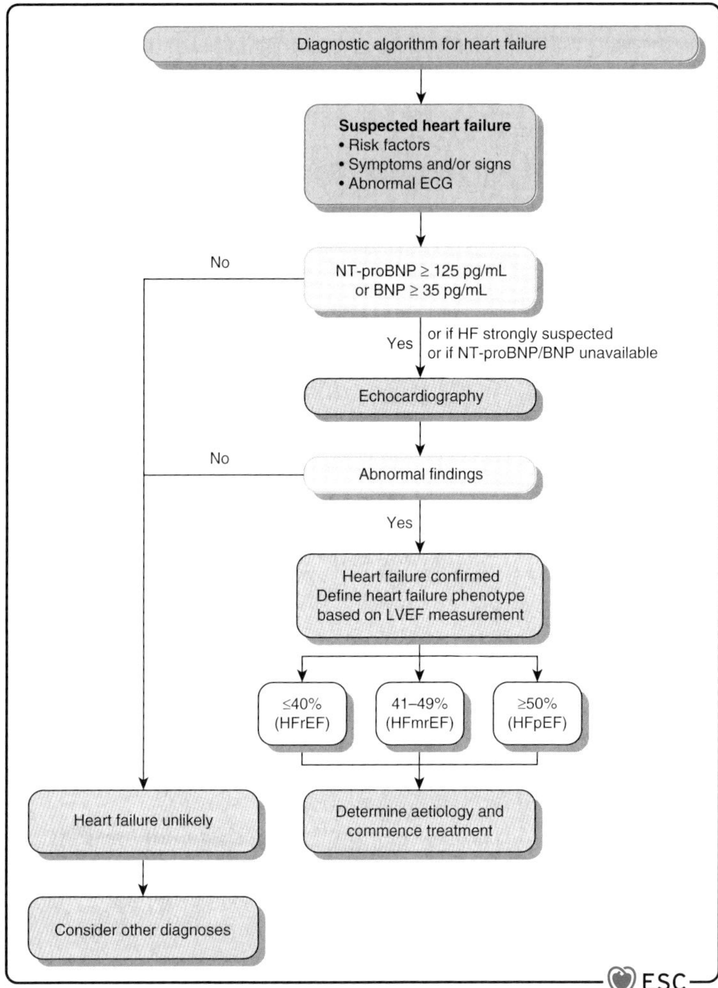

Fig. 10.1 The diagnostic algorithm for heart failure. *BNP,* B-type natriuretic peptide; *ECG,* electrocardiogram; *HF,* heart failure; *HFmrEF,* heart failure with mildly reduced ejection fraction; *HFpEF*, heart failure with preserved ejection fraction; *HFrEF,* heart failure with reduced ejection fraction; *LVEF,* left ventricular ejection fraction; *NT-proBNP,* N-terminal pro-B type natriuretic peptide. (European Society of Cardiology. (2021). ESC guidelines for the diagnosis and treatment of acute and chronic heart failure. Available at: https://www.escardio.org/Guidelines/Clinical-Practice-Guidelines/Acute-and-Chronic-Heart-Failure and Theresa A McDonagh et al., ESC Scientific Document Group, 2021 ESC Guidelines for the diagnosis and treatment of acute and chronic heart failure: Developed by the Task Force for the diagnosis and treatment of acute and chronic heart failure of the European Society of Cardiology (ESC) With the special contribution of the Heart Failure Association (HFA) of the ESC, European Heart Journal, 42 (36), 21 September 2021, 3599–3726, Figure 1. https://doi.org/10.1093/eurheartj/ehab368)

10.3.3 TREATMENT OF CHRONIC HEART FAILURE

The mainstay of treatment for CHF is medication and there are clear guidelines published by NICE (2023f) . Nonpharmacological treatments also have a place in HF management to improve blood flow to the heart, improve pumping or treat cardiac arrest (McDonagh et al., 2021) (Box 10.5).

BOX 10.5 ■ Nonpharmacological Treatment

- Revascularisation (coronary artery bypass graft surgery or PCI (percutaneous coronary intervention) for people with coronary artery disease will enhance blood flow to the heart.
- Cardiac resynchronisation therapy (CRT device) to resynchronise the electrical impulse through the ventricle and strengthen the pumping function of the heart. This device is a type of pacemaker and is sometimes implanted as a CRT-D, which is a combined CRT with defibrillator.
- Implantable Cardioverter-Defibrillator (ICD) device: People with heart failure are at an increased risk of cardiac arrest. An ICD may be appropriate for some patients with a low ejection fraction (EF). It internally defibrillates the heart if a serious ventricular arrhythmia is detected. Implantation of an ICD can be psychologically challenging for patients who may be anxious about device activation.

10.3.3.1 Cardiac Rehabilitation for People With Chronic Heart Failure

Cardiac rehabilitation (CR) is now recommended by NICE as an evidence-based intervention for people with stable HF (NICE, 2023f). CR interventions, which are often home based, are multifactorial and can be supported by HF community teams who may be visiting regularly during the CR programme (British Association for Cardiovascular Prevention and Rehabilitation, 2023). Exercise training forms an important component of CR and can improve physical fitness and quality of life (Taylor et al., 2019). Community nurses are well placed to support the rehabilitation process, by encouraging patients to engage with their exercise programme.

10.3.3.2 End-of-Life Care for People With Chronic Heart Failure

It is recognised that people with HF may not have their end-of-life needs appropriately met (McIlvennan & Allen, 2016). Community nurses are key in supporting and coordinating this vital care as they will have built up a good relationship with patients and their families often over many years of community care. It is important to have conversations with patients about their wishes, particularly regarding their desire to receive resuscitation or not.

10.3.4 THE ROLE OF THE COMMUNITY NURSE IN ENHANCING CARE OF PEOPLE WITH CHRONIC HEART FAILURE

- Ensure people understand their diagnosis and signpost to information online or provide written information if more appropriate. There is a wealth of information available from organisations such as the British Heart Foundation, Pumping Marvellous and Heart Failure Matters.
- Review their medication particularly on discharge from hospital as this will often change during an admission (Masters et al., 2019). If it looks wrong, highlight this to the general practitioner (GP) or community HF nursing team.
- Review symptoms during visits and report any worsening to specialist HF teams or GP. Any changes to symptoms could demand a sooner HF review or change in medication.
    - Observe swelling in ankles and sacrum if in bed and monitor skin integrity. Ensure pressure area care is carried out. This may involve noticing indentation on the feet from slippers or socks. Encourage the patient to elevate their feet on a stool when seated.
    - Talk to the patient about breathlessness and ask them to let you know if it worsens. This may be a subtle change, e.g., increased breathlessness on walking to the bathroom, or a change from breathlessness on activity to breathlessness at rest.

    - Encourage the patient to weigh themselves and report any sudden increases over 2–5 days which may indicate an increase in fluid retention.
    - Regularly check blood pressure and heart rate and rhythm by manual palpation and report any changes to the HF team.
- Encourage self-care and follow up on this during home visits. There is evidence that self-care is not well adhered to over time for people with CHF, so support and encouragement from a community nurse are vital.
    - Talk to the patient about taking their medication; noncompliance rates are high in people with CHF.
    - Encourage people to stay active, to plan travel and leisure activities according to physical ability and to participate in CR programmes.
    - Encourage healthy eating, particularly with low salt intake, good weight management to maintain a healthy weight.
- Work in partnership with other members of the multidisciplinary team (MDT) who also play a role in HF, e.g., specialist HF nurses who may also be visiting at home, occupational therapists who can support people with energy conservation and pacing, psychologists who can support psychological needs.
- Provide support and reassurance for people with an implantable Cardioverter-Defibrillator (ICD) and their families.
- Provide and support good end-of-life care, playing a pivotal role within the MDT. During end-of-life care, ensure that an ICD is deactivated when it becomes appropriate and agreed with the family and HF team.

REFLECTION

- Who do you have on your caseload with HF who you may be visiting for other reasons?
- What relationships could you build across the MDT to improve care of people with HF?
- As people with HF near the end of their lives, how can you best support them and advocate for their needs?

10.3.5 CONCLUSION

Evidence-based recommendations and clinical guidelines inform the discussion offering practical insights into the optimal management of HF. By understanding the complexities of HF and implementing multidisciplinary approaches to care, community nurses can improve patient outcomes and enhance quality of life for individuals living with this chronic condition.

10.4 Chronic Kidney Disease

10.4.1 INTRODUCTION

There is a global epidemic of chronic kidney disease (CKD), affecting 10%–15% of the population, and its prevalence is increasing (Levin et al., 2017). In the UK, CKD affects approximately 6% of the population, and 80% of those patients have multiple long-term conditions. £1 in every £77 of the NHS budget in England is spent on CKD. CKD is a general term for a myriad of disorders affecting either the structural and/or functional physiological role of the kidney (NICE, 2021).

The kidneys have a myriad of functions within the body, including fluid and electrolyte balance, acid–base balance, regulation of blood pressure, excretion of uraemic toxins, hormonal regulation of erythropoiesis, hydroxylation of vitamin D and gluconeogenesis and catabolism of filtered insulin (Mahon et al., 2013a).

10.4.2 CAUSES OF CHRONIC KIDNEY DISEASE

In the UK and other high-income countries, chronic kidney disease (CKD) is generally associated with old age, diabetes, hypertension, obesity and cardiovascular disease, with presumed pathological entities such as diabetic glomerulosclerosis and hypertensive nephrosclerosis. However, the cause and pathology, severity and rate of disease progression vary among individual patients, depending on age, ethnicity and socioeconomic factors (Freedman et al., 2018; Mahon et al., 2013b; Major et al., 2019) (Box 10.6). Jiang et al. (2023) pointed out that diabetic kidney disease is a major cause of kidney failure.

10.4.3 ASSESSMENT OF KIDNEY FUNCTION

NICE (2021) criteria for the definition of CKD is denoted by glomerular filtration rate (GFR) <60 mL/min per 1·73 m^2 or kidney damage (often indicated by the presence of proteinuria) for ≥3 months duration. GFR is the total volume of filtrate passing through the glomeruli (functional unit of the kidney) per minute. However, calculating GFR is challenging to assess in real-time as the process requires using an ideal, exogenous filtration marker. Subsequently, the two most widely used estimation equations

BOX 10.6 ■ The Risk Factors of CKD

- Susceptibility to kidney disease because of sociodemographic and genetic factors
  - Age
  - Ethnicity: People of ethnic minority heritage such as African Afro-Caribbean and Asians
  - Family history of CKD stage 5, or hereditary kidney disease
  - Low birth weight (2.5 kg or lower)
- Exposure to factors attributable to CKD
  - Hypertension
  - Diabetes mellitus
  - Cardiovascular disease
  - Current or previous history of acute kidney injury
  - Glomerular disease, e.g., acute glomerulonephritis
  - Potentially nephrotoxic drugs, e.g., aminoglycosides, angiotensin-converting enzyme (ACE) inhibitors, angiotensin-II receptor antagonists, bisphosphonates, calcineurin inhibitors (such as ciclosporin or tacrolimus), diuretics, lithium, mesalazine and nonsteroidal anti-inflammatory drugs (NSAIDs).
  - Conditions associated with obstructive uropathy, e.g., structural renal tract disease, neurogenic bladder, benign prostatic hypertrophy, urinary diversion surgery, recurrent urinary tract calculi
  - Obesity with metabolic syndrome (obesity alone is not a risk factor)
  - Gout
  - Solitary functioning kidney
  - Incidental finding of haematuria or proteinuria

TABLE 10.1 **Prognosis of Chronic Kidney Disease by Categorisation of Stage of Renal Impairment and Albuminuria**

- No CKD
- Moderate-risk CKD
- High-risk CKD
- Very high-risk CKD

				Albuminuria stages, description, and range (mg/g)				
				A1		A2	A3	
				Optimum and high-normal		High	Very high and nephrotic	
				<10	10–29	30–299	300–1999	≥2000
GFR stages, description, and range (mL/min per 1.73m^2)	G1	High and optimum	>105					
			90–104					
	G2	Mild	75–89					
			60–74					
	G3a	Mild-moderate	45–59					
	G3b	Moderate-severe	30–44					
	G4	Severe	15–29					
	G5	Kidney failure	<15					

(From Kidney Disease Improving Global Outcomes. (2013). Clinical practice guideline for the evaluation and management of chronic kidney disease. www.kdigo.org/clinical_practice_guidelines/pdf/CKD/KDIGO_2012_CKD_GL.pdf.).

are the Modification of Diet in Renal Disease (MDRD) and Chronic Kidney Disease Epidemiology Collaboration (CKD-EPI) creatinine equation; both equations incorporate correction factors for age, sex and race to provide an estimate (eGFR). Inherently, decreased GFR equations are based on serum estimation of creatinine (estimated GFR) but not by serum creatinine and confirmed measurement of GFR.

In view of this, the Kidney Disease Improving Global Outcomes (KDIGO, 2013) categorised the prognosis of CKD by the stage of renal impairment and albuminuria as shown in Table 10.1.

10.4.3.1 Impact of Race Coefficient on eGFR and Clinical Outcomes

Normal GFR in young adults is about 125 mL/min per 1·73 m^2; and GFR <15 mL/min per 1·73 m^2 is defined as end-stage renal disease. Until recently, standards of care included biological race as illustrated by different Black and White eGFR for kidneys (National Kidney Foundation, 2024). The use of race coefficient exacerbates disparities in kidney health by overestimating kidney function in Black patients. Hence, patients from Black and ethnic minority heritage are also more likely to be diagnosed late and therefore present late to renal services.

Yearby (2021) reported on the misuse of race in medicine and the identification of White population as the control group, which reinforces this racial hierarchy and subsequent health disparities, and limitations on access to equal treatment. This further impacts the likelihood of patients from Black and ethnic minority heritage experiencing poor cardiovascular health as well as the complications associated with progressive CKD; CKD is a major risk factor for cardiovascular disease (Major et al., 2019).

TABLE 10.2 ■ **Systemic Signs and Symptoms of CKD**

Organ System	Symptoms	Signs
General	Fatigue, weakness	Sallow appearance, chronically ill
Skin	Pruritus, easy bruised	Pallor, ecchymoses, excoriations, oedema
ENT	Metallic taste in mouth, epistaxis	Uraemic breath
Eye	—	Pale conjunctiva
Pulmonary	Shortness of breath	Rales, pleural effusion
Cardiovascular	Dyspnoea on exertion, retrosternal pain on inspiration (pericarditis)	Hypertension, cardiomegaly, friction rub
Gastrointestinal	Anorexia, nausea, vomiting, hiccups	
Genitourinary	Nocturia, impotence	Isosthenuria (excretion of urine whose specific gravity (concentration) is neither greater (more concentrated) nor less (more dilute) than that of protein-free plasma, typically 1.008–1.012
Haematologic	Lethargy, fatigue, weakness	Anaemia
Neuromuscular	Restless legs, numbness and cramps in legs	Uraemic neuropathy
Neurologic	Generalised irritability and inability to concentrate, decreased libido	Stupor, asterixis, peripheral neuropathy

CKD, Chronic kidney disease; *ENT,* ears, nose, throat.

The use of race coefficient has been criticised by numerous renal professionals which led to its removal in 2020 (Delgado et al., 2022; Shlipak et al., 2021). In the UK, NICE (2021) recommends the categorisation of stage of renal impairment and albuminuria as shown in Table 10.1.

10.4.4 SIGNS AND SYMPTOMS

Most importantly, CKD is often asymptomatic in the early stages, and it is detected during the assessment of comorbid disorders such as diabetes and hypertension. Rapidly progressive diseases can lead to kidney failure within months; however, most diseases evolve over decades and some patients do not progress during many years of follow-up (Mahon et al., 2013b). Most patients present with systemic signs and symptoms as shown in Table 10.2 when 70% of kidney function is lost.

10.4.5 COMPLICATIONS

A variety of complications evolve as eGFR declines to less than about 60 mL/min per 1.73 m^2. Complications include hypertension, anaemia, hyperparathyroidism, hyperphosphataemia, metabolic acidosis, hypocalcaemia and low serum albumin, fatigue, weakness, frailty and decreased health-related quality of life (HrQoL) (NICE, 2021).

10.4.6 MANAGEMENT

Interventions for CKD management can prevent development, slow progression, reduce complications of decreased GFR, reduce risk of cardiovascular disease and improve survival and HrQoL. These interventions include dietary, lifestyle, self-management and medicines optimisation (Dring & Hipkiss, 2015). However, timely diagnosis and a synergistic public health approach between primary and secondary healthcare for prevention, early detection and management are pivotal to overall patient outcomes.

Supporting patients with end-stage kidney disease costs the NHS more than £50,000 per patient per year. Interventions are available to reduce the risk of CKD progression and cardiovascular events (NHS Right Care, 2018); however, there is significant variation in self-care management and medicines optimisation, which is partly due to the multimorbidity associated with this patient group.

Community care nurses play a pivotal role in the management of patients with CKD. Helping and enabling people to be aware of their condition, providing individualised education to enable informed decision-making about long-term treatment and facilitating adherence have been reported as essential to the HrQoL (Cardol et al., 2023). Measures tailored towards optimal blood pressure (Cheung et al., 2017) and glycaemia control (NHS Right Care, 2018) have been highlighted as crucial towards preventing the decline of kidney function.

CASE STUDY 10.1

Uchenna is a 44-year-old African male living in London and has been on home haemodialysis following his CKD diagnosis 9 months ago. He speaks Igbo and limited English. He is known to have gout, an enlarged prostate, uncontrolled hypertension and diabetes. Uchenna is a married dad with 2 children. He is a heavy smoker and drinker.

Uchenna undergoes dialysis for 4 hours thrice weekly. He has been taught to insert his own needles, start and finish his treatment as well as IV medications administration since April 2023. You have visited Uchenna today and he is experiencing severe generalised headache and shortness of breath and feeling easily fatigued. He was recently seen by the diabetes nurse specialist during a routine appointment, and he was informed that his diabetes control was poor. His GP has added two more medications to his existing nine medicines. This has caused Uchenna to be very upset about his care. He believes that all the medications prescribed since the initial flare-up of his gout contributed to his kidney disease. He believes he developed kidney disease because he stopped going to church and praying.

He has been putting off going to see his GP with breathlessness because he does not want his kidney consultant to add any more medications and be referred to a dietitian as his previous encounter was poor. He alleges that the dietitian told him to stop eating Nigerian food.

Your observations are:

Blood pressure (BP) 162/102 mm Hg and 155/95 mm Hg (standing), pulse 87 bpm, respiratory rate 21 bpm, moderate bilateral pedal oedema.

PRESCRIPTION:

- Amlodipine 10 mg daily
- Atenolol 50 mg daily
- Candesartan 16 mg daily
- Dapagliflozin 10 mg daily
- Co-codamol 16/1000 mg every 4–6 hours PRN
- Insulin Lantus 10 units once per day
- Linagliptin 5 mg once daily
- Atorvastatin 40 mg daily
- Allopurinol 100 mg daily
- Bezafibrate 200 mg, 3 times a day

QUESTIONS:

1. What are some of the social factors contributing to Uchenna's ill-health?
2. How you could support Uchenna?
3. What services would you signpost Uchenna too?

Uchenna is experiencing a broad range of social determinants of health, including income, employment, education and diet, lifestyle, religious beliefs, culture and deprivation. Together, along with his underlying diabetes, hypertension and chronic disease, these factors are cumulatively making his overall health worse and reducing his access to healthcare services. Uchenna would benefit from a personalised care approach; personalised care means people have choice and control over the way their care is planned and delivered. It is based on 'what matters' to them and their individual strengths and needs. Use the triad of ideas, concerns, expectations (ICE) to explore and understand Uchenna's perspectives about his kidney health, treatment and underlying long-term conditions and medication adherence.

Uchenna may find it helpful to be:

- Offered access to health information including red flag symptoms and signs of worsening diabetes, hypertension and poor kidney treatment.
- Given information about what to tell health and social care professionals in a language of his preference.
- Medications clearly written down with uses, dose and side effects. Advocate for modified release of bezafibrate.
- Lifestyle change recommendations written down with their benefits.
- Information provided in plain language.
- It would also be helpful to signpost Uchenna to other services that might be helpful, including the Black kidney support groups and other support groups.

10.4.7 KIDNEY DISEASE AND HEALTH INEQUITY

Healthcare professionals have an important generic role in the early recognition, timely referral and/or management of a worsening kidney function. The incidence of kidney disease is higher among Afro-Caribbean people and adverse outcomes are higher among the most deprived populations. Box 10.7 offers a step-by-step guide on how community nurses can enable and facilitate health.

10.4.8 CONCLUSION

This section provides a comprehensive and informative overview of CKD, covering its causes, clinical manifestations, diagnosis, treatment modalities and preventive strategies. Furthermore, the impact and significance of CKD are examined, shedding light on its prevalence, socioeconomic implications and the need for concerted efforts to enhance awareness, education and access to quality care within the community.

10.5 Respiratory Disease

10.5.1 INTRODUCTION

Respiratory disease affects one in five people in the UK and is the third biggest cause of death in England (NHS England, 2023). Respiratory disease accounted for almost 20% of causes of death in the UK in 2013, with lung cancer, chronic obstructive pulmonary disease (COPD) and pneumonia accounting for the highest number of deaths (British Lung Foundation (BLF), 2023). England also has among the highest mortality rates related to respiratory conditions in Europe (Institute for Health Metrics and Evaluation

BOX 10.7 ■ Step-by-Step Guide on How Community Nurses Can Enable and Facilitate Health

Step 1: Be proactive—Early recognition of a CKD. Take opportunities to actively look out for patients presenting with CKD; be mindful of the inequalities more commonly experienced in patients who present from at-risk groups such as patients living in the most deprived areas and ethnic minority groups. Be familiar with the local policy and NICE guidance for the management of CKD. Remember to be especially vigilant for signs and symptoms of chest pain, dizziness, neurological events and fluid accumulation. If a diagnosis is made, making treatment plans or prescribing does not normally form part of a community nurse's role; it is therefore important to urgently highlight findings to a colleague with these skills. Contact a GP and/or diabetic team immediately for specialist advice. It is important to follow the individualised care plans in place for patients with diabetic kidney disease. Shared decision-making and applying the biopsychosocial approach are important to support tailored patient engagement with the management of CKD.

Step 2: Personalised care and culturally competent communication. Culturally competent communication refers to communicating with awareness and knowledge of healthcare disparities and understanding that sociocultural factors have important effects on health beliefs and behaviours, as well as having the skills to manage these factors appropriately. Respecting and understanding an individual's cultural and religious context help to build rapport and tailor your approach to best meet your patient's needs. Take some time to think about how to explain a diagnosis, rationale for monitoring and/or treatment. Personalising treatment for each patient's specific context and needs will bear the greatest success. Consider the patient's access to healthcare services: digital, phone, transport. Consider how you might be able to support mitigation against barriers.

Step 3: Treatment and follow-up. Optimisation of blood pressure and diabetes control.

TABLE 10.3 ■ **Leading Causes of Death Globally**

1	Ischaemic heart disease
2	Stroke
3	**Chronic obstructive pulmonary disease**
4	**Lower respiratory infections**
5	Neonatal conditions
6	**Trachea, bronchus, lung cancers**
7	Alzheimer disease and other dementias
8	Diarrhoeal diseases
9	Diabetes mellitus
10	Kidney diseases

(From World Health Organisation (WHO). (2020). The top 10 causes of death. https://www.who.int/news-room/fact-sheets/detail/the-top-10-causes-of-death#:~:text=The%20top%20global%20causes%20of,birth%20asphyxia%20and%20birth%20trauma%2C.)

(IHME), 2023). Hospital admissions are closely related to the incidence of respiratory disease, and this also has an impact on increased winter pressures on the NHS with almost double numbers of nonelective admissions in winter (NHS England, 2023).

Respiratory disease has a considerable health burden in the world (European Respiratory Society (ERS), 2013, 2017). Three respiratory conditions (Table 10.3) are among the top 10 leading causes of mortality in the world (WHO, 2020).

Additionally, five respiratory conditions account for the most common causes of illness and death. These include COPD, asthma, lower respiratory tract infections, tuberculosis and lung cancers (ERS, 2017). The high incidence rate of respiratory disease means that all nurses, including community nurses, will be providing care to patients with respiratory disease on many occasions. Of all respiratory conditions, COPD is the second most common cause of deaths after lung cancer in the UK (BLF, 2023) and will be the focus of the next section.

10.5.2 CHRONIC OBSTRUCTIVE PULMONARY DISEASE

Chronic Obstructive Pulmonary Disease (COPD) is defined as 'a heterogeneous lung condition characterized by chronic respiratory symptoms (dyspnoea, cough, expectoration, exacerbations) due to abnormalities of the airways (bronchitis, bronchiolitis) and/or alveoli (emphysema) that cause persistent, often progressive, airflow obstruction' (Global Initiative for Chronic Obstructive Disease (GOLD), 2023). The new definition emphasises the importance of looking at broader factors apart from tobacco smoking which can contribute to developing COPD (Box 10.8).

10.5.3 MANAGEMENT OF COPD IN PRIMARY CARE AND COMMUNITY SETTINGS

There is currently no cure for COPD (NICE, 2023b). Primary interventions should initially focus on health protection, prevention and promotion to prevent the development of COPD (NICE, 2019a). There are four main areas (Fig. 10.2) that community nurses need to focus on to support better management of patients with COPD.

BOX 10.8 ■ Common Symptoms of COPD

- Exertional breathlessness
- Chronic cough
- Regular sputum production
- Frequent winter 'bronchitis'
- Wheeze

(From National Institute for Health and Care Excellence (NICE). (2019). Chronic obstructive pulmonary disease in over 16s: Diagnosis and management. Available at: https://www.nice.org.uk/guidance/ng115.)

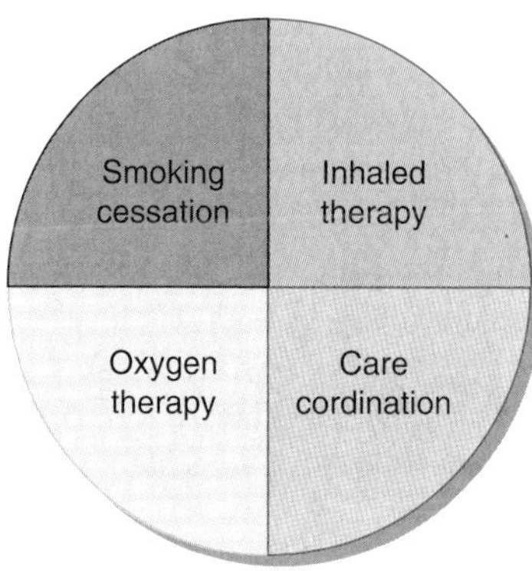

Fig. 10.2 Four areas of intervention for chronic obstructive pulmonary disease management.

10.5.3.1 Smoking Cessation

Smoking cessation for patients with COPD who are still smoking is the main protective factor to slow down the progression of disease (Gundry, 2020). Supporting patients living with COPD to quit smoking remains a challenge as smokers with COPD still report difficulties giving up smoking (Schmid-Mohler et al., 2020).

Smoking status should be assessed on a routine basis at initial assessment and reassessed if needed. This assessment should determine smoking behaviour, level of dependence and previous attempts to quit (NICE, 2023a). The National Centre for Smoking Cessation and Training (NCSCT) sets the training requirements for smoking cessation advisors (NCSCT, 2018; NICE, 2023a).

Each opportunity should be taken to provide very brief advice as well as supporting behavioural interventions (NICE, 2023a, 2023d) and where necessary to make referrals to local stop smoking services. In addition, eligible patients should be offered nicotine replacement therapy (NRT) and, if suitable, to also consider varenicline or bupropion. NICE (2023a) also recommends advice on nicotine-containing e-cigarettes and attending Allen Carr's in-person group seminars.

10.5.3.2 Inhaled Therapy

Inhaled medications are the frontline treatment drugs for managing COPD and other respiratory conditions. Advice and education on improving inhaler technique as well as concordance will enhance the efficacy of the drugs. Incorrect inhaler technique is common among patients with asthma and COPD (National Asthma Council Australia, 2016). NICE (2019a) states that all individuals can improve their inhaler technique with training and, additionally, different inhaler devices should be considered depending on the needs or ability of the patient. Nurses should be able to supervise and assist inhaler users with their technique and consider alternative delivery devices such as spacers if appropriate (Gundry, 2020; NICE, 2019a). Inhaler technique should be regularly assessed, and this can also include assessing usage of prescribed inhaled therapy; for example, overusage of salbutamol can suggest poor inhaler technique. Advice should also be given with the use of inhaled corticosteroids as side effects such as oral thrush can be an indication of poor inhaler technique. Users should be advised to rinse their mouth or brush their teeth after usage.

Videos on inhaler technique (suggested by British Thoracic Society (BTS), 2021) can be accessed at: https://www.asthma.org.uk/advice/inhaler-videos.

10.5.3.3 Oxygen Therapy

Long-term oxygen therapy (LTOT) can be recommended following careful assessment criteria (Box 10.9). LTOT is usually prescribed for patients with stable COPD and a persistent resting oxygen saturation of <92%.

Healthcare professionals and patients need to be aware that inappropriate use of oxygen can lead to respiratory depression in patients with COPD. Therefore it is essential for nurses to be aware of the oxygen prescription and range of oxygen saturations for the patients they are looking after. Oxygen is a prescribed medication (British National Formulary, 2023) and should be regarded as a drug, and therefore the same rigorous criteria for medication administration should be followed. Oxygen therapy can be delivered via three main ways, namely, (1) a nasal cannula via the nose, (2) a face mask positioned over the nose and mouth and (3) a mask attached to tracheostomy (Care Quality

BOX 10.9 ■ Criteria for Assessment of LTOT

- Very severe airflow obstruction (FEV1 below 30% predicted)
- Cyanosis (blue tint to skin)
- Polycythaemia
- Peripheral oedema (swelling)
- A raised jugular venous pressure
- Oxygen saturations of 92% or less breathing air

(From National Institute for Health and Care Excellence (NICE) (2016). *Chronic obstructive pulmonary disease in adults – Quality statement 3: Assessment for long-term oxygen therapy.* Available at: https://www.nice.org.uk/guidance/qs10/chapter/Quality-statement-3-Assessment-for-longterm-oxygen-therapy.)

BOX 10.10 ■ Functions of the MDT

- Assessment (including performing spirometry, assessing which delivery systems to use for inhaled therapy, the need for aids for daily living and assessing the need for oxygen)
- Care and treatment
- Advice on self-management
- Case identification and care coordination
- Education for patients and their carers

(From National Institute for Health and Care Excellence (NICE). (2019). Chronic obstructive pulmonary disease in over 16s: Diagnosis and management. Available at: https://www.nice.org.uk/guidance/ng115.)

Commission, 2022). Long-term oxygen therapy (LTOT) is usually provided via an oxygen concentrator in the patient's home and therefore safety issues such as preventing smoking and oxygen therapy should be carefully addressed (BTS, 2015). Other safety issues might also involve ensuring that there is enough tubing length to avoid falls and having backup oxygen cylinders in the event of electricity cuts.

10.5.3.4 Care Coordination and Multidisciplinary Management

Living with COPD or with other chronic respiratory conditions will require an MDT approach. This is particularly recommended for COPD by NICE (2019a) which identifies many functions (Box 10.10).

MDTs can be complex and extensive (NICE, 2023b). The Royal Pharmaceutical Society (2011) identifies several health and social care services who might be involved in providing care to patients (Box 10.11). Having a person coordinating care in managing and supporting the patient journey for patients with COPD is therefore helpful (Schmid-Mohler et al., 2020). The care coordinator can be a healthcare regulated person with expertise in respiratory care (Atwood et al., 2022; Chew & Mahadeva, 2018; NHS England, 2017a).

Patients living with COPD are more at risk of developing or are already living with other comorbidities (Primary Care Respiratory Society UK (PCRS-UK), 2016). Management of comorbidities and frailty also forms part of the priorities of optimisation (PCRS-UK, 2017). This will involve engaging with several other specialities to

BOX 10.11 ■ Other Services Available to Patients with COPD

- Physiotherapy
- Occupational therapy
- Social Services
- Hospital at home schemes
- District and community nursing services
- Specialist respiratory services
- Palliative care teams

provide optimum support for patients with COPD (Gustafsson & Nordeman, 2017). Whilst the community nurse might not be able to provide specialist respiratory care, it is essential that patients are referred to services such as physiotherapy (for lung exercises and if appropriate pulmonary rehabilitation), mental health support (to manage anxiety and depression) and occupational therapy (for equipment and home adjustments). The MDT approach is essential as living with a chronic long-term respiratory condition will have an impact on the ability of the patient to perform activities of daily living.

10.5.4 NUTRITIONAL SUPPORT

NICE (2019a) recommends referral to dietetics for patients with abnormalities (high or low or changing over time). Community nursing staff should monitor weight and pay attention to any changes especially if these are >3 kg (NICE, 2019b). Encouraging patients to exercise is also recommended as it not only improves respiratory outcomes but can also enhance the efficacy of nutritional supplements (NICE, 2023g). Weight loss can also be an indication of other causes such as asthma, HF and lung cancer (NICE, 2023b) and therefore thorough assessment and monitoring will be essential.

10.5.5 PALLIATIVE CARE

COPD has no cure and is a progressive illness, therefore disease progression follows a gradual course of decline which might lead to frequent exacerbations and eventually lead to death (NICE, 2023b).

The focus of palliative care needs to be on managing symptoms such as breathlessness, pain and cough. This will vary depending on the respiratory conditions.

10.5.6 CONCLUSION

Respiratory disease is a significant cause of death and contributes to many hospital admissions. Due to the high incidence of COPD which as yet has no cure, community nurses will often encounter patients with the condition. Areas for intervention include smoking cessation, inhaled therapy management, provision of oxygen therapy and case coordination. Care for patients with COPD can often be complex and challenging and requires a multidisciplinary approach to manage both the physical symptoms and emotional well-being. This is particularly pertinent when providing support during the palliative phase and end-of-life care.

10.6 Neurological Disorder

10.6.1 INTRODUCTION

The term 'neurological disorder' describes a broad constellation of physical conditions that affect the central and peripheral nervous systems, including the brain, spinal cord and muscles (WHO, 2016). These disorders can result from various factors, including congenital abnormalities, genetic predispositions, neurodegenerative processes and acquired brain injuries, occurring at any point during an individual's lifespan (Pugh et al., 2018). Recognising the global significance of neurological disorders as a challenge to healthcare services, the WHO identifies them as the leading nonfatal burden on healthcare provision, consuming substantial portions of healthcare budgets worldwide (WHO, 2017). In the UK, the prevalence of diagnosed neurological disorders is estimated at 1 in 6 individuals, with an additional 600,000 people diagnosed each year, highlighting the extensive impact of these conditions on healthcare services. Diagnoses are described across 16 condition categories and are included in 473 International Classification of Disease Codes (The Neurological Alliance, 2019).

Given the complex range of conditions that may be categorised under the umbrella of neurological disorder, nurses working in the community will play a significant role in both devising comprehensive care plans for these disorders and directly administering interventions aimed at treating comorbid symptoms (Pugh et al., 2018). The fact that in the UK 64% of people with neurological disorders who are admitted to the hospital do so because of a medical emergency emphasises the importance of high-quality community-based neurological health services (Pugh et al., 2018). Community service provision, however, faces several challenges including increasing levels of demand, chronicity of needs, cost and complexity. Furthermore, as there are over 250 recognised neurological conditions, needs-based service commissioning, design and delivery vary across the UK (NHS Wales, 2017).

10.6.2 INTEGRATED CARE

The presentation of neurological disorders varies in onset, complexity, severity and impact, and will therefore require a responsive multidisciplinary care pathway approach to meet the unique needs of patients (NHS Wales, 2022). For example, stroke, a medical emergency and the fourth leading cause of premature death in the UK, often leaves survivors with lifelong disabilities and chronic health needs (Malewezi et al., 2022). Integrated Community Stroke Services play a pivotal role in coordinating the care transition from hospitals to the community, offering specialised multidisciplinary rehabilitation services to stroke survivors (NHS, 2022). Community nurses assume a critical role in stroke rehabilitation and support, collaborating with MDT colleagues to develop and implement comprehensive care plans targeting physical impairments such as mobility issues, muscle weakness, and speech or swallowing difficulties. Additionally, they provide education to patients and their families on stroke prevention, risk factor management and lifestyle modifications to mitigate the risk of recurrence (Magwood et al., 2020).

10.6.3 THE ROLE OF COMMUNITY NURSING SERVICES

Community nurses provide care for individuals with degenerative and progressive neurological disorders characterised by the onset of symptoms and the presence of multiple comorbidities. For example, multiple sclerosis (MS) is a degenerative neurological condition affecting approximately 100,000 people in the UK (Strickland & Baguley, 2015). Whilst a definitive cause has not yet been established, it is thought that environmental and genetic factors create a pathological immune response leading to inflammation in the central nervous system (Waubant et al., 2019). Systemic causes mean that predicting the course of an individual's MS can be challenging, as diagnosis is complicated by the diverse onset and range of symptoms (Strickland & Baguley, 2015). Common symptoms can include fatigue, ataxia, muscle spasticity, visual and sensory impairments and cognitive decline (Mendes, 2016). Whilst MS itself is not thought to be life-limiting, premature death can arise from comorbid illnesses such as aspiration pneumonia, septicaemia or urinary tract infection (UTI) (Barnes, 2007). Historically, those diagnosed with MS have been cared for in hospitals however, placing greater emphasis on symptom detection, assessment, treatment and management means that those diagnosed with the condition can now enjoy a good quality of life at home or in a community setting (Strickland & Baguley, 2015). Community nurses play a central role in the care and support of people with MS and will be involved in delivering interventions which ameliorate needs arising from primary symptoms and secondary complications, for example, mobility and contractures, UTIs or constipation, tissue viability and palliative care (WHO, 2023).

Progressive motor neurodegenerative disorders, such as Parkinson disease or motor neuron disease, are incurable conditions that lead to chronic and complex physical disabilities which restrict the individual's activities of daily living and quality of life (Anestis et al., 2020). Nurses who provide care to individuals with motor neurodegenerative disorders such as Parkinson's disease will be expected to work within a competency framework which includes having a firm knowledge and understanding of symptoms, their presentation and management, person-centred assessment skills, collaborative care planning, outcome measurements and evaluation and teaching/mentorship skills (Parkinson UK, 2016). Nurses delivering care to individuals with motor degenerative disorders will require excellent communications skills and will need to demonstrate empathy and compassion, particularly when delivering a diagnosis and engaging with the individual and their family in decision-making regarding advanced care planning and end-of-life care (Anestis et al., 2020).

While some neurological disorders, such as epilepsy, are associated with higher mortality rates than the general population, effective treatment strategies can significantly reduce avoidable deaths and improve individuals' quality of life (Mbizvo et al., 2019). Epilepsy is a chronic condition that causes the individual to experience seizures. Whilst epilepsy can have major implications on health, well-being and life expectancy, antiepilepsy medication can control seizures in up to 70% of people (NICE, 2022e). Sudden unexplained death in epilepsy (SUDEP) is a phenomenon where people may die prematurely without a clear pathological aetiology; however, risks can be mitigated by empowering people with epilepsy and their carers with appropriate knowledge about the condition (Mesraoua et al., 2022). Good practice guidelines recommend that a risk assessment is carried out following a first unprovoked seizure (NICE, 2022). Epilepsy specialist nurses play a key role in completing risk assessments, developing and reviewing risk management plans and delivering interventions which support self-management strategies, thus promoting inclusion and participation (NICE, 2022).

10.6.4 CONCLUSION

Neurological disorders can often be progressive and present significant challenges to individuals. Due to these complexities, community nurses are often involved in patient care to help manage symptoms and provide support and education, which frequently involves collaboration with the wider MDT. National frameworks and guidelines are available to support care which needs to be delivered with compassion and an understanding of the physical and psychological impact on the patient's daily life.

CASE STUDY 10.2

Abigail is 35 years old and lives at home with her husband and 7-year-old daughter. She was diagnosed with MS 5 years ago after noticing a deterioration in her eyesight, balance and increasing feelings of fatigue. More recently, Abigail has experienced numbness in her lower limbs that has restricted her ability to walk independently. A deterioration in Abigail's mobility has led her to experience regular constipation.

- What services could you refer Abigail to for mobility support?
- What type of hydration and dietary advice would you provide regarding constipation?
- Are there any local charities that you could guide Abigail to for further support?

10.7 Frailty

10.7.1 INTRODUCTION

As a community nurse in the UK, understanding frailty and its management is crucial for providing optimal care and support to older individuals living with this condition. This section explains the clinical syndrome of frailty and offers advice on how community nurses can identify frailty, what the benefits of doing so are, and how they can assist and empower older adults with frailty to manage and navigate their daily lives more effectively.

10.7.2 UNDERSTANDING FRAILTY

Frailty is a complex medical syndrome, combining the effects of natural ageing with the outcomes of multiple long-term conditions, loss of fitness and reserve (Clegg et al., 2013). It commonly affects older adults and is associated with adverse health outcomes, including disability, hospitalisation and mortality. Frailty is not an inevitable consequence of aging but rather a distinct clinical syndrome. It is typically characterised by multiple physiological and functional impairments, including diminished strength, endurance, mobility, balance and cognitive function, and is often progressive (NHS England, 2017c). Older adults with frailty often experience fatigue, weight loss, slowed gait speed, reduced muscle strength and an increased susceptibility to falls and fractures (National Institute for Health Research (NIHR), 2017). Older people with frailty are more prone to developing complications from acute illnesses and are less resilient in recovering from them. Late recognition can impede choice around place of care (Perrels et al., 2014) and patient-centred decisions (Fleming et al., 2010). Recognising the signs and symptoms of frailty can help district nurses identify those at risk and initiate appropriate interventions.

10.7.3 IDENTIFYING FRAILTY

There is no agreed operational definition of frailty. There are various methods for identifying frailty, including the prognostic indicators described earlier which can be opportunistic or population based (NHS England, 2017c). The Clinical Frailty Scale (Rockwood et al., 2005), which was updated in 2020 (Mendiratta et al., 2023), is a commonly employed method in the UK that uses clinical descriptors and pictographs, with an easily applicable tool, to stratify older adults according to their level of frailty. Other validated tools include the Gait Speed Test, PRISMA-7 and the Timed Up and Go test (NHS England, 2017c).

10.7.4 BEST PRACTICE FOR SUPPORTING OLDER ADULTS WITH FRAILTY

As NHS England (2017c) highlighted, care and support can be optimised for adults with multimorbidity which can include anticipating crisis and ensuring an optimal recovery. The key to facilitating this is with a *Comprehensive Assessment.* This is vital to determine an individual's frailty status and identify their specific needs. This assessment should include physical, cognitive, psychosocial and practical aspects. Tools such as the Clinical Frailty Scale and the Comprehensive Geriatric Assessment can support identification of frailty and assessment (NHS England, 2017c). Within community nursing, it is important to be aware of the differences between these assessments and apply them using the online tools or access specialists within the local area. As the Royal College of Nursing (RCN, 2023) suggests, it is essential that nurses can direct patients and carers to supportive services and interventions. Once an accurate assessment has been conducted, then *person-centred care* will ensure that care is tailored to the unique needs and preferences of the older adult. It is vital to engage in open communication and encourage autonomy, respect choice and promote a sense of control and dignity (NIHR, 2017). When providing care for an individual at home, an approach that emphasises, 'what matters to you most?' is a useful guiding principle in assessment of need and evaluation of any intervention. People with frailty also retain considerable strengths and it is imperative that goal-oriented frailty care is guided by their values, priorities and preferences (Nicholson et al., 2023) (Table 10.4).

TABLE 10.4 **Benefits of Proactive Care for People with Frailty**

Benefit	Explanation
Enhanced quality of life	Proactive care empowers older individuals with frailty to manage their condition effectively, promoting independence and a higher quality of life. By addressing their specific needs, individuals can maintain their physical and cognitive function to the best of their abilities.
Reduced hospitalisations	Comprehensive and proactive care can help prevent unnecessary hospitalisations brought on by declines in health that could be effectively managed at home. Active management of frailty-related symptoms and early intervention by community nurses to address potential complications can help prevent hospital admissions and promote continuity of care at home.
Minimising functional decline	Proactive care strategies, including regular assessments, targeted interventions and collaboration with the multidisciplinary team, can help to limit further functional decline in individuals with frailty.
Improved care coordination	By fostering strong partnerships with other primary care providers, specialists and community services, community nurses can support care coordination for older adults with frailty. Regular communication and information sharing enhance the continuity and effectiveness of care.

For effective management of frailty, it is essential that *MDTs* work seamlessly including care professionals from health, social and voluntary care roles. Coordinated efforts enhance holistic care, enabling a comprehensive approach to managing frailty that supports effective management whereas disconnected services can create perceptions of care that are inconsistent and impersonal (Nicholson et al., 2023). When planning care for individuals at home, it is essential to scope the local area and identify the different teams and services that support older people with frailty. It can be useful to think about joint visits and understand each other's roles to avoid gaps in provision or duplication. Often, older adults with frailty have multiple comorbidities and take numerous medications. As NIHR (2017) identifies, *polypharmacy* is often associated with increasing the risk of unplanned hospital admissions and side effects of medications. Therefore it is important to ensure that older adults with frailty understand their medications, their purpose and potential side effects. Community nurses can promote safe medication practices, such as providing medication organisers and keeping an updated list of medications within the home, promote adherence through education and simplification supporting regular medication reviews.

As NICE (2019b) states, there is an undeniable link between a diagnosis of frailty and an increased risk of falls. For this reason, it is important for a community nurse to conduct a falls risk assessment and assess the home environment for hazards and refer on for adaptations if indicated. They are often in the best position to provide education on fall prevention strategies, such as maintaining good lighting, removing clutter and using assistive devices.

Ni Lochlainn et al. (2021) suggested that as nutrition can be a modifiable risk factor for frailty, dietary change could be one of the strategies recommended to prevent and treat it. Community nurses are often in the best place to discuss the benefits of a healthy balanced diet which is tailored to the individual's nutritional needs, is culturally appropriate and fits with their preferred eating and drinking practices. As the British Geriatric Society (2019) suggests, it can often be cost-effective to refer individuals to local dietetics services to manage poor nutrition if secondary causes have been excluded.

As NIHR (2017) identifies, the transition between older people living with frailty and those actively at the end of life is often unclear. Living with frailty makes people vulnerable to sudden deterioration, fluctuating capacity and uncertain recovery and increases their risk of morbidity and mortality (Clegg et al., 2013). Supporting the care of people with advancing frailty requires integrated care across the care continuum, including health, social and third sector input. Most older people with frailty want to live and die 'at home' and community nurses have a hugely important role to play in supporting older people to live and die well. Advance care planning is a helpful way to discuss an older person's wishes and desires at the end of life and guide care. The work of Combes et al. (2019) specifically on older people with frailty notes such conversations need to start early, focus on living well now as well as the future and seek to involve people who matter to the person whilst ensuring the older person with frailty and their choices are centre stage. Therefore community nurses are often best placed to speak to older people and their families and work with the local palliative care team for support as required (Box 10.12).

BOX 10.12 ■ Advice for Practice

- When talking about future wishes, it often helps to start with the now.
- If you are unsure about how a person will respond, try to understand what they have explored already, gain trust and be prepared for this to be a conversation over time rather than a one-off event.
- Gain support from colleagues, there will often be someone in your team with a practical interest and experience to support you.

10.7.5 CONCLUSION

Frailty is a clinical syndrome that significantly impacts the lives of older adults. Community nurses play a crucial role in supporting and empowering older adults with frailty to manage their condition effectively. Using the suggested strategies, community nurses can enhance quality of life, help to reduce unnecessary hospitalisations, and help limit functional decline in older adults living with frailty.

10.8 Dementia

Dementia is a general term used to describe a group of diseases which cause abnormal brain changes. Such changes affect a person's memory, language, problem-solving and other sensory and thinking abilities, and are severe enough to interfere in the person's daily life (WHO, 2023a). Dementia is considered the leading cause of death in England and Wales, accounting for 12.8% of all registered deaths (Social Care Institute of Excellence (SCIE), 2020). Furthermore, the SCIE (2020) reports that 92% of people with dementia will have at least one other health condition; 45% of people with dementia are reported to have four or more other health conditions. Dementia has become the most feared disease of people aged over 65 years (Alzheimer's Society, 2016).

It is worth noting the predicted impact of dementia with regards to prevalence related to severity (Table 10.5) and cost implications on health, social and unpaid care (Table 10.6).

Table 10.6 represents the cost in £million predicted for care. This includes statutory health and social care, the costs incurred by friends and family to care for a loved one and 'other' costs related to policy development, policing, advocacy and research.

Whilst dementia itself is a complex set of disease processes, navigating the UK health and social care system throughout the disease trajectory adds additional layers

TABLE 10.5 ■ **Prevalence of People Living with Dementia Related to Severity**

UK	2019	2020	2025	2030	2040	% Change
Mild	126,900	128,400	140,700	160,900	196,600	55%
Moderate	245,600	236,900	250,300	280,400	327,500	33%
Severe	510,600	510,600	542,600	792,100	1,066,000	109%
Total	883,100	907,900	1,060,100	1,233,400	1,590,100	80%

(From Care Policy and Evaluation Centre (CPEC). (2019). https://www.lse.ac.uk/cpec/assets/documents/cpec-working-paper-5.pdf.).

TABLE 10.6 **Cost Implications of Dementia on Health, Social and Unpaid Care**

UK	2019	2020	2025	2030	2040	% Change
Healthcare	4,900	5,000	6,300	7,900	12,500	155%
Social care	15,700	16,900	21,600	27,900	45,400	190%
Unpaid care	13,900	14,600	18,200	23,100	35,700	156%
Other	180	240	310	390	630	251%
Total	34,700	36,700	46,300	59,200	94,100	172%

(From Care Policy and Evaluation Centre (CPEC). (2019). https://www.lse.ac.uk/cpec/assets/documents/cpec-working-paper-5.pdf.)

of complexity and complications for the person with dementia and the people caring for them (Department of Health, 2009, 2015). Current guidance from NICE (Hayhoe et al., 2016) is that GPs should refer a person to memory services if they have symptoms likely to be related to dementia, after excluding any other modifiable causes. These services are run by mental health teams. This may increase the barriers to a person accessing and receiving a dementia diagnosis (Low & Purwaningrum, 2020).

Following a dementia diagnosis, the person's care will then be passed back to their GP, and currently fragmented, fragile postdiagnostic services. Some of the key issues related to people with dementia having access to good, lifetime support following a dementia diagnosis are an unsupported infrastructure; limited proactive reviews, no standardisation of what a dementia review should look like; limited capacity and capability to carry out postdiagnostic reviews; limited understanding of the person with dementia or their caregiver as to where to access postdiagnostic dementia services; living alone; and decreased health literacy in more deprived areas where health needs are often greater (Bamford et al., 2021; Cooper et al., 2017; Deckers et al., 2019; Giebel et al., 2021; Lane, 2022; Wheatley et al., 2021, 2022).

The lack of structured postdiagnostic services and lack of continuity of care for people with dementia will often lead to a person having unmet health and social care needs (Vestergaard et al., 2020). This may result in an increased need for urgent care including emergency department attendance, less access to elective healthcare interventions and increased speed of disease progression and mortality (Lane, 2022; Watson et al., 2020). The impact of dementia on other life-limiting conditions is further exacerbated in lower socioeconomic areas, where there is compelling evidence that there is an increased incidence of chronic disease, long-term conditions, vascular risks, frailty and malnutrition (Cooper et al., 2017; Lane, 2022; Vestergaard et al., 2020).

Whilst a person with dementia and their carer may need support adjusting to a new dementia diagnosis, over time these emotional and psychological needs are likely to change, leading to an increased risk of depression, anxiety and challenges within relationships, as family members struggle to cope with the increasing demands of being a carer (Bamford et al., 2021; Lane, 2022). This may result in the person with dementia having an increase in unmet needs and a decrease in their functional capability. In turn, this may lead to more rapid decline in physical and cognitive health, and an increased need for the person with dementia to enter a residential or nursing care facility (Lane, 2022; Read et al., 2021; Watson et al., 2020).

Whilst there remains no cure for dementia, it is recognised that there is a need for further research, with an emphasis on health promotion to reduce the risks of developing dementia (Livingston et al., 2020). Furthermore, there is a need to promote the value of psychosocial interventions and the use of technology, to improve the health outcomes and quality of life of people with dementia, enabling the person to remain well and live independently for longer in their own home (Stroka, 2021; Vernooij-Dassen et al., 2019).

Community and primary care services have a key role to play in the development of more robust, holistic and integrated care pathways that enables 'lifetime' support for people with dementia post diagnosis. Access to a named health or care coordinator to facilitate the navigation of a complex health and social care system and planning for future needs is required. This is essential for the management of other comorbidities and physical/sensory impairments that most people with dementia will experience through their disease trajectory (Lane, 2022; NICE, 2018a; Wheatley et al., 2020) (Table 10.7).

10.8.1 CONCLUSION

Dementia can be very complex and often has an impact on a person's daily life. One of the challenges includes navigating a fragmented healthcare system to access the care and support required. Community nurses are often best placed to facilitate this care through holistic assessment, person-centred care planning, crisis management (including respite), symptom management, providing education and supporting families to manage grief and loss.

10.9 Supporting Patients With Nutrition and Hydration Needs in the Community

Many people that community nurses care for have or are at risk of malnutrition (Malnutrition Task Force, 2023). Malnutrition and nutrition-related conditions include undernutrition, obesity, sarcopenia and micronutrient abnormalities (Cedarholm et al., 2017). As well as supporting people with existing nutritional issues, community nurses have a responsibility to ensure nutrition and hydration care are delivered effectively (Nursing and Midwifery Council, 2018). Community nurses ensure people they care for have adequate access to nutrition and hydration. In people living in their own homes, this is usually done by ensuring appropriate services and carer support are in place.

To ensure the provision of good nutritional care, community nurses screen for malnutrition, assess nutrition and hydration status and needs, develop an appropriate plan of care to meet the person's needs and then deliver the plan. An important step following this is to evaluate the plan of care and make any changes as required. The needs of the person may be to eat and drink to maintain comfort rather than to ensure nutritional requirements for that person's body weight and age are met (NICE, 2017).

10.9.1 MALNUTRITION

Screening for malnutrition should be undertaken using a validated and reliable screening tool such as the Malnutrition Universal Screening Tool (MUST) (British Association of Enteral and Parenteral Nutrition, 2023). This tool will identify those who are at risk

TABLE 10.7 **The Role of Community Nurses in Dementia Care: How This Aligns with the NHS Well Pathway for Dementia**

Preventing Well	Diagnosing Well	Supporting Well	Living Well	Dying Well
• Raising awareness of dementia and risk reduction within health and social care and the wider community. • Reducing the stigma associated with dementia, including the use of derogatory language, e.g., wandering. • Promoting good health—what's good for your heart is good for your brain. • Improved long-term condition management of other comorbidities. • Improved health literacy. • Community engagement especially in underrepresented communities, e.g., BAME, LGBTQIA+. • Risk reduction of falls decreased mobility, delirium, polypharmacy, malnutrition, dehydration, infections, incontinence, social isolation and depression.	• Supporting people to seek a timely dementia diagnosis. • Understanding and identifying the barriers to people seeking a dementia diagnosis—especially underserved and underreached communities. • Improving peridiagnosis support. • Supporting people to navigate a complex health and social care system. • Improving the education of health and social care professionals and the wider public about both typical and atypical signs and symptoms of dementia—to facilitate earlier recognition and diagnosis. • Early conversations about person-centred care planning. • Sharing information about research and clinical trials opportunities.	• Ensuring that the person has access to a holistic bio-psychosocial assessment. • Encouraging the person to remain as socially active as possible, including attending day centres, exercise classes, walking groups, etc. • Ensuring that family carers have access to a carer's assessment and psychosocial support. • Identification and effective management of any other long-term conditions or comorbidities. • Development of an advanced person-centred care plan. • Supporting the development of a crisis care plan, for example, if there was an untoward event that affected the main carer. • Encouraging the use of nonpharmacological interventions for the management of any reactive or emotional behavioural changes.	• Encouraging, within reason, positive risk taking to enable the person to remain active and independent for as long as possible. • Education and workshops to help the person with dementia and their families understand the changes that occur throughout the disease trajectory. • Building resilience in families. • Detailed advanced care planning including what to do in a crisis. • Symptom management of both an advancing dementia and other long-term conditions and comorbidities. • Relationship support. • Ensuring that family and carers have respite and a life beyond caring. • Ensuring that the person with dementia has equitable access to services and activities. • Managing grief, loss and bereavement which may start at the point of diagnosis. • Crisis prevention.	• Initiating and facilitating difficult conversations about advanced care planning and end of life. • Ensuring that the person has access to specialist palliative care services. • Being able to identify end of life for a person with dementia and ensuring that they are supported and have access to their preferred place of care. • Being able to recognise the dying phase and supporting the person to have a peaceful dignified death in their preferred place of care. • Delivering good, effective symptom management throughout end of life and the dying phase, including pain, distress and anxiety. • Emotional and psychological support for the family and carers pre and post bereavement. • Ensuring family and carers have access to counselling services.

BAME, Black, Asian and minority ethnic; *LGBTQIA+,* lesbian, gay, bisexual, transgender, queer, questioning, intersex or asexual. (From National Health Service. (2016). The well pathway for dementia. Available at: https://www.england.nhs.uk/mentalhealth/wp-content/uploads/sites/29/2016/03/dementia-well-pathway.pdf.)

of or have protein-energy undernutrition. As it calculates body mass index, it will also enable the nurse to identify if a person is overweight or obese. It cannot identify if a person has micronutrient deficiencies or other types of nutritional disorders. It will also not identify why a person may be malnourished or at risk of malnourishment, their normal dietary habits and their preferred diet. Therefore following screening an assessment of nutrition and hydration needs should be undertaken (British Association of Enteral and Parenteral Nutrition, 2022). This assessment may result in a plan to refer the person to the dietitian for a full assessment, the GP for medical review or to another appropriate healthcare practitioner such as the occupational therapist. Referral to social support activities, such as lunch clubs, may also be made to encourage good nutrition and hydration.

Community nurses are well placed to provide firstline nutrition and hydration advice. They can support the person to follow healthy eating guidelines using the UK Eatwell Guide (NHS, 2023a), lose weight by setting goals and signposting to resources (NHS, 2023b) and using a 'Making Every Contact Count' approach to supporting people to identify goals and associated actions (Health Education England, 2023). They also educate and work with salaried and unsalaried carers.

10.9.2 NUTRITIONAL SUPPLEMENTS

Nutrition support may be provided in the form of fortified diets, therapeutic diets, enteral nutrition by tube or parenteral nutrition (NICE, 2017). Fortifying the diet involves enhancing the nutritional quality of the existing diet. This can include adding commercial nutritional supplements to the daily dietary intake or changing the diet by addition of higher-energy and nutrient-dense food products such as cream, butter and cheese to the usual diet. The dietitian can provide expert advice and patient information on this aspect of nutritional support (British Dietetic Association, 2023).

10.9.3 ENTERAL FEEDING

The number of people with enteral feeding by tube at home is increasing. This can involve nutrition via a nasogastric tube, nasojejunal tube, gastrostomy or jejunostomy tubes. Generally, the overall management of the enteral nutrition and tube is undertaken by specialist teams which include home enteral nutrition teams and homecare services (Green et al., 2013). Management includes feed prescription, tube and stoma management, training the carer or person to manage the therapy and arrangements for replacement tubes. Community nurses in some areas may manage the tube without the support of a community enteral nutrition team. If this is the case, then they must be supported by the dietetics team and nutrition nurses in the acute setting. People with enteral tubes and their carers need intensive support from knowledgeable healthcare practitioners during the weeks following initial placement (Green et al., 2019a). Community nurses can reduce the burden associated with a new tube by providing support and advice consistent with the plan of care. With time the person with the tube and their carer become the expert in their tube management and may request support from community nurses with aspects such as equipment supply (Green et al., 2019b).

Parenteral nutrition may also be delivered at home. This therapy is complex and managed by homecare services and the nutrition support team in secondary care. Community nurses liaise with the specialist teams if any issues arise. Community nurses can signpost people with enteral nutrition by tube and parenteral nutrition and their carers to support groups such as 'PINNT' (patients on intravenous and naso-gastric nutrition treatment) (PINNT, 2023) to help them to adapt and manage their therapy.

10.9.4 CONCLUSION

People often live at home with complex nutrition and hydration requirements and for this reason community nurses often have an important role in supporting people they care for to meet these needs. This may include screening and assessments, providing advice and treatment, referring to other healthcare professionals and supporting the family and carers.

10.10 Wound Care in the Community

10.10.1 INTRODUCTION

The origins of skin health and wound care begin in the community setting. Nurses working in the community are at the forefront of delivering evidence-based wound care assessment, treatment and prevention. Skin health and wound care issues affect people from all walks of life, including older people, new mothers, people experiencing homelessness and people with health conditions or impairments (Cabinet Office, 2021). As a community nurse, preparation is key before attending to a patient; individuals living with a wound reside in a range of environments including their own home, residential or care setting, hostel or bed and breakfast. In essence, a community nurse needs to be prepared for the expected and unexpected and be able to adapt to work with the patients, their families and carers in a flexible manner, providing choice and person-centred care (Probst, 2021).

REFLECTION

Consider your knowledge of the anatomy and physiology of the human body:

- Integumentary system (see Fig. 10.3)
- Skeletal and muscular structures
- The vascular system

Among the body systems, mastering the pathophysiology of these three will be key to supporting work in tissue viability (Knight et al., 2020; Upton & Upton, 2015).

In recent years, there has been a focus on the economic impact of wound care in the UK with some important key points to consider (Swanson et al., 2019):

- The total annual cost of wound management to the NHS is £8.3 billion, of which 67% is spent on managing unhealed wounds.
- The NHS manages 3.8 million patients with a wound each year, which is equivalent to 7% of the adult population.
- 25% of all wounds lack a recorded differential diagnosis.
- The annual prevalence of wounds increased by 71% between 2012/2013 and 2017/2018, with patient management cost increasing by 47% in real terms.

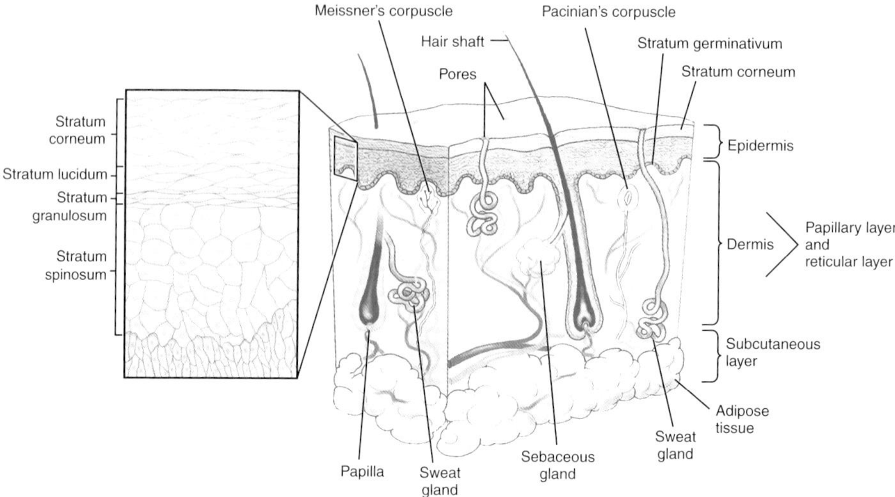

Fig. 10.3 Diagram of section of the skin. (From Zenith. (2050). Medical Assistant: Integumentary, Sensory Systems, Patient Care and Communication—Module A. Elsevier INC.)

- Annually, wound management resource use includes:
  - 54.4 million district/community nurse visits
  - 53.6 million healthcare assistant visits
  - 28.1 million practice nurse visits

Considering the impact of these figures on the caseload of community nursing, the cost to the NHS and the effect on the patient's quality of life, it is important that the following are prioritised:

- Patient engagement and concordance
- Assessment and differential diagnosis
- Referral and support systems for the patient and family
- The role of the patient in their care; choice and shared decision-making and prevention

The key to successful wound management is getting to know and understand the individual living with or at risk of a wound, how their physical emotional and psychosocial life has been affected and the prognostic factors of healing (diet, lifestyle, medication, mobility, sleep and well-being). It is important to support the assessment using an evidence-based clinical decision-support tool to promote consistent, holistic wound management (Atkin et al., 2019; National Wound Care Strategy Programme (NWCSP), 2023).

There are a variety of wound types, each with its own aetiology, clinical presentation and treatment pathways.

The NWCSP (2023) has developed recommendations which support excellence in preventing, assessing and treating people with wounds to optimise healing and minimise the burden of wounds for patients, carers and health and care providers (NHS England, 2023a). There are currently three clinical work streams that the NWCSP profiles:

1. Pressure ulcers (Box 10.13)
2. Lower limb: leg and foot ulcers
3. Surgical wounds

BOX 10.13 ■ Consider the Diagnosis of a Pressure Ulcer

- A diagnosis of pressure ulcer is typically obvious when a person with risk factors develops evidence of skin damage over a bony prominence. Pressure damage is supported by the presence of one of the following:
- An area of nonblanchable erythema. Note that nonblanchable erythema (redness) may present as colour changes or skin tone alterations, particularly in people with dark skin tones. It is important to feel the skin and observe for induration (hardness) or changes in texture, condition and temperature.
- Localised skin changes.
- A wound of varying severity on an anatomical site that is known (or suspected) to have previously been exposed to significant unrelieved pressure.

Further information can be found at National Institute for Health and Care Excellence (NICE) (2023). *Health topics A to Z: Chronic obstructive pulmonary disease: Scenario: End-stage chronic obstructive pulmonary disease.* Available at: https://cks.nice.org.uk/topics/chronic-obstructive-pulmonary-disease/management/end-stage-copd/#:~:text=For%20people%20with%20end%2Dstage,where%20appropriate)%20including%20advance%20decisions.

DEFINITION

The NICE (2023c), together with NHS England and a number of international organisations and centres of excellence, define a pressure ulcer as:

- A pressure ulcer is defined as localised damage to the skin and/or underlying tissue, as a result of pressure or pressure in combination with shear.
- They usually occur over a bony prominence but may also be related to a medical device or other objects.
- Pressure ulcers can range in severity, from patches of discoloured skin to extensive wounds filled with necrotic tissue and involving fascia, muscle and bone.
- Pressure ulcers most commonly occur over bony prominences but can develop on any part of the body, including mucosal surfaces.

REFLECTION

A pressure ulcer is normally located over a bony prominence; therefore consider the anatomical position and identify the bony prominence to ensure accuracy and document clearly in the required notes.

10.10.2 PRESSURE ULCERS

When reviewing a patient at risk of or living with a pressure ulcer it is important to consider the following:

- Risk factors that have predisposed the individual to the pressure ulcer, i.e., their physical condition, impaired mobility, neurological condition or stage of life (end-of-life care).
- What caused the pressure ulcer, where it occurred and the history and duration of the pressure ulcer. When investigating or exploring pressure ulcer development, it often feels like detective work; however, a chronological and factual history must be collected to help support healing and address any factors that may be preventing the pressure ulcer from healing. With permission from the patient and/or carer, it is useful to collect photographic evidence and measurements of the pressure ulcer dated and categorised—including anatomical position (Fig. 10.4).

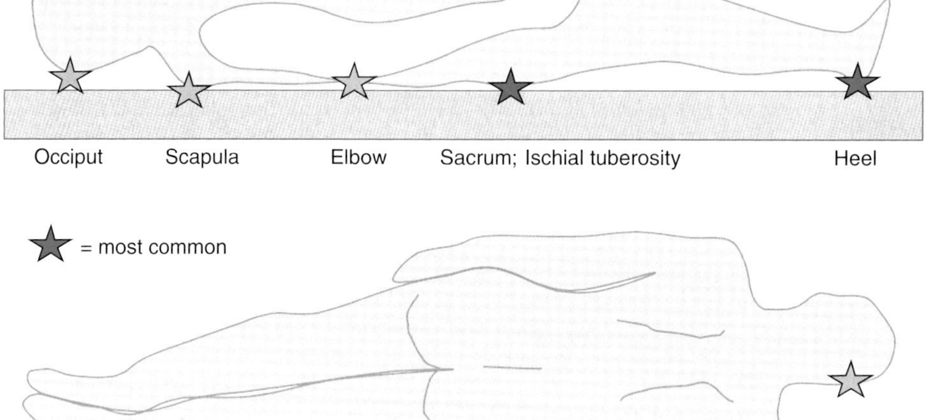

Fig. 10.4 Braden scale for the risk assessment of pressure ulcers. (From Mervis, J. S., & Phillips, T. J. (2019). Pressure ulcers: Pathophysiology, epidemiology, risk factors, and presentation. *Journal of the American Academy of Dermatology*, 81(4), 881–890.)

10.10.2.1 Bony Prominences

Common sites include the sacrum, heels, greater trochanter, ischial tuberosity, back of the head, ears, shoulders, elbows, inner knees or malleoli. Consider that pressure ulcers can also develop on mucosal surfaces and from devices for example, catheters, oxygen tubing, compression bandages and faecal containment devices.

- Associated comorbidities or factors that may affect or impair healing. For example, is the person malnourished (consider that this assessment is not just about weight and relates to the nutritional content of a person's diet)? Is there incontinence-associated dermatitis (IAD) and how can this be treated to prevent further skin breakdown? What is the overall health of the patient? Consider their stage and prognosis in life: is the individual immunosuppressed or taking substances that affect their physical healing, i.e., smoking, and/or their psychological well-being, i.e., illicit drugs or alcohol?

Remember anyone is potentially at risk of developing a pressure ulcer, and a validated risk assessment scale, such as the Braden or PURPOSE T risk assessment tool, should be used to support clinical judgement when assessing pressure ulcer risk (NICE, 2024).

10.10.3 LEG ULCERATION

A leg ulcer is defined as an open wound, a break in the skin below the knee, which originates on or above the malleolus that takes more than 2 weeks to heal (NWCSP, 2023).

TABLE 10.8 **Causes and Aetiologies of Leg Ulceration**

Aetiologies of Leg Ulceration	Differential Diagnosis
Venous insufficiency	• Superficial truncal reflux (varicosities) • Deep venous incompetence—thrombosis • Extrinsic compression (tumours)
Macrovascular arterial insufficiency	• Peripheral arterial disease (PAD) • Acute on chronic arterial disease • Vascular traumatic injury
Malignancy	• Basal cell carcinoma • Squamous cell carcinoma • Kaposi's sarcoma • Lymphoma • Mycosis fungoides
Skin infection/inflammation	• Cellulitis • Erysipelas
Vasculitis/microvascular insufficiency	• Microangiopathy • Raynaud's phenomenon • Buerger's disease
Lymphoedema/lipoedema	• Primary • Secondary
Haematologic disorders	• Anaemia (sickle cell) • Polycythaemia • Dysproteinaemia • Thrombophilia
Collagen vascular disorders	• Polymyalgia • Systemic lupus erythematous • Scleroderma • Polyarteritis nodosa • Wegener's granulomatosis
Excessive Pressure	• Diabetic neuropathy • Alcoholic neuropathy • Decubitus ulcers • Postoperative deformity • Bone spurs

(From Sidawy, A. N., & Perler, B. A. (2022.) *Rutherford's vascular surgery & endovascular therapy* (10th ed.). Elsevier.)

10.10.3.1 Differential Diagnosis

The differential diagnosis of leg ulceration should always include venous insufficiency (the most common), peripheral arterial disease (PAD) and mixed aetiology (PAD + venous), as well as excluding less frequent conditions including vasculitis, malignancies and ulcerating diseases such as pyoderma gangrenosum (Keller, 2018). Other potential causes and aetiologies of leg ulceration are reported in Table 10.8.

10.10.3.2 Patient Assessment and Diagnostic Process

The primary objective of the assessment is to reach the correct differential diagnosis, by establishing the underlying aetiology, and whether the leg ulceration is caused by incompetent veins (venous insufficiency) or narrowed/blocked arteries (PAD) in the lower limb, and to rule out any acute ischaemia or vascular injury. The secondary assessment should focus on the ulcer itself to establish the most appropriate treatment plan to promote healing. A structured approach to the ulcer assessment and wound bed preparation needs to be followed using the T.I.M.E concept; addressing the elements of **T**issue, **I**nfection and/or **I**nflammation, **M**oisture balance and the **E**dge of the wound (Swanson et al., 2019). (Fig. 10.5 and Box 10.14).

The baseline assessment for leg ulceration should include an ankle brachial pressure index (ABPI) and a toe brachial index (TBI) when the ABPI is abnormally high due to arterial wall calcification of the tibial arteries of the leg; calcifications are caused by atherosclerosis and are most often found in patients with diabetes or chronic kidney disease (CKD).

10.10.4 ARTERIAL LEG ULCERS

An ABPI <0.8 is suggestive of PAD. Arterial leg ulcer (i.e., tissue loss and PAD) is referred to as critical limb ischaemia (CLI) or chronic limb threatening ischaemia (CLTI). CLI–CLTI can rapidly progress to life-threatening sepsis and/or gangrene, ultimately leading to limb loss and death. Hence, an urgent specialist referral to the vascular service is warranted with the view of proceeding with further imaging (Duplex and computed tomography angiography (CTA)) and consideration for revascularisation (bypass surgery or endovascular treatment). The Vascular Society and NHS England (Commissioning for Quality and Innovation) recommend revascularisation to be performed within 14 days from the referral to the vascular team; this emphasises the importance of timely and accurate diagnosis by the primary care nursing team (Birmpili et al., 2022). Any compression therapy remains contraindicated until successful revascularisation is performed. Best medical therapy includes antiplatelet agents, statin and antibiotic therapy, if necessary (Conte et al., 2019).

10.10.5 VENOUS LEG ULCERS

Venous ulcerations represent the end-stage of venous hypertension. Clinical signs and symptoms of chronic venous insufficiency include hemosiderin pigmentation, venous eczema and truncal varicose veins.

Venous risk factors are:

- family history of varicose veins
- previous deep vein thrombosis (DVT), long bone fractures, orthopaedic surgery
- sedentary lifestyle

The gold standard treatment of venous leg ulcer is compression bandaging combined with endovenous treatment of the varicose veins (if suitable) (Gohel et al., 2018).

10.10.6 MIXED AETIOLOGY LEG ULCERS

More than 30% of leg ulcers are multifactorial, comprising both PAD and venous insufficiency (mixed aetiology). These are often particularly painful and hard to heal. The arterial component must be addressed first (as per the 'Arterial Leg Ulcers' section earlier) as a limb-salvaging procedure, prioritising surgical revascularisation prior to compression therapy.

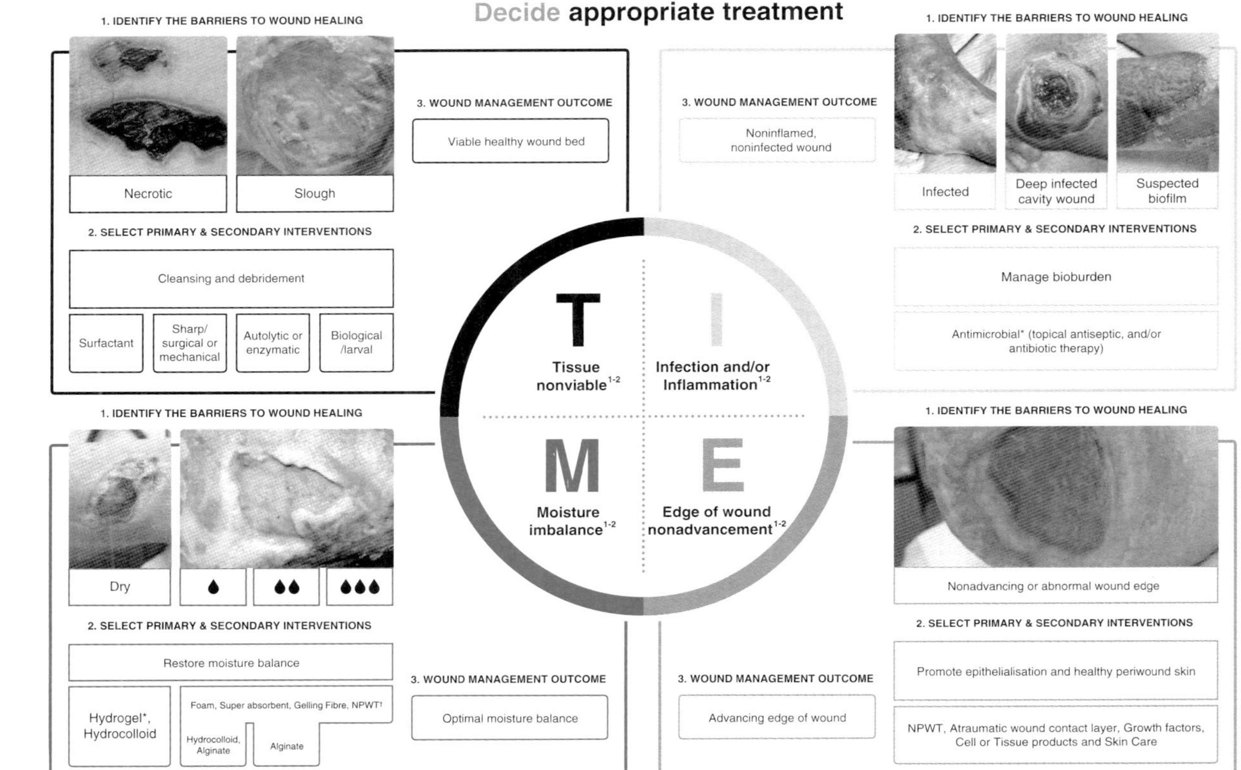

Fig. 10.5 T.I.M.E. clinical decision support tool. (Modified from T.I.M.E. clinical decision support tool; Swanson, T., Duynhoven, K., & Johnstone, D. (2019). Using the new T.I.M.E. Clinical Decision Support Tool to promote consistent holistic wound management and eliminate variation in practice at the Cambourne Medical Clinic, Australia: Part 1. *Wounds International, 10*(2), 28–39.)

BOX 10.14 ■ T.I.M.E. Concept

A structured approach to the ulcer assessment and wound bed preparation needs to be followed using the T.I.M.E concept, addressing the elements of **T**issue, **I**nfection and/or **I**nflammation, **M**oisture balance and the **E**dge of the wound (Swanson et al., 2019) (see Fig. 10.5).

- Look for a previous scan of their legs (venous, arterial) highlighting radiological evidence of venous insufficiency and/or PAD.
- Ensure there is adequate time to complete a full holistic assessment involving the patient at every stage of the decision.
- Explore if the person is experiencing pain with their leg ulceration and pharmacological and nonpharmacological strategies to address and alleviate their symptoms.
- Ask where the person sleeps—in their chair or in bed. This is because consistent leg elevation is an important part of alleviating symptoms of leg ulceration and associated swelling.
- Consider the impact of living with leg ulceration on the psychosocial well-being of the person and explore together what actions can be put in place to support the individual.

(From Swanson, T., Duynhoven, K. & Johnstone, D. (2019). Using the new T.I.M.E. Clinical Decision Support Tool to promote consistent holistic wound management and eliminate variation in practice at the Cambourne Medical Clinic, Australia: Part 1. *Wounds International, 10*(2), 28-39.)

All leg ulcerations should have an appropriate referral to the local vascular department for further investigations by the vascular team, which may include a venous/arterial duplex scan and in some instances both diagnostics.

10.10.7 SURGICAL WOUNDS

The majority of surgical wounds heal by primary intention. However, there are several reasons that a surgical wound may fail to heal and breakdown. The most common reason for delayed healing is a surgical site infection (SSI), defined as an 'infectious process present at the site of surgery' (NWCSP, 2021). Infection can result in wound dehiscence where the separation of the margins of a surgically closed wound when wound closure materials are removed.

It is important to identify the signs and symptoms of wound infection and collaborate and refer to the most suitable clinician as appropriate, i.e. team lead, tissue viability nurse, GP and/or surgical team.

- Pain in the affected area
- Swelling
- Redness that is spreading across the skin around the wound
- The wound and/or skin surrounding feeling hot to touch
- Discharge from the wound which can be malodourous and be green or yellow in colour

Other signs of infection in the body can include feeling generally unwell and/or having a temperature (fever).

The NWCSP (2024) have identified a number of early red flags for ongoing care of surgical wounds as provided in Fig. 10.6.

If the patient has a suspected wound infection, then medical advice should be sought as antibiotic therapy and further investigations and referrals may be needed. In the

Early Red Flags: Treat as an emergency situation
- Haemorrhage
- Newly exposed viscera

Intermediate Red Flags: Immediate Treatment
- Systemic signs of infection/sepsis

Immediate Referral
- Spreading infection

24 hour referral
- Local Infection
- Dehiscence if: surgery involved Implants
- Aesthetically or functionally important surgical site
- Exposed Implant

72 Hour Referral
- Dehiscence with newly exposed subcutaneous layers and fascia
- Suspected sinus/fistula/tunnelling
- Draining seroma's
- Stoma within wound boundaries

Fig. 10.6 Early red flags in post operative wound care. (Adapted from the National Wound Care Strategy Programme (NWCSP) (2024))

meantime: The key recommendations for prevention of SSIs and treatment of infected wounds and those healing by secondary intention in the postoperative phase are:

Changing dressings

- Use an aseptic nontouch technique for changing or removing surgical wound dressings.
- Monitor pain and offer appropriate analgesia.
- Encourage fluids to keep hydrated.

Postoperative wound cleansing

- Use sterile saline for wound cleansing up to 48 hours after surgery.
- Advise patients that they may shower safely 48 hours after surgery.
- Use potable tap water for wound cleansing after 48 hours if the surgical wound has separated or has been surgically opened to drain pus.

Dressings for wound healing by secondary intention

- Do not use Eusol and gauze, moist cotton gauze or mercuric antiseptic solutions to manage surgical wounds that are healing by secondary intention.
- Use an appropriate interactive dressing to manage surgical wounds that are healing by secondary intention.

BOX 10.15 ■ Practical Tips to Manage Wound Care in the Community

1. Be prepared and organised: read the patient's notes beforehand and prepare your time and dressings to maximise the time you spend with the patient.
2. Wound assessment and dressing changes are time consuming: when appropriate, ring ahead and ensure your patient is ready and comfortable and, if appropriate, analgesia is timed alongside the dressing change.
3. Dressings can be painful, embarrassing and distressing for patients: a positive, caring mindset, taking time to listen, is key to engagement and concordance with your patient in their wound treatment. If a patient does not have a positive experience with their wound care dressing, they are more likely than not to disengage.
4. Explain your assessment and involve the patient in their care and decision-making. When measuring the wound and photographing with consent, ask the patient if they would like to see their wound and explain the progress of the current condition and what can be done to optimise healing or manage the symptoms.
5. Document your assessment and plan carefully ensuring that colleagues follow your plan of care, optimising consistency and patient confidence.
6. Find out who your local tissue viability and vascular nurse contacts are locally and arrange to meet the teams to build networks; this will support communication and onward referral of patients.

There are several key national and international resources that can be referred to for further information on how to support patients living with wounds or lower limb and foot vascular conditions in the community.

- The Leg Club Foundation—https://www.legclub.org/
- Legs Matter Campaign—https://legsmatter.org/
- The British Lymphology Society—https://www.thebls.com/
- The Society of Tissue Viability—https://societyoftissueviability.org/
- European Wound Management Association—https://ewma.org/
- European Pressure Ulcer Advisory Panel—https://epuap.org/

There are also other areas of wound assessment and care that are provided by community nurses where levels of complexity need to be considered, such as inclusion, homeless health and individuals who experience mental health problems' (Geraghty, 2023; Mental Health Foundation, 2022)· Community nurses are often asked to review patients with wounds as a consequence of self-harm, or those who have a history of injecting in the lower limbs who have leg ulceration or injecting related wounds. It is important to consider the appropriate language when engaging with people from all walks of life to ensure that individuals are not stigmatised or labelled by their medical history, lifestyle or social circumstance (Mitchell, 2021; Public Health England, 2021). Community nurses will also encounter a variety of wounds at the end of a person's life, including malignant fungating wounds and skin failure, which can predispose the person to pressure ulcers and other conditions such as moisture-associated skin damage (MASD) (Fletcher et al., 2020) (Box 10.15).

10.10.8 CONCLUSION

Wound care is one of the most diverse and complex areas of clinical care in the community. When competently delivered, in a person-centred manner, it is one of the most rewarding parts of the job. This area of practice demands that nurses continuously keep up to date with their clinical skills and knowledge.

Community nurses need to ensure that their patients have received a thorough and up-to-date assessment and that differential diagnosis has been discussed with the MDT where appropriate. Patients need to receive evidence-based treatment and community nurses need to ensure that they are informed, involved and confident with their care. Both physical and psychological aspects must be considered for holistic patient care which should be delivered with compassion, kindness and positivity.

10.11 Continence Care

Continence care is an important, but an often overlooked, aspect of community nursing (Bakan et al., 2021; Trueland, 2022). The impact of incontinence on an individual includes physical and mental health, such as loss of skin integrity, independence, self-esteem, quality of life, negativity on sexual health and relationship issues (Kehinde, 2016; NHS England, 2018). These also influence the wider family and include an increase in workload such as laundry and the cost of purchasing continence aids, causing a financial burden. Sometimes, incontinence can be the last determinant in a person being admitted to a care home setting (King's Fund, 2014; Talley et al., 2021). Incontinence is often viewed as an inevitable part of life caused by childbirth, menopause and ageing (Fu et al., 2023; NICE, 2019c). However, incontinence is preventable and there are many treatments that can improve the outcome for a person with incontinence (NHS England, 2018). With the increasing complexity and frailty of the health of the population, the number of patients with continence problems will increase.

DEFINITION

Incontinence is defined as the accidental loss or leaking of urine or faeces which cannot be controlled (National Collaborating Centre for Women's and Children's Health UK, 2013).

A community nurse is in a prime position to identify patients who could benefit from preventable or active approaches to continence care (NHS England, 2018). However, community nurses often state they have had little or no training in assessing a patient's continence issues (McCann et al., 2021; Trueland, 2022). Yet they are often faced with complex patients and have challenges in identifying suitable remedies, particularly in patients with neurological conditions such as stroke, multiple sclerosis (MS), Parkinson disease and spinal injury (Yates, 2019).

This section aims to offer a brief overview of the options available to community nurses for preventative care and treatment options for patients with bladder and/or bowel problems.

REFLECTION

- Consider a patient you have seen in your nursing practice recently who has been affected by incontinence. What was the impact of this on their physical and mental health and on their family/carers?
- How did you ensure the patient was cared for appropriately? What assessments did you complete?
- How did you communicate with the patient regarding any changes to their lifestyle to support improving or managing their continence problem?

All patients under the care of a community nurse should have a holistic assessment. Continence care must be included in this assessment as problems with bladder and bowel function can have a significant impact on the patient in many ways (Trueland, 2022). A patient with incontinence has an increased risk of breakdown in their skin integrity, infections due to faecal contamination of the urinary tract or soiling of bandaging, for example, to leg ulcer dressings (NHS England, 2018; Talley et al., 2021). Incontinence can affect the patient's mental health as they can lose their self-esteem. Some patients may hide their incontinence for fear of their family not wanting to manage this or from embarrassment or belief that nothing can be done to resolve/improve the problem (Fu et al., 2023; NHS England, 2018). Community nurses need the skills to be able to help patients manage their symptoms using suitable treatment options (Bakan et al., 2021; Trueland, 2022; Yates, 2019).

10.11.1 CONTINENCE MANAGEMENT

Where an issue with incontinence has been identified, a patient should have an appropriate assessment to ensure 'getting it right the first time' (NHS Improvement, 2017). A successful assessment can lead to avoidance of hospital admissions, prevention of deterioration in their health and a reduction in the use of continence products which are costly and have a negative environmental impact. Indwelling catheters have a high risk of infection and complications including mortality (NHS England, 2018). An appropriate assessment should include identifying and excluding red flags such as bladder cancer, a physical assessment including urinalysis, bladder scanning (to identify a raised residual urine), examination of genitalia to exclude prolapse or conditions of the foreskin in men, and per rectal examination may be required to identify the presence of stool (CKS/NICE, 2019c, 2023a, 2023b). Once an assessment has been completed, the patient and/or carer should be informed of the likely cause of the problem and appropriate treatment options (NICE, 2012). This should be shared in simple-to-understand terms and any treatment should be proportional and tailored to the condition, agreeable to the patient and discussion of how long this may take to help. For example, pelvic floor exercise regimes can take weeks to help (Table 10.9).

Treatment options are wide and variable and often include simple measures (Colley, 2020; Palmer et al., 2022; Trueland, 2022) (Table 10.10).

Medication is available, but consideration needs to be given to the potential for side effects, particularly with those that have an anticholinergic burden that could affect a patient's cognition. Medication can be offered to patients who have an overactive bladder and in catheterised patients who may expel their catheter (CKS/NICE, 2023a). For constipation which cannot be improved with a change in dietary and fluid intake, increased activity or a change in medication, laxatives, suppositories or enemas may be required. However, it would not be recommended to use enemas long term, and consideration needs to be given to the risk in frail/elderly patients (CKS/NICE, 2023b).

There are multiple aids to support the management of incontinence. These include sheaths, urinals, commodes or other toileting aids, intermittent and indwelling catheters, transanal irrigation, reusable or disposable incontinence products and 'Just can't wait cards' (Bladder and Bowel Community, n.d.). Newer aids are being developed all the time, including suction devices, artificial intelligence and device monitors (Innovate UK KTN, 2023; Robson, 2017; Zavodnik et al., 2020).

TABLE 10.9 **Types of Incontinence**

Stress incontinence	Is when urine leaks due to exertion such as coughing and sneezing.
Urge incontinence	Is when urine there is an urgent desire to pass urine and the person leaks urine before they can get to the toilet. This is often associated with frequency and urgency and can be caused by an overactive bladder.
Overflow incontinence	Is when the bladder does not completely empty. This can cause frequency, urgency, symptoms of urge and stress incontinence and can increase the risk of urine infections. The person may strain to empty their bladder and feel discomfort.
Mixed incontinence	Is when there are symptoms of both stress and urge incontinence.
Functional incontinence	Is caused by issues outside the bladder such as disease process and mobility issues.

Colley, W. (2020). Urinary continence assessment, treatment and management. https://www.continenceassessment.co.uk/colley_model/; NICE. (2024a). LUTS in men. Available at: https://cks.nice.org.uk/topics/luts-in-men. NICE. (2024b). Incontinence—urinary, in women. Available at: https://cks.nice.org.uk/topics/incontinence-urinary-in-women/.

TABLE 10.10 **Treatment Options**

Urinary Treatments	**Bowel Treatments**
Fluid intake—type and amount	Dietary intake—increase or decrease fibre, regular mealtimes
Urge suppression techniques	Exercise regime
Just Can't Wait cards	Just Can't Wait cards
Pelvic floor exercises	Pelvic floor exercises
Bladder emptying techniques	Nonstraining bowel emptying techniques
Timed voiding	Medication—oral. Also review if current medication may be aggravating the problem
Medication. Also review if current medication is causing side effects	Medication—rectal
Devices—toileting aids, external collection devices, intermittent or indwelling catheter	Devices such as toileting aids, collection devices, plugs or irrigation
Continence pads	Continence pads

(From https://cks.nice.org.uk/topics/luts-in-men/; https://cks.nice.org.uk/topics/incontinence-urinary-in-women/; https://cks.nice.org.uk/topics/constipation/; Colley, W. (2020). Urinary continence assessment, treatment and management. https://www.continenceassessment.co.uk/colley_model/; https://www.nice.org.uk/guidance/cg148; Palmer, C., Richardson, D., Rayner, J., Drake, M. J., and Cotterill, N. (2022). Professional perspectives on impacts, benefits and disadvantages of changes made to community continence services during the COVID-19 pandemic: Findings from the EPICCC-19 national survey. *BMC Health Services Research, 22*, 783.; Trueland, J. (2022). Good continence care: Tips for nurses working in any setting. *Nursing Standard, 38*(9).)

TABLE 10.11 **HOUDINI**

H	Haematuria
O	Obstruction
U	Urology surgery
D	Decubitus ulcer (pressure ulcer)
I	Input and output measurement
N	Nursing end-of-life care
I	Immobility

Adams, D., Bucior, H., Day, G., & Rimmer, J. (2012). HOUDINI: Make that urinary catheter disappear – Nurse-led protocol. *Journal of Infection Prevention, 13*(2), 44–46.

Indwelling catheters should ideally be one of the last options when treating continence problems. This is due to the high risk of infection and other complications such as bladder spasm, by-passing, discomfort and pain. When considering the option of an indwelling catheter, the community nurse should consider the option of intermittent self-catheterisation if there is a high residual or difficulty in passing urine (Woodward, 2014). This is due to the lower risk of infection and complications. If this option is not appropriate, the community nurse should consider the HOUDINI acronym approach to ascertain if an indwelling catheter should be used. Where none of the listed conditions apply to the patient, the catheter should be removed/not inserted (Table 10.11).

There are different types of catheters that can be used, including different materials, and sizes. Some catheters are for short-term use only and others can be used in the long term. The community nurse must check for relevant allergies including latex and local anaesthetics. Most catheters have a balloon that is filled with water and 10 mL should be sufficient. A greater balloon size can cause trauma to the bladder neck (particularly if the catheter is expelled due to spasm) and increase the volume of urine that is left in the bladder (below the eyelets) which could increase the risk of urine infections (Simpson, 2017). The larger Charriere size (diameter) can cause greater trauma to the urethra. Catheter length is also important, and a standard length must be used for all men. Using a female length catheter can cause trauma if the balloon is inflated in the male urethra. However, some female patients may prefer the standard-length catheter as this may reduce the risk of the bifurcation being too close to the perineal area or rubbing on the inner thigh (National Patient Safety Agency, 2009; Zavodnik et al., 2020) (Table 10.12).

The community nurse could also consider the options of free drainage bags or catheter valves and maintain a closed drainage system to reduce the risk of infection. The benefits of catheter valves include being able to allow the bladder to behave as close to normal physiology as possible, by filling and emptying at regular periods which may reduce the risk of infection and help to maintain bladder tone (Holroyd, 2021; Simpson, 2017). There is a large selection of different drainage bags that are available. Fixation devices are essential and need to be fitted correctly. If used correctly, these can help to reduce the risk of trauma to the bladder neck and urethral cleaving due to the friction or pull of the catheter and/or drainage bag (Woodward, 2014) (Table 10.13).

Once the correct catheter has been selected, the nurse must follow procedures to ensure valid consent has been obtained with the benefits and risks and ensure that the

TABLE 10.12 ■ **Catheter Types**

Materials	Length	Charriere Size	Design
Latex Hydrogel catheters have a latex core.	Standard 40–45 cm With 10 mL balloon, 30 mL balloon should never be used routinely and are only used if a plan of care is directed by the urology team	Male 12ch–16ch (good practice 14ch) Female 10ch–14ch (good practice 12ch)	Most patients can be catheterised using a standard-tipped catheter. Open-tipped catheters or a Tiemann catheter (has a curved tip designed to negotiate the urethra in men with prostatic hypertrophy) may sometimes be prescribed following specialist review.
All silicone catheters must be used in patients with a latex allergy.	Standard	As above	Standard. Need to check manufacturer's details for use for suprapubic catheters.
Silver coated catheters: There is insufficient evidence to use silver coated or antimicrobial catheters. However, they may be prescribed for a specific patient following a specialist review.	Standard	As above	May need to be changed more regularly. Need to check manufacturer's details.

(From Royal College of Nursing. (2021). *Catheter care: RCN guidance for healthcare professionals*. RCN, London.)

patient/carer can care for the device (Table 10.14). This includes patients being able to drink adequate fluids, empty the catheter bag, reduce the risk of trauma, identify when there are problems and when to ask for help/assistance (Table 10.15).

Inserting a catheter must be completed using an aseptic technique (Simpson, 2017). First time urethral catheter policies may vary in different settings with considerations needing to be given to medical history such as prostate, bladder and pelvic cancers as these patients may have increased complications. Some of these patients may not be suitable to have their catheters changed in a domiciliary setting, particularly if they have had problems with significant bleeding with catheter insertion/change. Where a urethral catheterisation is not possible, some patients may need to be referred to urology for a suprapubic catheter. These may be preferable for patients with neurological disease, patients who are wheelchair users or where there has been trauma to the urethra. The selection of a catheter for suprapubic catheters is slightly different and the district nurse must use a catheter that is licensed for suprapubic use. Some catheters have cuffing concerns when the balloon is deflated which can cause trauma to the channel and cause discomfort and pain.

Once the catheter has been inserted, the patient should be provided with a catheter passport with the relevant details of the catheter type and contact numbers included for any concerns. An appointment should be booked for changing the catheter. Most catheters are changed at least 12-weekly according to manufacturers' guidelines for use, this will depend on the catheter material and clinical presentation. However, this could depend on

TABLE 10.13 ■ **Considerations for Choice of Bags, Valves and Fixation Devices**

Accessories	Comments
Leg bags	Changed weekly. Can be connected to a night bag overnight to avoid disruption at night
Overnight bags	Changed daily or weekly With tap to drain/tear off edge to empty bag
Sport bags	To hide under shorts. Will need emptying more frequently
Large bags	For use for patients in wheelchairs when unable to empty bag
Body worn bags	Risk to not draining correctly due to being above bladder and not draining using gravity
Materials	Consider potential allergies from drainage bags
Catheter valves	Changed weekly. Ensure patient/carer is aware of regular emptying of bladder. Able to leave open with night drainage bag at night if preferred
Night bag stand	To ensure night bag is secured to prevent kinking of tubing and keep bag below the level of the bladder
Straps to support leg bags with Velcro	Ensure threaded through correctly to allow urine to drain freely and not occlude connection between bag and catheter tubing. Ensure strapping does not rub/cause pressure issues/swelling on leg. Secured, but not tight
Stocking/sleeving	To secure leg bag without straps. Ensure measured to fit and not to cause pressure issues/swelling
Straps or fixation devices	For abdomen (suprapubic) or thigh. Ensure fixation does not cause pressure issues/swelling and is changed as per manufacturer's guidelines or visibly soiled

Holroyd, S. (2021). Catheter valves: Appropriate use and reduction of risk to bladder. *Journal of Community Nursing, 35*(5), 52–56; Simpson, P. (2017). Long-term urethral catheterisation: Guidelines for community nurses. *British Journal of Nursing, 26*(9), S22–S26; Woodward, S. (2014). Community nursing and intermittent self-catheterisation. *British Journal of Community Nursing, 19*(8), 388, 390–393.

TABLE 10.14 ■ **Risks and Benefits of Catheterisation**

Risks	**Benefits**
Infection, sepsis, bleeding, bladder spasm, bypassing, discomfort, bladder/bowel/urethral/prostate trauma	Comfort, reduce skin integrity risk, accurate fluid output, reduce symptoms of retention

NICE. (2018). Urinary tract infection (catheter-associated): Antimicrobial prescribing. Available at: https://www.nice.org.uk/guidance/ng113.

the guidance from the medical companies and nursing/medical decisions. Some patients may need to have their catheter changed more frequently such as those with a suprapubic catheter, or where there are issues with blockages or track issues with a suprapubic catheter.

There are a significant number of complications that occur with catheters. The nurse needs to be aware of the possible options in dealing with these to avoid unnecessary hospital admissions (Table 10.16).

Where issues with emptying the bladder are transitory, the nurse should arrange a trial without catheter (TWOC).

TABLE 10.15 **Advice for Patients and Reasoning**

Advice for Patients	Reasoning
All patients with an indwelling urinary catheter must be advised to ensure at least daily hygienic care of the genital area with soap and water and must be supported to do so if they are unable to do this for themselves. It is important to wash under the foreskin (if present) and replace after cleaning to avoid any complications such as paraphimosis.	To reduce the risk of infection or skin excoriation.
A dependant free drainage bag on free drainage must only be used if clinically required, or if a patient cannot manage a catheter valve.	Can cause loss of bladder tone and a reduction in bladder capacity. Increased risk of infection. Possible sphincter/bladder neck damage due to the weight of the drainage bag once it is full of urine and not supported appropriately.
If a drainage bag is required, this must be positioned below the level of the bladder and should not be in contact with the floor. The bag must be held on a designated single-patient use catheter stand. A supporting device such as a sleeve, strap or an adhesive dressing (following an assessment of skin integrity) should be used. Leg bags require to be changing every 7 days. A night bag must also be changed every 7 days and rinsed through every morning and left to dry with the cap in place (unless it is a single use night bag which is changed daily).	To reduce the risk of infection.
Catheter valves are an excellent alternative to drainage bags. They are discreet and more comfortable.	They can reduce the risk of trauma and offer potential maintenance of bladder function, capacity and tone, mimicking normal bladder function. They may promote a successful trial without catheter in the future. Care needs to be taken with patients who have ureteric reflux.
If a catheter is blocked, this can cause a great deal of discomfort. The catheter and any drainage tubing must be checked to ensure that it is not kinked and that no straps/support are restricting the drainage of the urine. The drainage bag must be below the level of the bladder. Ensure that the patient is not constipated and has had sufficient oral intake.	There is insufficient evidence to recommend the use of catheter maintenance installations to minimise the risk of blockages and encrustations. There is some evidence to suggest that if blockages do occur, they may dissolve the blockage. However, they must not be used regularly unless as a management plan that has been prescribed by a urology team. Frequent use can cause side effects and increase the risk of infection as the closed system is broken.

10.11.2 AUTONOMIC DYSREFLEXIA

Nurses should also be aware of the life-threatening condition of autonomic dysreflexia (AD) with care of catheters or bowels. This is a condition that usually affects patients with spinal cord injury above T6 (but not exclusively, other conditions can also have this complication, such as Parkinson disease) which can cause symptoms of increased blood pressure. (Please note the patient with a spinal cord injury may have a lower blood pressure, therefore the patient's baseline observations are required before making any clinical judgements.) The patient with an impacted bowel, distended bladder/blocked catheter or full drainage bag may present with a pounding headache, flushing above the level of injury, sweating, goosebumps and nasal congestion. When this occurs, the patient needs urgent treatment which will have been prescribed on an individual basis by their spinal cord injury unit. This normally includes medication to lower their blood pressure. The nurse also needs to be aware of the importance of resolving the trigger and support prophylaxis to avoid AD (Linsenmyerm et al., 2020; NHS Improvement, 2018; NICE, 2022; Wan & Krassioukov, 2014).

TABLE 10.16 **Troubleshooting for Urinary Catheterisation**

Issue	Possible Reason/Resolution
Catheter not draining	Catheter may not have been correctly inserted. Consider recatheterising Patient may be dehydrated Tubing may be kinked Drainage bag above the level of the bladder Constipation/impaction Blocked catheter
Bladder spasm/ catheter being expelled	Consider medication to resolve spasm Treat constipation If balloon has been perforated, refer to urology as likely cause from bladder stones
Bleeding	Can be caused due to trauma on insertion or if catheter has been pulled If speck of blood, monitor and reassure. Consider increasing fluids if appropriate If significant, dial 999 to obtain medical assistance Patients on anticoagulation medication are at higher risk of bleeding If patient has complications, consider alternative management plan/referral to urology and catheter changes to be completed in an environment where there is more medical support If brown urine, consider if this could be fecaluria from perforated bowel in patients catheterised with suprapubic catheter. Urgent assistance would be required
Pain	Analgesia Can be caused by bladder spasm Irritation/sensitivity to catheter material Infection If related to erection, consider Charriere size and trial a smaller one. Consider alternative methods of management such as intermittent catheterisations or suprapubic
Infection	Dipstick urinalysis is not advised in catheterised patients If patient is symptomatic, take catheter sample of urine from catheter port and consider if antibiotics are required while maintaining antibiotic stewardship (NICE, 2018b) Consider if catheter can be removed Educate the patient/carer on prevention of infections Consider increasing fluid intake Refer to other professionals if issues continue
Blocking/by-passing	Keep a catheter diary Ensure patient is drinking adequate fluids Check tubing is not kinked Ensure the Charriere size, material and length of catheter are appropriate Check for constipation/impaction If encrustation is an issue: If possible, consider higher citric acid diet and fluids Catheter maintenance solutions (citric acid based) may help. However, these can increase the risk of infection and can irritate the bladder If issues continue, refer to urology

TABLE 10.16 **Troubleshooting for Urinary Catheterisation—cont'd**

Issue	Possible Reason/Resolution
Colour of urine not yellow	Patient dehydrated Related to food intake, e.g., beetroot Side effects of medication, e.g., sulfazalazine, B vitamins Purple urine syndrome due to sulphates and phosphates in the urine
Phimosis/ paraphimosis	Phimosis (tight foreskin) can make catheterisation difficult. Anaesthetic gel may help, but consider referral to GP/urology Paraphimosis foreskin has been retracted and not repositioned/pulled forward after catheterisation/hygiene. Patient needs referral to GP/urology dependent on severity
Difficulty removing catheter	Balloon not deflating—leave for a time and try again. Try a different syringe. DO NOT CUT the catheter. Can be caused if water drained too quickly and valve collapses. 'Milk' tubing above bifurcation. Insert 1–2 mL of sterile water into channel to release/clear blockage. Connect needle to syringe and insert into catheter tubing directly above the inflation valve (below the bifurcation). Gently withdraw water from the balloon. If successful, inspect balloon for any faults to ensure no debris has been left in the bladder. If unsuccessful, arrange urgent medical attention If faulty catheter, keep catheter and contact manufacturer for next steps Cuffing issue with suprapubic catheters. Select different catheter

NICE. (2018). Urinary tract infection (catheter-associated): Antimicrobial prescribing. Available at: https://www.nice.org.uk/guidance/ng113.

10.11.3 ONGOING REVIEW

Patients with continence problems should have regular reviews to offer physical and emotional support. Treatment options may need adjusting, particularly in patients with long-term deteriorating conditions as their condition can deteriorate and cause complications (NICE, 2012).

10.12 Social Isolation, Loneliness and Health

10.12.1 INTRODUCTION

Nearly 1 in 10 people in the UK feel lonely often or always (Office for National Statistics, 2023). Loneliness is a negative emotion that is a result of feeling alone although it is curiously unrelated to the number of people around us. As Peplau and Perlman (1982) described in their classic work, it is possible to be alone and content or surrounded by people and still feel a lack of social connection.

As the population is ageing, so is the number of people living with complex health needs (Maybin et al., 2016). The COVID-19 pandemic highlighted this issue and recent research confirms that those most at risk of loneliness include those who have a long-term condition and those who live alone (Department for Digital, Culture, Media and Sport, 2022). Therefore the patient group seen by a community nursing team are at high risk of loneliness.

10.12.2 THE EFFECT OF LONELINESS ON HEALTH

It is well recognised that loneliness has a significant negative impact on health outcomes (Czaja et al., 2021; WHO, 2021). Holt-Lunstad et al. (2015) investigated the links with mortality and suggested that loneliness can increase mortality risk by 30%, while others have drawn links with increased morbidity in relation to specific conditions. For example, Freak-Poli et al. (2022) point to systematic reviews of cardiovascular disease which demonstrate poorer outcomes for those with poor social health. Following the peak of the COVID-19 pandemic, loneliness was found to have been associated with as high a risk of hospitalisation as hypertension and other preexisting conditions (Wang, 2023).

The effect of loneliness on mental health was assessed through a qualitative study by Overend et al. (2015). It is known that loneliness is an independent risk factor for depression (Wakefield et al., 2020); however, Overend et al. (2015) suggest that this may be 'hidden' among the elderly who are likely to attribute their low mood as a side effect of the physical health need and are less likely to speak to their GP about this. She suggests that loneliness is an important and often overlooked factor in assessing depression in older adults.

10.12.3 ASSESSMENT OF LONELINESS

Community nurses are in an ideal position to detect and respond to loneliness although psychological health is often treated as lower priority than care planning for physical needs. Chana et al. (2016) suggest high workloads and lack of training are the cause of this barrier and go on to suggest that the use of an assessment tool may help. This is supported by the Campaign to End Loneliness (2023) and the government strategy policy aimed at tackling loneliness (Department for Digital, Culture, Media and Sport, 2018).

Various tools are available such as the De Jong Gierveld Loneliness Scale (De Jong-Gierveld & Kamphuis, 1985) or the widely used UCLA 3-point scale first developed in 1978 by Ferguson, Russell and Peplau (Fergusson et al., 1978). However, the ethical complexities of assessing loneliness should be considered as there is a concern that asking about this area of life can appear judgemental and highlight loneliness for those who do not want to address the issue. As with other screening the implications of detection must be balanced with the provision of services to meet the need.

10.12.4 PROVIDING SUPPORT

Social prescribing has long been recognised as a nonmedical strategy that community nurses use informally to build social connections (Howarth, 2020) and is also now formally recognised within the NHS (2019a) Long Term Plan. The Universal Personal Care Report (NHS, 2019b) provides principles for how social prescribing can be implemented although the challenges for housebound patients are not addressed and community nurses need to remain creative in how they can use the local social prescribing networks to support their patients.

Digital exclusion contributes to social isolation (Department for Digital, Culture, Media and Sport, 2022). Mistry and Jabbal (2023) report that 14 million people in the UK have low digital capability, and of these, 30% find this limits their access to NHS services. New projects to reduce this inequity of access are being introduced among the elderly housebound community and despite the challenges of equipment and limited people resources these have reduced loneliness for those involved (Surrey Coalition for the Disabled, 2023).

In addition to social prescribing pathways and technological solutions, there are local community initiatives such as friendship or lunch clubs organised by established charities such as Age Concern which can support the lonely. Community nursing initiatives such as leg clubs providing wound care can also alleviate loneliness as well as promote physical healing (Box 10.16).

BOX 10.16 ■ Community Nurses Can Make a Difference When They

- Prioritise loneliness within their initial patient assessment.
- Include social prescribing within their care plan.
- Build up networks with community organisations that encourage social connections.
- Encourage technological based solutions where possible.
- Remember the value of the nurse–patient relationship.

CASE STUDY 10.3

Background: Mr Kennett is an 80-year-old widower living alone in a suburban community. Mr Kennett's family are scattered across the country, and he is currently housebound as his leg ulcers have contributed to reducing his mobility and he is embarrassed to go outside with visible leg bandaging. Mr Kennett's loneliness became more pronounced after his wife died as she was his main source of companionship.

Community nurse assessment: Mr Kennett shows signs of depression, and his physical health is declining. The UCLA loneliness scale indicated that he often felt lonely. He said he felt invisible and had little hope for the future.

Intervention: The community nurse liaised with her local branch of Age UK who were able to offer a befriending service. Mr Kennett was suitable to attend a leg ulcer clinic and the community nurse organised community transport to facilitate this. She encouraged him to discuss his feelings with his children and to consider using a tablet to set up regular video calls with his family.

Outcome: Over time, Mr Kennett's loneliness decreased as he gained social support, improved mental well-being and gained a sense of purpose. Alongside this, his physical health improved as the leg ulcer began to improve and he valued meeting other members of the community at the leg ulcer clinic.

10.12.5 CONCLUSION

When community services are stretched, it is a challenge to meet the mental health needs of patients but when consideration can be given to assessing, reporting and planning to improve the social health of community patients, this will maximise their physical health outcomes.

References

Adams, D., Bucior, H., Day, G., & Rimmer, J. (2012). HOUDINI: Make that urinary catheter disappear – Nurse-led protocol. *Journal of Infection Prevention*, *13*(2), 44–46. Available at https://tinyurl.com/5n995y8j Accessed on: 30.9.23.

Alzheimer's Society. (2016). *Over half of people fear a dementia diagnosis, 62 per cent think it means 'life is over'*. Available online https://www.alzheimers.org.uk/news/2018-05-29/over-half-people-fear-dementia-diagnosis-62-cent-think-it-means-life-over.

American Diabetes Association. (2021). Classification and diagnosis of diabetes: Standards of medical care in diabetes—2021. *Diabetes Care*, *44*(Supplement 1), S15–S33. https://doi.org/10.2337/dc21-s002. [online].

American Diabetes Association. (2024). Hyperglycemia (high blood glucose). *ADA*. [online] diabetes.org. Available at https://diabetes.org/living-with-diabetes/treatment-care/hyperglycemia. [Accessed 19 January 2024].

Anestis, E., Eccles, F., Fletcher, I., French, M., & Simpson, J. (2020). Giving and receiving a diagnosis of a progressive neurological condition: A scoping review of doctors' and patients' perspectives. *Patient Education and Counselling*, *103*(9), 1709–1723. https://doi.org/10.1016/j.pec.2020.03.023.

Atkin, L., Bućko, Z., Montero, E. C., Cutting, K., Moffatt, C., Probst, A., et al. (2019). Implementing TIMERS: The race against hard-to-heal wounds. *Journal of Wound care*, *28*(3 Suppl 3), S1–S49.

Atwood, C. ,E., Bhutani, M., Ospina, M. ,B., Rowe, B. ,H., Leigh, R., et al. (2022). Optimizing COPD acute care patient outcomes using a standardized transition bundle and care coordinator: A randomized clinical trial. *Chest*, *162*(2), 321–330.

Bain, A., Kavanagh, S., McCarthy, S., & Babar, Z. (2019). Assessment of insulin-related knowledge among healthcare professionals in a large teaching hospital in the United Kingdom. *Pharmacy (Basel)*, *30;7*(1), 16.

Bakan, A. B., Aslan, G., & Yildiz, M. (2021). Effects of the training given to older adults on urinary incontinence. *Ageing International*, *46*, 324–336. Available at https://link.springer.com/article/10.1007/s12126-020-09390-x#:~:text=Conclusion,with%20medicine%20or%20surgical%20treatments Accessed on 24.9.23.

Bamford, C., Wheatley, A., Brunskill, G., Booi, G., Allan, L., Banerjee, S., & on behalf of the PriDem study team., et al. (2021). Key components of post-diagnostic support for carers: A qualitative study. *PLoS One*, *16*(12):e0260506.

Barnes, F. (2007). Care of people with multiple sclerosis in the community setting. *British Journal of Community Nursing*, *12*(12), 552–557. https://doi.org/10.12968/bjcn.2007.12.12.27741.

Birmpili, P., Atkins, E., Boyle, J. R., Sayers, R. D., Blacker, K., Williams, R., et al. (2022). The Vascular PAD-QIF CQUIN: What is it, why is it important, what does it mean for vascular units. *J. Vasc. Soc. G.B. Irel.*, *1*(3), 63–64.

Bladder & Bowel UK. (n.d.). https://www.bbuk.org.uk/. Accessed on 27.9.23.

Bladder and Bowel Community, n.d. FREE Just Can't Wait Toilet Card. Available at: https://www.bladderandbowel.org/help-information/just-cant-wait-card/.

British Association for Cardiovascular Prevention and Rehabilitation (BACPR). (2023). *Standards and core components for cardiovascular disease prevention and rehabilitation*. https://www.bacpr.org/__data/assets/pdf_file/0021/64236/BACPR-Standards-and-Core-Components-2023.pdf.

British Association of Enteral and Parenteral Nutrition. (2022). *Nutritional assessment*. [Online] Available at https://www.bapen.org.uk/nutrition-support/assessment-and-planning/nutritional-assessment. [Accessed 12 April 2023].

British Association of Enteral and Parenteral Nutrition. (2023). *'MUST' calculator*. [Online] Available at https://www.bapen.org.uk/screening-and-must/must-calculator. [Accessed 12 April 2023].

British Dietetic Association. (2023). *About dietetics*. [Online] Available at https://www.bda.uk.com/about-dietetics.html. [Accessed 2 June 2023].

British Geriatric Society. (2019). *CGA in primary care settings: Weight loss and nutrition issues*. Available from: https://www.bgs.org.uk/resources/17-cga-in-primary-care-settings-weight-loss-and-nutrition-issues.

British Heart Foundation. (2020). Heart failure: A blueprint for change. Building a better future for heart failure together. *BHF*. https://www.bhf.org.uk/what-we-do/policy-and-public-affairs/transforming-healthcare/heart-failure-report.

British Lung Foundation (BLF). (2023). *Lung disease in the UK – big picture statistics*. Available at https://statistics.blf.org.uk/lung-disease-uk-big-picture. [Accessed 6 July 2023].

British National Formulary. (2023). *Oxygen*. Available at https://bnf.nice.org.uk/treatment-summaries/oxygen/. [Accessed 17 July 2023].

British Thoracic Society. (2015). *BTS guidelines for home oxygen use in adults*. Available at https://www.brit-thoracic.org.uk/document-library/guidelines/home-oxygen-for-adults/bts-guidelines-for-home-oxygen-use-in-adults/. [Accessed 10 September 2023].

British Thoracic Society (BTS). (2021). *BTS information: Respiratory inhalers*. Available at https://www.brit-thoracic.org.uk/document-library/quality-improvement/covid-19/bts-information-respiratory-inhalers/. [Accessed 17 July 2023].

Cabinet Office. (2021). *Guidance: Inclusive language: words to use and avoid when writing about disability*. Available at https://www.gov.uk/government/publications/inclusive-communication/inclusive-language-words-to-use-and-avoid-when-writing-about-disability.

Campaign to End Loneliness. (2023). *The state of loneliness 2023*. https://tacklinglonelinesshub.org/resources/the-state-of-loneliness-ons-data-on-loneliness-in-britain/#:~:text=Campaign%20to%20End%20Loneliness%2C%202023&text=The%20data%20shows%20the%20number,million%20people%20were%20chronically%20lonely.

Cardol, C.K., van Middendorp, H., Dusseldorp, E., van der Boog, P.J.M., Hilbrands, L.B., Navis, G., et al., & E-GOAL Study Group. (2023). eHealth to improve psychological functioning and self-management of people with chronic kidney disease: A randomized controlled trial. *Psychosomatic Medicine*, *85*(2), 203–215. https://doi.org/10.1097/PSY.0000000000001163.

Care Quality Commission. (2022). *Managing oxygen in care homes*. Available at https://www.cqc.org.uk/guidance-providers/adult-social-care/managing-oxygen-care-homes. [Accessed 17 July 2023].

Cedarholm, T., Barazzoni, R., Austin, P., Ballmer, P., Biolo, G., Bischoff, S.C., et al. (2017). ESPEN guidelines on definitions and terminology of clinical nutrition. *Clinical Nutrition*, *36*(1), 49–64. https://doi.org/10.1016/j.clnu.2016.09.004.

Chana, R., Marshall, P., & Harley, C. (2016). The role of the intermediate care team in detecting and responding to loneliness in older clients. *British Journal of Community Nursing*, *21*(6), 292–298. https://doi.org/10.12968/bjcn.2016.21.6.292.

Cheung, A.K., Rahman, M., Reboussin, D.M., Craven, T.E., Greene, T., Kimmel, P.L., et al., & SPRINT Research Group. (2017). Effects of intensive BP control in CKD. *Journal of the American Society of Nephrology*, *28*(9), 2812–2823. https://doi.org/10.1681/ASN.2017020148.

Chew, J., & Mahadeva, R. (2018). The role of a multidisciplinary severe chronic obstructive pulmonary disease hyperinflation service in patient selection for lung volume reduction. *Journal of Thoracic Disease*, *10*(Suppl. 27), S3335–S3343.

CKS/NICE. (2019). *Lower urinary tract symptoms in men*. Available at https://cks.nice.org.uk/topics/luts-in-men/. Accessed: 26.9.23.

CKS/NICE. (2023a). *Incontinence – urinary, in women*. Available at https://cks.nice.org.uk/topics/incontinence-urinary-in-women/. Accessed: 26.9.23.

CKS/NICE. (2023b). *Constipation*. Available at https://cks.nice.org.uk/topics/constipation/. Accessed: 26.9.23.

Clegg, A., Young, J., Iliffe, S., Rikkert, M. O., & Rockwood, K. (2013). Frailty in elderly people. *The Lancet*, *381*(9868), 752–762.

Colley, W. (2020). *Urinary continence assessment, treatment and management*. Available at https://www.continenceassessment.co.uk/colley_model/. Accessed on 27.9.23.

Combes, S., Nicholson, C. J., Gillett, K., & Norton, C. (2019). Implementing advance care planning with community-dwelling frail elders requires a system-wide approach: an integrative review applying a behaviour change model. *Palliative Medicine*, *33*(7), 743–756.

Conte, M. S., Bradbury, A. W., Kolh, P., White, J. V., Dick, F., Fitridge, R., & GVG Writing Group., et al. (2019 Jun). Global vascular guidelines on the management of chronic limb-threatening ischemia. *Journal of vascular surgery cases*, *69*(6S), 3S–125S.e40. https://doi.org/10.1016/j.jvs.2019.02.016. Epub 2019 May 28. Erratum in: J Vasc Surg. 2019 Aug;70(2):662.

Cooper, C., Lodwick, R., Walters, K., Raine, R., Manthorpe, J., Iliffe, S., & Peterson, I. (2017). Inequalities in receipt of mental and physical healthcare in people living with dementia. *Age and Ageing*, *46*, 393–400.

Czaja, S. J., Moxley, J. H., & Rogers, W. A. (2021). Social support, isolation, loneliness, and health among older adults in the PRISM randomized controlled trial. *Frontiers in Psychology, 12*. https://www.frontiersin.org/articles/10.3389/fpsyg.2021.728658.

De Jong-Gierveld, J., & Kamphuis, F. (1985). De Jong-Gierveld Loneliness Scale. *American Psychologists Association* Washington.

Deckers, K., Cadar, D., Van Boxtel, M. P. J., Verhey, F. R. J., Steptoe, A., & Kohler, S. (2019). Modifiable risk factors explain socioeconomic inequalities in dementia risk: Evidence from a population-based prospective cohort study. *Journal of Alzheimer's Disease, 71*, 549–557.

Delgado, C., Baweja, M., Crews, D.C., Eneanya, N. D., Gadegbeku, C.A., Inker, L.A., et al. (2022). A unifying approach for GFR estimation: Recommendations of the NKF-ASN task force on reassessing the inclusion of race in diagnosing kidney disease. *American Journal of Kidney Diseases, 79*(2), 268–288.e1. https://doi.org/10.1053/j.ajkd.2021.08.003.

Delves-Yates, C. (2022). *Essentials of nursing practice* (3rd ed.). Los Angeles, London, New Delhi, Singapore, Washington DC, Melbourne: Sage.

Department for Digital, Culture, Media and Sport. (2018). *A connected society: A strategy for tackling loneliness*. London: HM Government.

Department for Digital, Culture, Media and Sport. (2022). *Investigating factors associated with loneliness amongst adults in England during the pandemic*. https://www.gov.uk/government/publications/factors-associated-with-loneliness-in-adults-in-england-during-the-pandemic/investigating-factors-associated-with-loneliness-amongst-adults-in-england-during-the-pandemic.

Department of Health. (2009). *Living well with dementia: A national dementia strategy*. Available online https://www.gov.uk/government/publications/living-well-with-dementia-a-national-dementia-strategy.

Department of Health. (2015). *Prime Minister's challenge on dementia 2020*. Available online https://www.gov.uk/government/publications/prime-ministers-challenge-on-dementia-2020.

Diabetes UK. (2021). *Diabetes diagnoses double in the last 15 years*. [online] Diabetes UK. Available at https://www.diabetes.org.uk/about-us/news-and-views/diabetes-diagnoses-doubled-prevalence-2021. [Accessed 19 January 2024].

Diabetes UK. (2022a). *What is insulin?*. [online] Diabetes UK. Available at https://www.diabetes.org.uk/guide-to-diabetes/managing-your-diabetes/treating-your-diabetes/insulin/what-is-insulin. [Accessed 19 January 2024].

Diabetes UK. (2022b). *Hyperglycaemia*. [online] Diabetes UK. Available at https://www.diabetes.org.uk/Guide-to-diabetes/Complications/hypers. [Accessed 19 January 2024].

Diabetes UK. (2023). *Research on preventing amputations*. [online] Diabetes UK. Available at https://www.diabetes.org.uk/our-research/about-our-research/our-impact/preventing-amputations. [Accessed 23 January 2024].

Diggle, J. (2022). How to minimise insulin errors. DiabetesontheNet. *Diabetes & Primary Care, [online], 24*, 181–182. Available at https://diabetesonthenet.com/diabetes-primary-care/how-to-minimise-insulin-errors-2022/. [Accessed 19 January 2024].

Dring, B., & Hipkiss, V. (2015). Managing and treating chronic kidney disease. *Nursing Times*, 111(7), 16–19.

European Respiratory Society. (2013). *Respiratory diseases in the world. Realities of today – Opportunities for tomorrow*. Available at https://www.thoracic.org/about/global-public-health/firs/resources/firs-report-for-web.pdf. [Accessed 6 July 2023].

European Respiratory Society. (2017). *The global impact of respiratory disease* (2nd ed.). Available at. https://static.physoc.org/app/uploads/2019/04/22192917/The_Global_Impact_of_Respiratory_Disease.pdf. [Accessed 6 July 2023].

European Society of Cardiology. (2021). *ESC guidelines for the diagnosis and treatment of acute and chronic heart failure*. Available at: https://www.escardio.org/Guidelines/Clinical-Practice-Guidelines/Acute-and-Chronic-Heart-Failure.

Fleming, J., Zhao, J., Farquhar, M., Brayne, C., Barclay, S., & Collaboration CCO-sCS. (2010). Place of death for the 'oldest old': ≥ 85-year-olds in the CC75C population-based cohort. *Br J Gen Pract*, *60*(573), e171–e179.

Ferguson, M., Russell, D., & Peplau, L. (1978). *The Loneliness Scale*. University of California.

Fletcher, J., Beeckman, D., Boyles, A., Fumarola, S., Kottner, J., McNichol, L., et al. (2020). International best practice recommendations: Prevention and management of moisture-associated skin damage (MASD). *Wounds International*. Available from https://multimedia.3m.com/mws/media/2155609O/3m-masd-wounds-international-recommendation-us-version.pdf.

Forum for Injection Technique (FIT). (2016). *The UK injection technique recommendations* (4th ed.). Oxford, UK: FIT. Available at. https://www.diabetesincontrol.com/wp-content/uploads/2017/06/FIT-UK-Forum.SMALL_.pdf.

Freak-Poli, R., Hu, J., Zaw, A., & Barker, F. (2022). Does social isolation, social support or loneliness influence health or well-being after a cardiovascular disease event? A narrative thematic systematic review. *Health and Social Care in the Community*, *30*(1), 16–18.

Freedman, B.I., Limou, S., Ma, L., & Kopp, J.B. (2018). APOL1-associated nephropathy: A key contributor to racial disparities in CKD. *American Journal of Kidney Diseases*, *72*(5 Suppl 1), S8–S16. https://doi.org/10.1053/j.ajkd.2018.06.0202. (Accessed 13 June 2023).

Fu, Y., Jackson, C. ,A., Nelson, A., Iles-Smith, H., & McGowan, L. (2023). Exploring support, experiences and needs of older women and health professionals to inform a self-management package for urinary incontinence: A qualitative study. *British Medical Journal*, *13*:e071831. Available at https://bmjopen.bmj.com/content/13/7/e071831.full Accessed on 26.9.23.

Geraghty, J. (2023). Misunderstood and Overlooked webinar: Addressing leg ulceration as a physical health need for people experiencing homelessness. *Single Homeless Project*. Available from https://www.shp.org.uk/news/addressing-leg-ulceration-as-a-physical-health-need-for-people-experiencing-homelessness.

Giebel, C., Robertson, S., Beaulen, A., Zwakhalen, S., Allen, D., & Verbeek, H. (2021). "Nobody seems to know where to even turn to": Barriers in accessing and utilising dementia care services in England and the Netherlands. *International Journal of Environmental Research and Public Health*, *18*(12233).

Gohel, M. S., Heatley, F., Liu, X., Bradbury, A., Bulbulia, R., Cullum, N., & EVRA Trial Investigators., et al. (2018 May 31). A randomized trial of early endogenous ablation in venous ulceration. *N Engl J Med*, *378*(22), 2105–2114.

GOLD. (2023). *Global strategy for the diagnosis, management, and prevention of chronic obstructive pulmonary disease (2023 report)*. Global Initiative for Chronic Obstructive Lung Disease.

Green, S. M., Dinenage, S., Gower, M., & Van Wyk, J. (2013). Home enteral nutrition: Organisation of services. *Nursing Older People*, *25*(4), 14–18.

Green, S. M., Townsend, K., Jarrett, N., & Fader, M. (2019a). The experiences and support needs of people living at home with an enteral tube: a qualitative interview study. *Journal of Human Nutrition and Dietetics*, *32*(5), 646–658.

Green, S. M., Townsend, K., Jarrett, N., Westoby, C., & Fader, M. (2019b). People with enteral tubes and their carers' views of living. *Journal of Clinical Nursing*, *28*, 3710–3720.

Gregory, S., & Curtis, K. (2022). Embedding flash glucose monitoring technology within neighbourhood nursing teams. *Journal of Diabetes Nursing, [online]*, *26*(2), 235. Available at https://diabetesonthenet.com/journal-diabetes-nursing/flash-neighbourhood-nursing/. [Accessed 3 January 2024].

Gundry, S. (2020). COPD 2: Management and nursing care. *Nursing Times*, *116*(5), 48–51.

Gustafsson, T., & Nordeman, L. (2017). The nurse's challenge of caring for patients with chronic obstructive pulmonary disease in primary health care. *Nursing Open*, *4*, 292–299.

Hayhoe, B., Majeed, A., & Perneczky, R. (2016). General practitioner referrals to memory clinics: Are referral criteria delaying the diagnosis of dementia? *Journal of Royal Society of Medicine*, *109*(11), 410–415.

Health Education England. (2023). *About the Making Every Contact Count programme*. [Online] Available at https://www.e-lfh.org.uk/programmes/making-every-contact-count/. [Accessed 17 April 2023].

Hicks, D., & James, J. (2023). *Correct injection technique in diabetes care best practice guideline*. [online] Trend Diabetes. Available at https://trenddiabetes.online/wp-content/uploads/2023/10/Guideline_ITM_2023-1.pdf. [Accessed 2 January 2024].

Holt-Lunstad, J., Smith, T., Baker, M., Harris, T., & Stephenson, D. (2015). Loneliness and social isolation as risk factors for mortality: A meta-analytic review. *Perspectives on Psychological Science*, *10*(2), 227–237.

Holroyd, S. (2021). Catheter valves: Appropriate use and reduction of risk to bladder. *Journal of Community Nursing*, *35*(5), 52–56. Available at https://tinyurl.com/2s3na96e Accessed 10.10.23.

Howarth, M., Griffiths, A., Da Silva, A., & Green, R. (2020). Social prescribing: A 'natural' community-based solution. *British Journal of Community Nursing*, *25*(6), 294–298. https://doi.org/10.12968/bjcn.2020.25.6.294.

Innovate UK KTN. (2023). *AI-enabled portable incontinence management device*. Available at https://iuk.ktn-uk.org/projects/healthy-ageing-challenge-community-of-practice/ai-enabled-portable-incontinence-management-device/. Accessed on 27.9.23.

Institute for Health Metrics and Evaluation (IHME). (2023). *Health data – United Kingdom – England*. Available at https://www.healthdata.org/united-kingdom-england. [Accessed 6 July 2023].

Jiang, S., Fang, J., & Li, W. (2023). Protein restriction for diabetic kidney disease. The Cochrane Database of Systematic Reviews, 1(1), CD014906. https://doi.org/10.1002/14651858.CD014906.pub2.

Kehinde, O. (2016). Common incontinence problems seen by community nurses. *Journal of Community Nursing*, *30*(4), 46–55. Available at https://web-p-ebscohost-com.chain.kent.ac.uk/ehost/pdfviewer/pdfviewer?vid=10&sid=32c06f84-9215-402f-8c14-5cf034b89a58%40redis Accessed 24.9.23.

Keller, J. J. (2018). Leg Ulcers: Expanding the differential. *Current Dermatology Reports*, *7*(3), 180–189.

Kidney Disease Improving Global Outcomes (KDIGO). (2013). Clinical practice guideline for the evaluation and management of chronic kidney disease. www.kdigo.org/clinical_practice_guidelines/pdf/ CKD/KDIGO_2012_CKD_GL.pdf.

King's Fund. (2014). *Admission to a nursing home can never become a 'never' event*. King's Fund. Available at https://www.kingsfund.org.uk/insight-and-analysis/blogs/admission-nursing-home-never-become-never-event#:~:text=But%20care%20homes%20can%20never,living%20in%20their%20own%20homes. (Accessed on 4 July 2024).

Knight, J., Nigam, Y., & Cutter, J. (2020). *Understanding anatomy & physiology in nursing*. London: Learning Matters.

Kumar, P., & Clark, M. (2020). *Clinical Medicine* (10th ed.). London: Elsevier Health Sciences.

Lacy, M. E., Gilsanz, P., Eng, C., Beeri, M. S., Karter, A. J., & Whitmer, R. A. (2020). Severe Hypoglycemia and cognitive function in older adults with type 1 diabetes: The Study of Longevity in Diabetes (SOLID). *Diabetes Care*, *43*(3), 541–548. https://doi.org/10.2337/dc19-0906. [online].

Lane, J. C. (2022). *An exploration of clinical literature: How the evidence could influence policy and care pathways – To improve the health and care outcomes of people living with dementia in the four nations of the United Kingdom*. Unpublished Academic Paper; University of Hull.

Leung, E., Wongrakpanich, S., & Munshi, M. N. (2018). Diabetes management in the elderly. *Diabetes Spectrum*, *31*(3), 245–253. https://doi.org/10.2337/ds18-0033. [online].

Levin, A., Tonelli, M., Bonventre, J., Coresh, J., Donner, J.A., Fogo, A.B., et al., & ISN Global Kidney Health Summit participants. (2017). Global kidney health 2017 and beyond: A roadmap for closing gaps in care, research, and policy. *Lancet*, *390*(10105), 1888–1917. https://doi.org/10.1016/S0140-6736(17)30788-2.

Linsenmyerm, T. ,A., Gibbs, K., & Solinsky, R. (2020). Autonomic dysreflexia after spinal cord injury: Beyond the basics. *Current Physical Medicine and Rehabilitation Reports*, *8*(4), 1–9. Available at https://link.springer.com/article/10.1007/s40141-020-00300-5 Accessed on 5.11.23.

Livingston, G., Huntley, J., Sommerlad, A., Ames, D., Ballard, C., Banerjee, S., et al. (2020). Dementia prevention, intervention, and care: 2020 report for the Lancet Commission. *The Lancet*, *369*, 413–446.

Loveday, H. ,P., Wilson, J. ,A., Pratt, R. ,J., Golsorkhi, M., Tingle, A., et al. (2014). Epic3: National evidence-based guidelines for preventing healthcare-associated infections in NHS hospitals in England. *Journal of Hospital Infection*, S1–S70. Available at https://tinyurl.com/5bnhyky8 Accessed on 10.10.23.

Low, L. F., & Purwaningrum, F. (2020). Negative stereotypes, fear and social distance: A systematic review of depictions of dementia in popular culture in the context of stigma. *Bio Med Central Geriatrics*, *20*(477).

Magwood, G. S., Nichols, M., Jenkins, C., Logan, A., Qanungo, S., Zigbuo-Wenzler, E., & Ellis, C. (2020). Community-based interventions for stroke provided by nurses and community health workers: A review of the literature. *Journal of Neuroscience Nursing*, *52*(4), 152–159. https://doi.org/10.1097/jnn.0000000000000512.

Mahon, A., Jenkins, K., & Burnapp, L. (2013a). Renal pathophysiology. In A. Mahon, K. Jenkins, & L. Burnapp (Eds.), *Oxford handbook of renal nursing, Oxford handbooks in nursing*. Oxford: Oxford Academic. https://doi.org/10.1093/med/9780199600533.003.0002. (Accessed 13 June 2023). (Online edition).

Mahon, A., Jenkins, K., & Burnapp, L. (2013b). Clinical assessment of the chronic kidney disease patient. In A. Mahon, K. Jenkins, & L. Burnapp (Eds.), *Oxford handbook of renal nursing, Oxford handbooks in nursing*. Oxford: Oxford Academic. https://doi.org/10.1093/med/9780199600533.003.000. (Online edition).

Major, R.W., Shepherd, D., Medcalf, J.F., Xu, G., Gray, L.J., & Brunskill, N.J. (2019). The kidney failure risk equation for prediction of end stage renal disease in UK primary care: An external validation and clinical impact projection cohort study. *PLoS Medicine*, 16(11), e1002955.

Malewezi, E., O'Brien, M. R., Knighting, K., Thomas, J., & Jack, B. (2022). A different way of life: A qualitative study on the experiences of family caregivers of stroke survivors living at home. *British Journal of Community Nursing*, *27*(11), 558–566. https://doi.org/10.12968/bjcn.2022.27.11.558.

Malnutrition Task Force. (2023). *Malnutrition in England factsheet*. [Online] Available at https://www.malnutritiontaskforce.org.uk/malnutrition-england-factsheet. [Accessed 18 April 2023].

Masters, J., Barton, C., Blue, L., & Welstand, J. (2019). Increasing the heart failure nursing workforce: recommendations by the British Society for Heart Failure Nurse Forum. *British Journal of Cardiac Nursing*, *14*(11), 1–12.

Maybin, J., Charles, A., & Honeyman, M. (2016). *Understanding quality in district nursing*. London: King's Fund.

Mbizvo, G. K., Bennett, K., Simpson, C. R., Duncan, S. E., & Chin, R. F. M. (2019). Epilepsy-related and other causes of mortality in people with epilepsy: A systematic review of systematic reviews. *Epilepsy Research*, *157*:106192. https://doi.org/10.1016/j.eplepsyres.2019.106192.

McCann, M., Kelly, A., Eustace-Cook, J., Houlin, C., & Daly, L. (2021). Community nurses' attitudes, knowledge, and educational needs in relation to urinary incontinence assessment and management: A systematic review. *Journal of Clinical Nursing*, *31*(7-8), 1041–1060. https://onlinelibrary.wiley.com/doi/full/10.1111/jocn.15969. Accessed on 27.9.23.

McDonagh, T.A., Metra, M., Adamo, M., Gardner, R.S., Baumbach, A., Böhm, M., et al., & ESC Scientific Document Group. (2021). ESC guidelines for the diagnosis and treatment of acute and chronic heart failure. *European Journal of Heart Failure*, *24*(1), 4–131.

McIlvennan, C. K., & Allen, L. A. (2016). Palliative care in patients with heart failure. *British Medical Journal*, *353*.

Mendes, A. (2016). Community management and pioneering treatments in MS. *British Journal of Community Nursing*, *21*(2). https://doi.org/10.12968/bjcn.2016.21.2.107. pp. 107–107.

Mendiratta, P., Schoo, C., & Latif, R. (2023). Clinical Frailty Scale. In *StatPearls [Internet]*. Treasure Island (FL): StatPearls Publishing. Available from: https://www.ncbi.nlm.nih.gov/books/NBK559009/.

Mental Health Foundation. (2022). *Talking about mental health*. Available from https://www.mentalhealth.org.uk/explore-mental-health/a-z-topics/talking-about-mental-health.

Mesraoua, B., Tomson, T., Brodie, M., & Asadi-Pooya, A. A. (2022). Sudden unexpected death in epilepsy (SUDEP): Definition, epidemiology, and significance of education. *Epilepsy & Behavior*, *132*. :108742. https://doi.org/10.1016/j.yebeh.2022.108742.

Mistry, P., & Jabbal, J. (2023). *Moving from exclusion to inclusion in digital health and care*. The King's Fund. Retrieved from https://www.kingsfund.org.uk/publications/exclusion-inclusion-digital-health-care.

Mitchell, A. (2021). Self-harm wounds: assessment and management. *British Journal of Nursing*, *30*(12), S16–S20.

National Asthma Council Australia. (2016). *Inhaler technique for people with asthma or COPD*. Available at https://extranet.who.int/ncdccs/Data/AUS_D1_Inhaler_Technique_Infopaper-FULL-UPDATED-11-1.pdf. [Accessed 11 July 2023].

National Collaborating Centre for Women's and Children's Health UK. (2013). *Urinary incontinence in women: The management of urinary incontinence in women*. London: Royal College of Obstetricians and Gynaecologists (UK). PMID: 25340217.

National Health Service. (2019a). *NHS Long Term Plan*. https://www.longtermplan.nhs.uk/.

National Health Service. (2019b). Universal personalised care. *Implementing the comprehensive model*. Accessed at https://www.england.nhs.uk/wp-content/uploads/2019/01/universal-personalised-care.pdf.

National Health Service. (2020). *Low blood sugar (hypoglycaemia)*. [online] NHS. Available at https://www.nhs.uk/conditions/low-blood-sugar-hypoglycaemia/. [Accessed 19 January 2024].

National Health Service. (2023a). *Eat well*. [Online] Available at https://www.nhs.uk/live-well/eat-well/. [Accessed 13 April 2023].

National Health Service. (2023b). *Lose weight*. [Online] Available at https://www.nhs.uk/better-health/lose-weight/. [Accessed 2023 April 2023].

National Institute for Health and Care Excellence (NICE). (2012). *Urinary incontinence in neurological disease: Assessment and management (CG148)*. NICE. Available at https://www.nice.org.uk/guidance/cg148. Accessed on 24.09.2023.

National Institute for Health and Care Excellence (NICE). (2015a). Checking your own blood glucose, and target levels. Information for the public. Type 1 diabetes in adults: diagnosis and management. *Guidance. NICE*. [online]. Available at https://www.nice.org.uk/guidance/ng17-/ifp/chapter/Checking-your-own-blood-glucose-and-target-levels. [Accessed 19 January 2024].

National Institute for Health and Care Excellence (NICE). (2015b). *Diabetes (type 1 and type 2) in children and young people: diagnosis and management NICE guideline*. [online] Available at https://www.nice.org.uk/guidance/ng18/resources/diabetes-type-1-and-type-2-in-children-and-young-people-diagnosis-and-management-pdf-1837278149317. [Accessed 19 January 2024].

National Institute for Health and Care Excellence (NICE). (2017). *Nutrition support for adults: Oral nutrition support, enteral tube feeding and parenteral nutrition*. London: National Institute for Health and Care Excellence. Available at https://www.nice.org.uk/guidance/cg32. [Accessed 22 March 2023].

National Institute for Health and Care Excellence (NICE). (2018a). *Dementia: Assessment, management and support for people living with dementia and their carers*. Available online https://www.nice.org.uk/guidance/ng97.

National Institute for Health and Care Excellence. (NICE). (2018b). *Urinary tract infection (catheter-associated): antimicrobial prescribing*. Available at https://www.nice.org.uk/guidance/ng113. Accessed on: 30.9.23.

National Institute for Health and Care Excellence (NICE). (2018c). *Chronic heart failure in adults: Diagnosis and management NICE guideline*. NG106. https://www.nice.org.uk/guidance/ng106.

National Institute for Health and Care Excellence [NICE]. (2019a). *Chronic obstructive pulmonary disease in over 16s: Diagnosis and management*. Available at https://www.nice.org.uk/guidance/ng115/resources/chronic-obstructive-pulmonary-disease-in-over-16s-diagnosis-and-management-pdf-66141600098245 (Accessed: 10 July 2023).

National Institute for Health and Care Excellence. (NICE). (2019b). *CKS. Falls – risk assessment*. Available from: https://cks.nice.org.uk/topics/falls-risk-assessment/.

National Institute for Health and Care Excellence. (NICE). (2019c). *Urinary incontinence and pelvic organ prolapse in women: Management (NG123)*. https://www.nice.org.uk/guidance/ng123. Accessed on 27.9.23.

National Institute for Health and Care Excellence (NICE). (2021). *Chronic kidney disease: Assessment and management*. Available at: https://www.nice.org.uk/guidance/ng203.

National Institute for Health and Care Excellence (NICE). (2022a). *Epilepsies in children, young people and adults (NG217)*. Available at https://www.nice.org.uk/guidance/ng217. [Accessed 16 June 2023].

National Institute for Health and Care Excellence (NICE). (2022b). *Hypoglycaemia*. [online] NICE. Available at https://bnf.nice.org.uk/treatment-summaries/hypoglycaemia/. [Accessed 3 January 2024].

National Institute for Health and Care Excellence (NICE). (2022c). *Overview. Type 2 diabetes in adults: Management. Guidance*. NICE [online]. Available at https://www.nice.org.uk/guidance/ng28. [Accessed 19 January 2024].

National Institute for Health and Care Excellence. (NICE). (2022d). *Rehabilitation after traumatic injury. C3 specific programmes and packages in spinal cord injury for people with complex rehabilitation needs after traumatic injury. NICE guideline NG211. Evidence review underpinning recommendations 1.15.1 to 1.15.37 and research recommendations in the NICE guideline*. Available at https://tinyurl.com/mry7d3c4. Accessed on 5.11.23.

National Institute for Health and Care Excellence. (NICE). (2023a). *Clinical knowledge summaries – Smoking cessation*. Available at https://cks.nice.org.uk/topics/smoking-cessation/. [Accessed 10 July 2023].

National Institute for Health and Care Excellence. (NICE). (2023b). *Health topics A to Z: Chronic obstructive pulmonary disease: Scenario: End-stage chronic obstructive pulmonary disease*. Available at https://cks.nice.org.uk/topics/chronic-obstructive-pulmonary-disease/management/end-stage-copd/#:~:text=For%20people%20with%20end%2Dstage,where%20appropriate)%20including%20advance%20decisions. [Accessed 18 July 2023].

National Institute for Health and Care Excellence (NICE). (2023c). *Pressure ulcers: What is a pressure ulcer?* Available from https://cks.nice.org.uk/topics/pressure-ulcers/background-information/definition/.

National Institute for Health and Care Excellence. (NICE). (2023d). *Tobacco: Preventing uptake, promoting quitting, and treating dependence*. Available at https://www.nice.org.uk/guidance-/ng209/resources/tobacco-preventing-uptake-promoting-quitting-and-treating-dependence-pdf-66143723132869. [Accessed 10 July 2023].

National Institute for Health and Care Excellence. (NICE). (2023e). *Urinary tract infections in adults*. NICE Standard (QS 90). Available at https://www.nice.org.uk/guidance/qs90. Accessed on 24.10.23.

National Institute for Health and Care, Excellence. (2023f). *NICE CKS heart failure – Chronic*. https://cks.nice.org.uk/topics/heart-failure-chronic/.

National Institute for Health and Care Excellence. (NICE). (2023g). *Chronic obstructive pulmonary disease in adults – Quality statement 3: Assessment for long-term oxygen therapy*. Available at https://www.nice.org.uk/guidance/qs10/chapter/Quality-statement-3-Assessment-for-long-term-oxygen-therapy. [Accessed 17 July 2023].

National Institute for Health and Care Excellence. (NICE). (2024) CKS: How should I assess a person's risk of developing a pressure ulcer? Available at: https://cks.nice.org.uk/topics/pressure-ulcers/diagnosis/risk-assessment/.

National Institute for Health Research. (2017). *Comprehensive care: Older people living with frailty in hospitals*. Available from https://evidence.nihr.ac.uk/wp-content/uploads/2020/03/Comprehensive-Care-final.pdf.

National Kidney Foundation. (2024). *Understanding why eGFR laboratory reports include African American and non-African American results*. Available at: https://www.kidney.org/atoz/content/race-and-egfr-what-controversy.

National Patient Safety Agency. (2009). *Rapid response report NPSA/2009/RRR02: Female urinary catheters causing trauma to adult males* https://www.cas.mhra.gov.uk/ViewandAcknowledgment/ViewAttachment.aspx?Attachment_id=100861. [Accessed 24 October 2023].

National Wound Care Strategy Programme. (2024). *Recommendations for surgical wounds*. Available from https://www.nationalwoundcarestrategy.net/surgical-wounds/.

National Wound Care Strategy Programme. (2023). *National wound care strategy programme. An NHS England programme being delivered by the AHSN Network*. Available from https://www.nationalwoundcarestrategy.net/.

NCSCT. (2018). *NCSCT training standard – Learning outcomes for training stop smoking practitioners*. Available at https://www.ncsct.co.uk/publications/ncsct-training-standard-learning-outcomes-for-training-stop-smoking-practitioners. [Accessed 11 July 2023].

NHS England. (2017a). *RightCare pathway: COPD*. Available at https://www.england.nhs.uk/rightcare/wp-content/uploads/sites/40/2017/12/nhs-rightcare-copd-pathway-v18.pdf. [Accessed 10 September 2023].

NHS England. (2017b). *The safe use of insulin and you*. https://www.england.nhs.uk/improvement-hub/wp-content/uploads/sites/44/2017/11/Safe-use-of-insulin-and-you-patient-info-booklet.pdf.

NHS England. (2017c). *Toolkit for general practice in supporting older people living with frailty*. NHS England.

NHS England. (2018). *Excellence in continence care: Practical guidance for commissioners and leaders in health and social care*. Available at https://www.england.nhs.uk/publication/excellence-in-continence-care/. Accessed on 24.9.23.

NHS England. (2019). *Improving insulin administration in a community setting*. https://www.england.nhs.uk/atlas_case_study/improving-insulin-administration-in-a-community-setting/.

NHS England. (2022). *National service model for an integrated community stroke service*. [Accessed on: 23/06/23]. Available at https://www.england.nhs.uk/publication/national-service-model-for-an-integrated-community-stroke-service/.

NHS England. (2023a). *elfh: elearning for healthcare. Wound care education for the health and care workforce*. Available from https://www.e-lfh.org.uk/programmes/wound-care-education-for-the-health-and-care-workforce/.

NHS England. (2023b). *Respiratory disease*. Available at https://www.england.nhs.uk/ourwork/clinical-policy/respiratory-disease/#:~:text=Respiratory%20disease%20affects%20one%20in,the%20biggest%20causes%20of%20death. [Accessed 6 July 2023].

NHS Improvement. (2017). *Getting it right first time*. Available at https://improvement.nhs.uk/news-alerts/getting-it-right-frst-time-recruits-new-clinical-leads/. Accessed on 27.9.23.

NHS Improvement. (2018). *Patient Safety Alert, Resources to support safer bowel care for patients at risk of autonomic dysreflexia*. Available at: https://www.england.nhs.uk/wp-content/uploads/2019/12/Patient_Safety_Alert_-_safer_care_for_patients_at_risk_of_AD.pdf.

NHS RightCare. (2018). *NHS RightCare scenario: The variation between sub-optimal and optimal pathways*. Available at: https://www.england.nhs.uk/rightcare/wp-content/uploads/sites/40/2018/02/abduls-story-progressive-chronic-kidney-disease-full-narrative-1.pdf.

NHS Wales. (2017). *Neurological conditions delivery plan*. [Accessed on: 23/06/23]. Available at https://www.gov.wales/sites/default/files/publications/2019-02/neurological-conditions-delivery-plan-july-2017.pdf.

NHS Wales. (2022). *The quality statement for neurological conditions*. [Accessed on: 23/06/23]. Available at https://www.gov.wales/quality-statement-neurological-conditions-html.

Ni Lochlainn, M., Cox, N.J., Wilson, T., Hayhoe, R.P.G., Ramsay, S.E., Granic, A., et al. (2021). Nutrition and frailty: Opportunities for prevention and treatment. *Nutrients*, *13*(7), 2349. https://doi.org/10.3390/nu13072349.

Nicholson, C. J., Combes, S., Mold, F., King, H., & Green, R. (2023). Addressing inequity in palliative care provision for older people living with multimorbidity. Perspectives of community-dwelling older people on their palliative care needs: A scoping review. *Palliative Medicine*, *37*(4), 475–497. https://doi.org/10.1177/02692163221118230.

Nursing and Midwifery Council. (2018). *The Code: Professional standards of practice and behaviour for nurses, midwives and nursing associates*. London: Nursing and Midwifery Council.

Office for National Statistics. (2023). *UK measures of national well-being dashboard*. at https://www.ons.gov.uk/peoplepopulationandcommunity/wellbeing/articles/ukmeasuresofnationalwellbeing/dashboard. Accessed on 26/7/23.

Overend, K., Bosanquet, K., Bailey, D., Foster, D., Gascoyne, S., & Lewis, H. (2015). Revealing hidden depression in older adults: A qualitative study within a randomised controlled trial. *BMC Family Practice*, *16*(142), 1–8.

Palmer, C., Richardson, D., Rayner, J., Drake, M. ,J., & Cotterill, N. (2022). Professional perspectives on impacts, benefits and disadvantages of changes made to community continence services during the COVID-19 pandemic: Findings from the EPICCC-19 national survey. *BMC Health Services Research*, *22*, 783. Available at https://bmchealthservres.biomedcentral.com/articles/10.1186/s12913-022-08163-3 Accessed on 24.9.23.

Parkinson's UK. (2016). *A competency framework for nurses working in Parkinson's disease management* (3rd ed.). [Accessed on: 23/06/23]. Available at. https://www.parkinsons.org.uk/professionals/resources/competency-framework-nurses-working-parkinsons-disease-management-3rd.

Peplau, L., & Perlman, D. (1982). *Perspectives on loneliness in Loneliness: A sourcebook of theory, research and therapy*. New York: Wiley and Sons.

Perrels, A. J., Fleming, J., Zhao, J., Barclay, S., Farquhar, M., Buiting, H. M., et al. (2014). Place of death and end-of-life transitions experienced by very old people with differing cognitive status: retrospective analysis of a prospective population-based cohort aged 85 and over. *Palliative Medicine*, *28*(3), 220–233.

Phillips, A., Edmonds, M., Holmes, P., Robbie, J., Odiase, C., & Grumitt, J. (2020). ACT NOW in diabetes and foot assessments: an essential service. *Practice Nursing*, *31*(12), 516–519. https://doi.org/10.12968/pnur.2020.31.12.516.

PINNT. (2023). *Friendship and support for patients receiving artificial nutrition*. [Online] Available at https://pinnt.com/Home.aspx. [Accessed 21 April 2023].

Plewa, M. C., Bryant, M., & King-Thiele, R. (2021). *Euglycemic diabetic ketoacidosis*. [online] PubMed. Available at https://www.ncbi.nlm.nih.gov/books/NBK554570/.

Probst, S. (Ed.). (2021). *Wound care nursing: A person-centred approach* (3rd ed.) London: Elsevier Limited.

Public Health England. (2021). *Guidance. Wound aware: A resource for commissioners and providers of drug services*. Available from https://www.gov.uk/government/publications/wound-aware-a-resource-for-drug-services/wound-aware-a-resource-for-commissioners-and-providers-of-drug-services.

Pugh, J. D., McCoy, K., Williams, A. M., Bentley, B., & Monterosso, L. (2018). Rapid evidence assessment of approaches to community neurological nursing care for people with neurological conditions post-discharge from acute care hospital. *Health & Social Care in the Community, 27*(1), 43–54. https://doi.org/10.1111/hsc.12576.

Read, S., Hu, B., Wittenberg, R., Brimblecombe, N., Robinson, L., & Banerjee, S. (2021). A longitudinal study of functional unmet need among people with dementia. *Journal of Alzheimer's Disease, 84*(2), 705–716.

Robson, M. (2017). The squeezy pelvic floor muscle exercise app: User satisfaction survey. *Journal of Pelvic, Obstetric, and Gynaecological Physiotherapy, 121*, 64–68. Available at https://thepogp.co.uk/_userfiles/pages/files/11_14301024_0.pdf Accessed on 27.9.23.

Rockwood, K., Song, X., MacKnight, C., Bergman, H., Hogan, D. B., McDowell, I., & Mitnitski, A. (2005). A global clinical measure of fitness and frailty in elderly people. *CMAJ, 173*(5), 489–495.

Royal College of Nursing. (2021). *Catheter care: RCN guidance for healthcare professionals.* London: RCN.

Royal College of Nursing. (2023). RCN new definition of nursing background research and rationale. London: Royal College of Nursing.

Royal Pharmaceutical Society. (2011). *Supporting patients with chronic obstructive airways disease (COPD).* Available at https://www.rpharms.com/Portals/0/Documents/Old%20news%20documents/news%20downloads/copd-qrg-1-.pdf. [Accessed 18 July 2023].

Schmid-Mohler, G., Clarenbach, C., Brenner, G., Kohler, M., Horvath, E., Spielmanns, M., & Petry, H. (2020). Advanced nursing practice in COPD exacerbations: The solution for a gap in Switzerland? *ERJ Open Research*, 6, 00354-2019. https://doi.org/10.1183/23120541.00354-2019.

Schwinger, R. H. (2021). Pathophysiology of heart failure. *Cardiovascular Diagnosis & Therapy, 11*(1), 263–276.

Shlipak, M.G., Tummalapalli, S.L., Boulware, L.E., Grams, M.E., Ix, J.H., Jha, V., et al., & Conference Participants. (2021). The case for early identification and intervention of chronic kidney disease: Conclusions from a Kidney Disease: Improving Global Outcomes (KDIGO) Controversies Conference. *Kidney International, 99*(1), 34–47. https://doi.org/10.1016/j.kint.2020.10.012.

Sidawy, A. N., & Perler, B. A. (2022). *Rutherford's vascular surgery & endovascular therapy* (10th ed.). Elsevier.

Simpson, P. (2017). Long-term urethral catheterisation: Guidelines for community nurses. *British Journal of Nursing, 26*(9), S22–S26. Available at https://tinyurl.com/38dpujra Accessed on 10.10.23.

Smith, M., Clapham, L., & Strauss, K. (2017). UK lipohypertrophy interventional study. *Diabetes Research and Clinical Practice, 126*, 248–253. https://doi.org/10.1016/j.diabres.2017.01.020.

Social Care Institute of Excellence. (2020). *Dementia.* Available online https://www.scie.org.uk/dementia/about/.

Standl, E., Stevens, S. R., Lokhnygina, Y., Bethel, M. A., Buse, J. B., Gustavson, S. M., et al. (2019). Confirming the bidirectional nature of the association between severe hypoglycemic and cardiovascular events in type 2 diabetes: Insights from EXSCEL. *Diabetes Care, 43*(3), 643–652. https://doi.org/10.2337/dc19-1079. [online].

Stratton, I. M., Adler, A., Neil, A., Matthews, D., Manley, S., Cull, C., et al. (2000). Association of glycaemia with macrovascular and microvascular complications of type 2 diabetes (UKPDS 35): Prospective observational study. *BMJ, 321*(7258), 405–412. https://doi.org/10.1136/bmj.321.7258.405. [online].

Stroka, M. (2021). Psychosocial interventions for patients with dementia: Here's what works. *Neurology Advisor*. Available on line: https://www.neurologyadvisor.com/topics/alzheimers-disease-and-dementia/psychosocial-interventions-dementia-quality-of-life-cognitive-function/.

Strickland, K., & Baguley, F. (2015). The role of the community nurse in care provision for people with multiple sclerosis. *British Journal of Community Nursing*, *20*(1), 6–10. https://doi.org/10.12968/bjcn.2015.20.1.6.

Surrey Coalition for the Disabled (2023). https://surreycoalition.org.uk/

Swanson, T., Duynhoven, K., & Johnstone, D. (2019). Using the new T.I.M.E. Clinical Decision Support Tool to promote consistent holistic wound management and eliminate variation in practice at the Cambourne Medical Clinic, Australia: Part 1. *Wounds International*, *10*(2), 28–39.

Talley, K. M. C., Davis, N. J., Peden-McAlpine, C., Martin, C. L., Weinfurter, E. V., & Wyman, J. F. (2021). Navigating through incontinence: A qualitative systematic review and meta-aggregation of the experiences of family caregivers. *International Journal of Nursing Studies*, *123*, 1–12. Available at https://www.sciencedirect.com/science/article/abs/pii/S0020748921002091 Accessed on 25.9.23.

Taylor, R. S., Walker, S., Ciani, O., Warren, F., Smart, N. A., Piepoli, M., & Davos, C. H. (2019). Exercise-based cardiac rehabilitation for chronic heart failure: The EXTRAMATCH II individual participant data meta-analysis. *Health Technol Assess*, *23*(25), 1–98.

The Neurological Alliance. (2019). *Neuro numbers 2019*. [Accessed on 16.06.23]. Available at https://www.neural.org.uk/publication/mental-health-rightcare-pathways-proposal-2/.

The Primary Care Respiratory Society UK. (2016). Diagnosis and management of COPD in primary care. *Sutton Coldfield: PCRS-UK.*

The Primary Care Respiratory Society UK. (2017). *Right Care Pathway: COPD*. Available at https://www.england.nhs.uk/rightcare/wp-content/uploads/sites/40/2017/12/nhs-rightcare-copd-pathway-v18.pdf. [Accessed 18 July 2023].

Trueland, J. (2022). Good continence care: Tips for nurses working in any setting. *Nursing Standard*, *38*(9). Available at https://rcni.com/nursing-standard/newsroom/analysis/good-continence-care-tips-nurses-working-any-setting-187821. Accessed on 24.9.23.

Upton, D., & Upton, P. (2015). *Psychology of wounds and wound care in clinical practice*. London: Springer.

Vernooij-Dassen, M., Moniz-Cook, E., Verhey, F., Chattat, R., Woods, B., Meiland, F., et al. (2019). Bridging the divide between biomedical and psychosocial approaches in dementia research: the 2019 INTERDEM manifesto. *Aging and Mental Health*, *25*(2), 206–212.

Vestergaard, A. H. S., Sampson, E. L., Johnson, S. P., & Peterson, I. (2020). Social inequalities in life expectancy and mortality in people with dementia in the United Kingdom. *Alzheimer's Disease and Associated Disorders*, *34*(3), 254–261.

Wakefield, J. R. H., Bowe, M., Kellezi, B., Butcher, A., & Groeger, J. (2020). Longitudinal associations between family identification, loneliness, depression, and sleep quality. *British Journal of Health Psychology*, *25*(1), 1–16.

Wan, D., & Krassioukov, A. V. (2014). Life-threatening outcomes associated with autonomic dysreflexia: A clinical review. *The Journal of Spinal Cord Medicine*, *37*(1), 2–10. Available at https://tinyurl.com/bdft9xr9 Accessed on 24.10.23.

Wang, S., Quang, L., Chavorro, J., & Roberts, A. (2023). Depression, worry, and loneliness are associated with subsequent risk of hospitalization for COVID-19: A prospective study. *Psychological Medicine*, *53*(9), 4022–4031. https://doi.org/10.1017/S0033291722000691.

Watson, J., Giebel, C., Green, M., Darlington-Pollock, F., & Akpan, A. (2020). Use of routine and cohort data globally in exploring dementia care pathways and inequalities: A systematic review. *International Journal of Geriatric Psychiatry*, *36*, 252–270.

Waubant, E., Lucas, R., Mowry, E., Graves, J., Olsson, T., Alfredsson, L., & Langer-Gould, A. (2019). Environmental and genetic risk factors for MS: An integrated review. *Annals of Clinical and Translational Neurology*, *6*(9), 1905–1922. https://doi.org/10.1002/acn3.50862. Epub 2019 Aug 7. PMID: 31392849; PMCID: PMC6764632.

Wheatley, A., Bamford, C., Brunskill, G., Booi, L., Dening, K. H., Robinson, L., & on behalf of the PriDem study team. (2021). Implementing post diagnostic support for people living with dementia in England: a qualitative study to barriers and strategies used to address these in practice. *Age and Ageing*, *10*(50), 2230–2237.

Wheatley, A., Bamford, C., Brunskill, G., Dening, K. H., Allan, L., Rait, G., Robinson, L., & The PriDem Study project team. (2020). Task-shifted approaches to post diagnostic dementia support: a qualitative study exploring professional views and experiences. *British Medical Journal Open*, *10*:e040348.

Wheatley, A., Poole, M., Robinson, L., & on behalf of the PriDem study team. (2022). Changes to post diagnostic dementia support in England and Wales during the COVID-19 pandemic: A qualitative study. *British Medical Journal Open*, *12*:e059437.

Woodward, S. (2014). Community nursing and intermittent self-catheterisation. *British Journal of Community Nursing*, *19*(8), 388. p 390-393 Available at https://tinyurl.com/572psj3b Accessed on 10.10.23.

World Health Organisation. (2016). *What are neurological disorders?*. [Accessed on: 23/06/23]. Available at http://www.who.int/features/qa/55/en/.

World Health Organisation. (2017). *Atlas: Country resources for neurological disorders* (2nd ed.). [Accessed on 16.06.23]. Available at. https://www.who.int/publications/i/item/9789241565509.

World Health Organisation (WHO). (2020). *The top 10 causes of death*. Available at https://www.who.int/news-room/fact-sheets/detail/the-top-10-causes-of-death#:~:text=The%20top%20global%20causes%20of,birth%20asphyxia%20and%20birth%20trauma%2C. [Accessed 6 July 2023].

World Health Organisation. (2021). *Advocacy brief: Social isolation and loneliness*. Accessed at https://www.who.int/teams/social-determinants-of-health/demographic-change-and-healthy-ageing/social-isolation-and-loneliness.

World Health Organisation. (2023a). *Dementia*. Available online https://www.who.int/news-room/fact-sheets/detail/dementia.

World Health Organisation. (2023b). *Diabetes*. [online] World Health Organisation. Available at https://www.who.int/news-room/fact-sheets/detail/diabetes. [Accessed 27 December 2023].

Yates, A. (2019). Basic continence assessment: 'What community nurses should know'. *Journal of Community Nursing*, *33*(3), p52–55. Available at https://www.jcn.co.uk/journals/issue/06--2019/article/basic-continence-assessment-what-community-nurses-should-know Accessed on 24.9.23.

Yearby, R. (2021). Race based medicine, colorblind disease: How racism in medicine harms us all. *The American Journal of Bioethics*, *21*(2), 19–27. https://doi.org/10.1080/15265161.2020.1851811.

Zavodnik, J., Harley, C., Zabriskie, K., & Brahmbhatt, Y. (2020). Effect of a female external urinary catheter on incidence of catheter-associated urinary tract infection. *Cureus*, *12*(10):e1113. https://www.ncbi.nlm.nih.gov/pmc/articles/PMC7682542/ Accessed on 27.9.23.

CHAPTER 11

Mental Health in Community Nursing

Alyson Price ■ Maria Cozens

LEARNING OUTCOMES

After reading this chapter you should be able to:

- Gain a deeper understanding of the mental health impact on patients living with long-term conditions
- Appreciate the core skills required to effectively assess and support mental health needs for patients with long-term conditions
- Gain an understanding of the needs of patients who have a diagnosis of serious mental illness (SMI) presenting with comorbidities or multimorbidities in the community
- Understand the challenges of caring for the physical health needs of patients with a learning disability (LD)

11.1 The Mental Health Impact of Living With a Physical Long-Term Condition

11.1.1 INTRODUCTION

Healthcare professionals when providing effective care for chronic and long-term conditions (LTCs) must recognise the importance of mental health (Naylor et al., 2012). The government identified the importance of considering this in 'No Health Without Mental Health' (Department of Health (DH), 2011), identifying that people with LTCs are two to three times more likely to experience poor mental health compared to the general population. Almost one-third of those with LTCs also have a mental health problem, and the presence of a mental health problem not only complicates but also exacerbates a patient's physical condition by reducing adherence to treatment, reducing ability to manage their conditions and ultimately resulting in them spending more time in hospital, with poorer clinical outcomes and reduced quality of life (Nicol & Hollowood, 2023).

There is recognition that despite changes in nurse education raising awareness and encouraging parity of esteem (Nursing and Midwifery Council (NMC), 2018), it can be challenging and stressful to ensure that both the mental health and physical needs of the patients that are cared for are met. This section aims to provide an understanding of the issues patients are likely to face, the knowledge and skills required to assess those needs and how to build therapeutic relationships and refer on to additional services.

11.1.2 CONSIDERATIONS AND SKILLS FOR COMMUNITY NURSES

There are mental health services and specialists to refer to when there are concerns about a patient's mental health, well-being and safety to ensure they receive more in-depth support and assessment. However, there are certain skills and abilities all nurses should possess, no matter what field or specialism they are aligned to.

Depression and anxiety in particular are mental health conditions that are common features of many LTCs (Centre for Mental Health & National Voices, 2021; Naylor et al., 2012). Furthermore, suicidality is also linked to long-term chronic, painful conditions due to the impact on quality of life, economic stability, self-esteem, feelings of hopelessness, perceived burdensomeness and increased isolation/social disconnection (Rogers et al., 2021; Willard-Virant, 2021). It is therefore important not only to understand the symptoms and impact of depression and anxiety (see the following Reflection) but also, crucially, not to ignore them. To know how to engage with someone experiencing these symptoms, support them effectively and to know when they may need to seek more specialist support.

REFLECTION

Using the following documents:

- NICE (2022)—Depression in adults: treatment and management.
- NICE (2020)—Generalised anxiety disorder and panic disorder in adults: management.
- ICD-11—International Classification of Diseases 11th Revision: The global standard for diagnostic health information, https://icd.who.int/en.

Consider how you would recognise the symptoms of depression and anxiety in your patients and how you would support them.

In 2021, the Centre for Mental Health and National Voices published research regarding the impact of LTCs on mental health and the experiences of the care they received. The research also considered a patient's access to information and further mental health support, how they were supported to come to terms with the illness and its effects and their emotional and relational well-being. The research identified many barriers and system-wide issues to be addressed such as better continuity of care between services, support and advice between appointments, longer appointments, holistic health checks and integrated care systems. However, the overarching message was simple: show care and compassion in every interaction, reduce mental health stigma, signpost effectively and take every opportunity to ask about emotional well-being—'Ask Me How I Am' (Centre for Mental Health & National Voices, 2021).

11.1.3 BUILDING THERAPEUTIC RELATIONSHIPS

Peplau (1952/1991) identified that one of the most powerful tools that nurses have across all fields, and the foundation of everything they do, is the ability to communicate and build therapeutic relationships with patients.

DEFINITION OF UNCONDITIONAL POSITIVE REGARD

'UPR involves as much feeling of acceptance for the client's expression of negative, 'bad', painful, fearful, defensive, abnormal feelings as for his expression of 'good', positive, mature, confident, social feelings, as much acceptance of ways in which he is inconsistent as of ways in which he is consistent… It means caring for the client, but not in a possessive way or in such a way as simply to satisfy the therapist's own needs. It means caring for the client as a separate person, with permission to have his own feelings, his own experiences' (Rogers, 1957, p. 22).

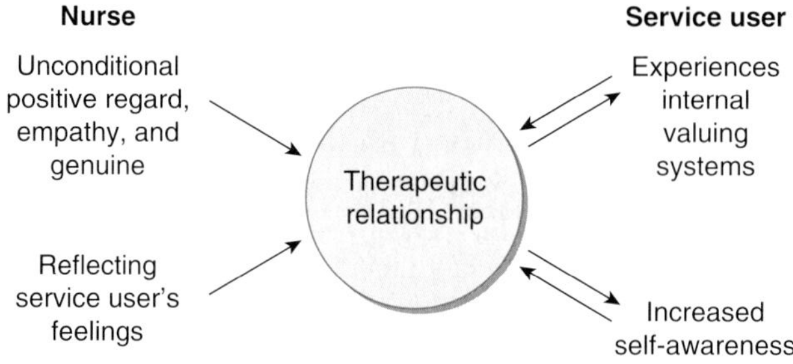

Fig. 11.1 Elements of therapeutic relationships.

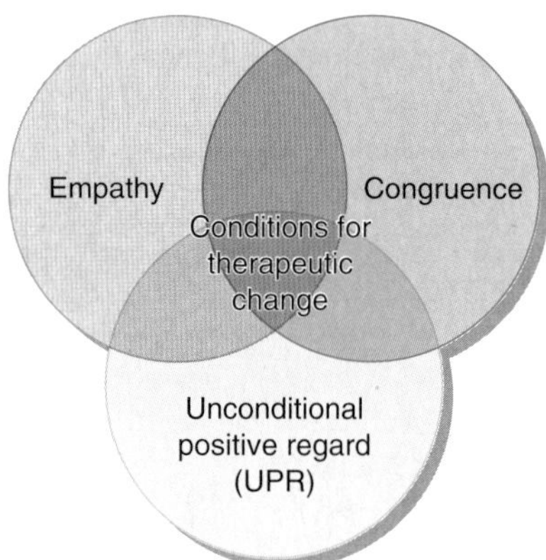

Fig. 11.2 Conditions for therapeutic change.

Further to this, Carl Rogers emphasised the need to look at the whole person and the uniqueness of each individual (McLeod, 2023). This approach and emphasis on empathy, unconditional positive regard (UPR) and active listening, authentic communication and understanding have significantly influenced how nurses develop interpersonal relationships, promote empathy and develop person-centred care. The value of this within building relationships and promoting therapeutic change is illustrated in Figs 11.1 and 11.2.

11.1.3.1 Showing Genuineness, Empathy and Listening to the Person

By demonstrating kindness, acceptance, warmth, nonjudgement and empathy, the patient–nurse relationship becomes one whereby trust replaces fear, gentleness replaces anger, clarity replaces bewilderment, connection replaces aloneness and caring replaces feelings of vulnerability (Gil, 2020).

The following may provide some guidance for community nurses when discussing mental health concerns with their patients.

- *Time and space* to communicate—thoughts, feelings and emotions can be difficult to relay, and patients may feel anxious, fearful and unsure about how this will be received (significant stigma still exists in relation to mental health despite numerous campaigns by the National Health Service (NHS) and third sector organisations).

- Show *congruence in communication* between the words that are used, tone and pitch of voice and nonverbal communication (body language and facial expression); think about eye contact. If the message is relayed through nonverbal communication and the tone is incongruent with the message being relayed verbally, the patient will repudiate what is being said and instead believe what the nonverbal communication is relaying.
- Listen to understand, do not listen to reply.
- *Active listening skills*—Listening which involves paying full attention to what is being relayed and demonstrating this through verbal and nonverbal communication.

It involves the aforementioned skills as well as:

- ✓ Not making judgements or taking a position
- ✓ Not interrupting
- ✓ Therapeutic use of silence to process and formulate thoughts on both sides of the interaction
- ✓ Make appropriate eye contact to show attention and utilise appropriate facial expressions—e.g., smile if it is appropriate
- ✓ Paraphrase or repeat what has been relayed—it checks understanding is accurate and shows the patient is being listened to
- ✓ Ask questions to clarify if required, or to allow for expansion
- ✓ Summarise
- ✓ If needed collaboratively problem-solve together

(Covey, 2020; Grande, 2020)

11.1.4 REFERRAL TO MENTAL HEALTH SERVICES

Different services are accessible via a range of referral pathways, and secondary services such as charities are also available, which provide invaluable advice and support (for example, 'Mind').

GP/primary care is a common referral route for mental health as it is often seen as the first point of contact within healthcare for many (even when acutely unwell), particularly if individuals already have a LTC diagnosed and are being supported. Most hospitals will also have a Psychiatric Liaison Team or Service to refer patients to if they are admitted.

NHS Talking Therapies are available and include counselling, cognitive behavioural therapy (CBT) and guided self-help. Referral to these services does not require an individual to have a diagnosed mental health problem or necessarily require a referral from a doctor or health professional as self-referral is accepted. The NHS 'Every Mind Matters' website also provides self-care tips to improve mental well-being.

High-risk individuals or those who may be acutely unwell should attend an emergency department (ED) for assessment or be referred to Common Point of Entry/Single Point of Access service for an urgent assessment.

Services for mental health are structured differently depending on the geographical area that the patient resides in, and different regions will have various types and levels of specialist services available depending on the needs of the population. An example is demonstrated in Fig. 11.3. All Mental Health Trusts will have a website that clearly identifies the services available in the region, how to access these services and actions to take including contact numbers for an emergency.

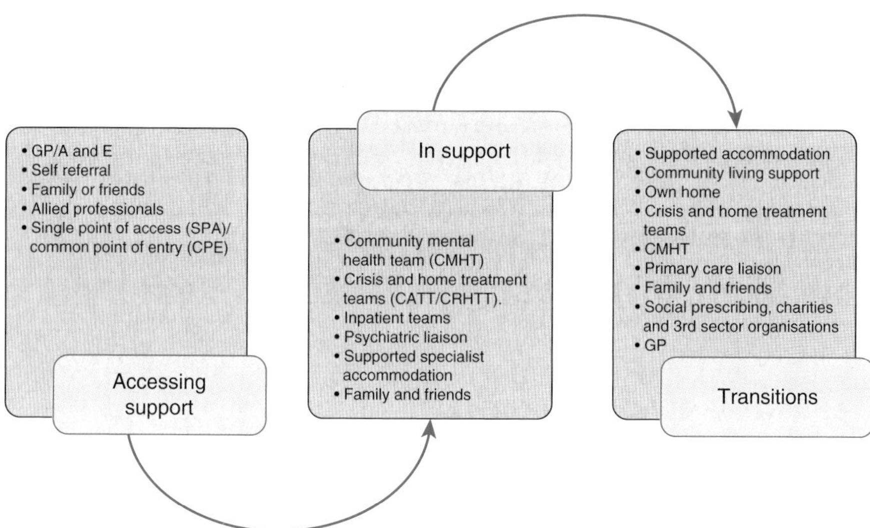

Fig. 11.3 Mental health services at different stages of care.

Once someone is engaged in services, there are a variety of services that may be provided either in hospital or at home and include general inpatient, specialist inpatient wards, supported living, rehabilitation placements, crisis resolution and home treatment teams (CRHTTs/crisis teams), assertive outreach teams (AOTs) and community mental health teams (CMHTs).

11.1.5 CONCLUSION

For effective care within community nursing, there is a need to work collaboratively and in a person-centred way with all patients. Build relationships, trust and rapport and take time to listen to every aspect of what the patient may be communicating. Ask them how they are and provide them with a safe environment in which to talk about how they are feeling, how their condition may be impacting them and work with them to find the solutions that best meet their needs. Show care and compassion in every interaction and take every opportunity to ask about the patient's emotional well-being.

11.2 Mental Illness and Concurrent Physical Health Issues

11.2.1 INTRODUCTION

Within the community nursing context, there will likely be a wide range of individuals with varying degrees of mental illness (MI). For contextual purposes and reflecting on the predominant subgroup, with the highest physical healthcare needs, this section will focus on individuals with severe mental illness (SMI). Community nurses are often at the forefront of holistic assessment and care delivery for individuals with both complex and often dual long-term physical and mental health diagnoses. The aim of this section is to focus on critical knowledge for working with individuals who have a diagnosis of SMI presenting with comorbidities or multimorbidities in the community.

DEFINITIONS

Mental health: According to the World Health Organization (2022), mental health is a 'state of mental well-being' in which people can cope with everyday (ambient) stress, understand their abilities, learn and develop whilst adding value to society.

Mental health problems: Mind (2017) describes mental health problems as 'common and normal experiences'; again, there is a spectrum of challenges from, for example, mild depression and anxiety to more specific and longer-term mental health problems such as bipolar and schizophrenia, which fall into our next category of SMI.

Serious mental illness (SMI): refers to individuals with psychological challenges that are often so debilitating that their ability to engage in functional or occupational activities is severely impaired (DH, 2018).

11.2.2 BACKGROUND AND CONTEXT

It is vital to conceptualise the broad spectrum of mental health challenges to gain a better understanding of the various difficulties people may experience, which can depend on a wide range of variables. The mental health spectrum (MHS) offers insight into the vast array of challenges that one can experience. The MHS aims to positively reframe mental health and mental illness through a more positive lens, suggesting that mental health represents a 'spectrum of experiences' ranging from excellent mental health on one end to more severe and enduring functional impairment at the other end.

11.2.3 PRINCIPLE STATISTICS

Within the sphere of general MI, it is broadly accepted that one in four people will experience some type of mental health issue each year (Mind, 2020). Data also suggest that one in six people will experience a mental health issue in any given week (McManus et al., 2016). A recent study by the Office of National Statistics (2022) suggested that 1 in 6 adults over the age of 16 reported moderate to severe depression symptoms. Approximately 1 in 5 people will experience suicidal thoughts in their lifetime, 1 in 14 people will engage in self-harm and approximately 1 in 15 people attempt suicide (Mind, 2020). Within the SMI category, current prevalence rates of schizophrenia suggest that it affects 1 in 300 people worldwide (0.32%) (Institute of Health Metrics and Evaluation (IHME), 2019). People with schizophrenia are likely to die two to three times earlier than the general population (Laursen et al., 2014). Statistics relating to bipolar disorder suggest that in the year of 2019, approximately 40 million people worldwide had a diagnosis (IHME, 2019).

11.2.4 HEALTH DISPARITIES

Despite efforts on multiple fronts including government policy, guidelines and public health approaches, people with SMI continue to experience 15 to 20 years shorter life expectancy than the general population (Thornicroft, 2013). This is related to a wide range of variables such as access to services, psychoactive medications, limited education and occupational opportunities. Evidence suggests that the life expectancy gap has not improved; conversely, some research is indicative of a widening gap (Royal College of Nursing, 2018). Research shows that people with SMI are more likely to experience lifestyle-related conditions such as respiratory, circulatory and digestive disorders in comparison to the general population (Gamble & Brennan, 2023).

11.2.5 PARITY OF ESTEEM

One of the core working frameworks within current health policies is centred around placing equal importance between mental health and physical health or parity of esteem (Department of Health, 2011). Parity of esteem has evolved since its initial introduction in 2012; the current meaning is to describe a range of approaches taken to redress gaps between physical and mental health issues.

11.2.6 ASSESSMENT APPROACHES

Coupland, cited in Gamble and Brennan (2023, p. 111), suggests that the provision of good physical healthcare for people with SMI should always have a multidisciplinary approach. It should adopt a public health approach inclusive of health promotion and health education. In addition, Coupland, cited in Gamble and Brennan (2023, p. 112), suggested that professional curiosity should be central to any assessment conducted when working with individuals with complex presentations. Engel's (1977) biopsychosocial model of assessment continues to provide the most comprehensive framework for conceptualisation of challenging presentations. This involves looking at any biological markers of ill health, an exploration of the psychological factors and finally any social elements which are impacting on the person.

11.2.7 MAKE EVERY CONTACT COUNT

Working in a community nursing role offers a unique opportunity to support individuals with complex needs. The public health initiative of Make Every Contact Count (MECC) (National Institute for Health and Care Excellence (NICE), 2019) is especially applicable within the context of supporting individuals with SMI through encouraging and/or facilitating health behavioural changes that may be having an impact on the individual's well-being. Reference to Prochaska et al.'s (1993) Transtheoretical Model of Behaviour Change is critical here in staging one's readiness for change. Finally, within any healthcare episode, there is the opportunity to positively influence the individual's ability to access and receive equitable care utilising The Equality Act (2010).

11.2.8 TRAUMA-INFORMED CARE PRINCIPLES

'Trauma results from an event, series of events, or set of circumstances that is experienced by an individual as harmful or life threatening' (Office for Health Improvement and Disparities, 2022). It is both unique to the individual who has experienced this and can have a lasting and significant impact on all aspects of a person's well-being.

Trauma-informed care (TIC) has received increased traction in recent years in response primarily to the recognition of the strong correlation between trauma and the development of long-term mental health issues (Musket, 2014). TIC principles are starting to expand and permeate many health and social care policies. Trauma is complex and has many variables; however, working within the core principles of a trauma informed approach for all can enable a more inclusive and proactive approach (Collin-Vézina et al., 2020). Originally, the principles of TIC emerged from the US Substance Abuse and Mental Health Services Administration (SAM-HAS).

The following highlight the six core principles towards delivering a TIC within day-to-day care delivery:

1. Trustworthiness and transparency
2. Security and safety
3. Peer support and empowerment
4. Collaborating and mutuality
5. Empowerment and choice
6. Culturally informed and responsive service offer

11.2.8.1 Be Trauma Informed

It may not be the responsibility to treat the trauma-related problems that would be the remit of specialist trauma services, however, there are ways in which you can be trauma-informed in your practice:

- Recognise that trauma can impact a person, group or community in many different ways—including physiologically, psychologically and socially and ensure our healthcare interventions are cognisant of that.
- Understanding and recognising the signs and symptoms of trauma and providing services which are sensitive to the needs of those individuals.
- Avoid retraumatisation: retriggering previous trauma and thoughts, feelings and sensations which might have been experienced at the time; reminders of previous trauma by events/situation(s) which may or may not be traumatic in themselves.

CASE STUDY 11.1

Rose is a 45-year-old female with a diagnosis of paranoid schizophrenia and type 2 diabetes. During and post the peak of the COVID-19 pandemic, Rose had been finding managing her physical and mental healthcare needs increasingly challenging. Rose was discharged by her local Community Mental Health team 6 years ago following a period of mental health stability, although she remains open for a 6 month psychiatry review.

Rose does not attend her GP surgery frequently and feels she can 'manage her own health'. Rose has one sister, Neha, who helps when she can. Rose has been on 15 mg of olanzapine for over 10 years for the management of her schizophrenia. She was diagnosed with type 2 diabetes 5 years ago which was detected incidentally following admission for a broken arm. Rose is currently prescribed metformin 500 mg, three times a day.

Rose had a recent visit to the accident and ED for a wound on her leg; the hospital referred Rose to the community nursing service for monitoring of a diabetic leg ulcer and for being housebound for wound management support.

During the first home visit, the community nurse explored how the leg ulcer developed using TIC principles exploring Roses' current understanding of her type 2 diabetes diagnosis and management. Through conversation and exploration, it is clear that Rose does not understand her type 2 diabetes diagnosis and also does not understand the significance of taking her diabetes medication at the prescribed time.

The community nurse makes a referral to the local authority for an Urgent Care and Support Needs Assessment for social support (under the Social Care Act, 2012). The community team also contact Rose's community mental health team requesting a mental health review. A blister pack for ease of medication management is requested via Rose's local pharmacy. The community nurse arranges with Neha to support Rose with her medication management for the present time. An SMI review (annual health review) is requested between Rose and her GP. Finally, the community nursing team will continue to visit Rose regularly for wound management support.

REFLECTION

- How would you assess a person's knowledge of their LTC? Would you know who to contact?
- Have you heard of the term Urgent Care and Support Needs Assessments?
- Where would you be able to gather this information?
- Do you know how to contact the community mental health nurses in your area?

11.2.9 CONCLUSION

It is evident that community nurses have a vital role in supporting the physical health needs of individuals with SMI in the community. There are core approaches such as the use of MECC and TIC which can be utilised within any care context but are of notable help in the context of supporting complex multimorbidity issues within the SMI population. Putting the person at the centre of their care is an ever-important guiding principle as well as retaining a multidisciplinary and partnership focused approach.

11.3 Learning Disabilities: Key Considerations for Community Nurses

11.3.1 INTRODUCTION

Working in partnership with individuals with learning disabilities (LDs), their families and carers is a critical part of the role of the community nurse. Community nurses hold a unique position to identify, assess and escalate health-related issues for the LD population. The principles of Make Every Contact Count (DH, 2016) should be at the forefront of any healthcare professional. However, with the LD population, it has perhaps even more reverence given the ongoing life health disparities and marked reduced life expectancy rates (University of Bristol Norah Fry Centre for Disability Studies, 2017).

DEFINITION

One of the most used definitions in the UK today remains as one that was produced by the Department of Health in 2001. It provides an overview of the three key areas in which people with LDs can experience challenges. It is defined as follows: 'a significantly reduced ability to understand new or complex information, to learn new skills (impaired intelligence), with a reduced ability to cope independently (impaired social functioning) which started before adulthood, with a lasting development' (DH, 2001, p. 14).

11.3.2 STATISTICS

In the UK, current numbers suggest that there are approximately 1.5 million individuals living with a LD; a breakdown of the numbers suggests that there are approximately 1.2 million adults and approximately 300,000 children (Office of National Statistics, 2020). The word approximate is of significance here, and it is widely accepted that many people in the community could meet the LD definition, however, have not been through the diagnostic process for a number of reasons.

11.3.3 CONCEPTUAL APPROACHES

Broadly speaking, there are two main conceptual approaches in operation within the LD field, namely, the medical model of disability and the social model of disability, the latter highlighting current contemporary approaches.

The medical model of disability focuses on what is 'wrong with the person' and as such how this can be 'fixed'. It is important to state that this is an outdated approach; however, this approach does still appear to covertly resonate in some parts of healthcare to the present day. The social model of disability emerged from the Fundamental Principles of Disability, a document first published in 1976 (Union of the Physically Impaired Against Segregation (UPIAS), 1976), which argued that people are not disabled by their impairments but the disabling barriers within society (Oliver, 2013). Barriers faced by individuals with disabilities such as physical, social and economic, place limitations on one's ability to fully participate in society (Northway, 1998). The overarching premise of the Social Model of Disability is that the system should flex and adapt to meet the needs of the individual.

11.3.4 CLASSIFICATION OF LEARNING DISABILITIES

An LD can broadly be classified into two main categories: genetic or environmental (Gates & Mafuba, 2016). Genetic causes tend to occur predominantly at the point of conception or within early foetal development. Environmental causes could include a range of variables which could affect foetal development in the preconceptual, perinatal or postnatal time periods. It is also widely accepted that in some cases, the cause of LD may be unknown (Gates & Mafuba, 2016).

11.3.5 DEGREE OF LEARNING DISABILITY

A brief note on the degree of LD is paramount to the understanding and approaches within community nursing. Intelligence testing is a contentious area of debate; however, to understand some of the parameters from a community nursing context, it can be beneficial (Box 11.1).

11.3.6 HEALTH DISPARITIES

It is widely accepted that people with LD experience health disparities at a higher rate than the general population (McMahon & Hatton, 2020). People with LD experience increased rates of respiratory disease, sensory impairments and epilepsy (Emerson & Baines, 2011). One of the core disparities remains in life expectancy, standing currently at between 15 and 20 years earlier for people with LD when compared to the general population (O'Leary et al., 2018; University of Bristol Norah Fry Centre for Disability Studies, 2017). People with LD also experience increased morbidities and increased incidence of hospital admissions compared to the general population (Wilson & Charnock, 2017). One of the most prevalent and recurrent barriers affecting health disparities within the LD population is that of access to timely and appropriate healthcare (McCormick et al., 2020). Many reports have identified challenges in accessing healthcare such as the Mencap (2007) 'Death by Indifference', followed by the Michael Inquiry

BOX 11.1 ■ Definitions of Learning Disability

The World Health Organization (1992) classifies the degree of LD in accordance with the distance one moves away from the normal IQ for the general population.

IQ of 71–84 is indicative of borderline learning disability (not eligible for LD services)

IQ of 50–69 is indicative of a mild LD (eligible for LD services, likely have care and support needs, possibly living independently)

IQ of 35–59 is indicative of a moderate LD (eligible for LD services, highly likely to have care and support needs, likely to need supervised accommodation)

IQ of 20–34 is indicative of a severe LD (eligible for LD services, will have care and support needs and will require 24/7 supervision)

IQ of >20 refers to individuals with an IQ which is likely to be >20 with complex additional disabilities. Individuals who fall within this category can present with complex needs requiring 24/7 support to ensure that activities of daily living are achieved and maintained

in 2008 (Michael, 2008). In 2013 a report commissioned to explore the causative factors in the premature deaths of people with LD found delayed diagnoses and timely referrals to secondary care to be a major issue (Heslop et al., 2013). This report also found challenges in terms of healthcare staff failing to implement reasonable adjustments under The Equality Act (2010).

11.3.7 THE MENTAL CAPACITY ACT

Within the context of The Mental Capacity Act (2005), one must always start from the positions where one assumes that the person has capacity. Healthcare staff have a legal duty to assess capacity should any queries arise during their interactions to obtain informed consent where possible (The Mental Capacity Act, 2005). From complex investigations/treatments, capacity assessments will require a multidisciplinary approach and should include the person with a LD, next of kin, family members, any formal/informal carers and care team where applicable. In the absence of family members or next of kin, a referral to an independent mental capacity advocate (IMCA) should be considered, who can advocate on the service user's behalf where required or appropriate (MCA, 2005).

11.3.8 DIAGNOSTIC OVERSHADOWING

Any commentary when reflecting on the needs of people with LD would not be complete without exploring the concept of diagnostic overshadowing. Diagnostic overshadowing is a phenomenon where a possible physical or psychological emerging issue is credited to the person's LD, resulting in delayed diagnosis and subsequent treatment being offered (Ali et al., 2013). In the LD population, the individual may not present with clear signs and symptoms in a traditional sense; instead, they may present with behavioural changes and a presentation that is outside of their usual baseline. It is vital to explore and rule out any potential physical health issues first, then move to potential psychological as well as social care needs (Javaid, 2019). Community nurses are in a prime position to observe these presentations and raise concerns and escalate through their usual pathways.

CASE STUDY 11.2

Tom is a 35-year-old male with profound LD residing in a residential care home. He has complex additional needs inclusive of autism, behaviours that challenge and a visual impairment in his left eye. Tom has no verbal communication; however, he can communicate through nonverbal methods through eye contact and an augmented form of Makaton. Tom can mobilise with support of one staff either side. Tom had a complex childhood and was taken into care at the age of 6 when his parents expressed that they could no longer manage his needs. Tom started head-banging at the age of 4 and as such he wears a helmet to the present day to minimise the impact. Tom enjoys going out for drives with staff, loves cups of tea and has a healthy and varied diet. Tom has a mental health diagnosis of depression and anxiety. Tom has tried many medications over the years and is currently on olanzapine 10 mg (BD), 2 mg diazepam (TDS). Over time, Tom's presentation in terms of challenging behaviour has escalated to include skin picking and punching himself in the head, which resulted in a number of open wounds on his body. This resulted in Tom requiring 2:1 staffing for his personal safety. Recently, Tom started to refuse food and fluids; Tom is also presenting as more distressed and as such the incidents of head-banging and skin picking have intensified. This has resulted in a recent hospital admission for possible sepsis (wound related). Tom is now back in the care home and a referral has been made to community nurse for wound management and review.

REFLECTION

- Do you regularly visit residential care homes registered for people with a LD?
- Do you have LD-specific training?
- What would be your priorities for Tom's care?
- Where would you look to help guide your decision-making?

There are a number of areas where the community nurse can support the care home in addressing Tom's needs holistically.

- Provision of person-centred care, talk to Tom as an individual, speak to the staff to take a history, try to get a baseline of Tom's usual presentation and what has recently changed.
- Speak to family members, next of kin, friends, formal and informal carers.
- Utilise the principles of collaborative decision-making (NICE, 2021).
- Consider The Equality Act (2010); consider what reasonable adjustments the individual requires to access primary/secondary care including diagnostic tests/treatment to rule out a potential biological issue.
- Check current support plans such as care plan, hospital passport, communication passport.
- Check if Tom is known to the local community LD team, and if not, make a referral where required.
- Check with residential home staff to see if Tom has attended his annual health check; if not, can this be arranged and what adjustments might be required.
- Check if Tom has an allocated social worker; consider if a needs assessment review from Social Care is needed (Health and Social Care Act, 2012).
- Consider if Tom's needs can be met though his current accommodation, for example, does he need regular nursing care due to his physical health needs?

- Review notes where possible from primary care inclusive of hospital admissions.
- For any decision specifics relating to treatment complete a Capacity Assessment.
- Consider referrals to other relevant healthcare professionals such as dietician or occupational therapist.
- Present Tom's case within team meetings, any complex case presentations forums and within Integrated Care Network meetings/forum.

11.3.9 CONCLUSION

Community nurses have critical expertise in taking a considered holistic approach to meeting complex needs. Community nurses have excellent communication and teamworking skills which can foster and develop positive working relationships with LD staff and/or family members to provide optimum support for the LD population. For people with LD, community nurses can make use of and understand some of the soft signs of deterioration using their knowledge and experience as part of the clinical decision-making process. Overall, community nurses play a vital role in enhancing the quality of care and quality of life for people with LD.

References

Ali, A., Scior, K., Ratti, V., et al. (2013). Discrimination and other barriers to accessing health care: perspectives of patients with mild and moderate intellectual disability and their carers. *PLoS One*, *8*(8):e70855.

Centre for Mental Health & National Voices. (2021). *'Ask me how I am'.* https://www.nationalvoices.org.uk/project/ask-how-i-am/.

Collin-Vézina, D., Brend, D., & Beeman, I. (2020). When it counts the most: trauma-informed care and the COVID-19 global pandemic. *Developmental Child Welfare.*

Covey, S. (2020). *The 7 habits of highly effective people* (30th ed.). UK: Simon & Schuster.

Department of Health. (2001). *Valuing people: A new strategy for learning disability for the 21st Century.* London: The Stationary Office. CM5086.

Department of Health. (2011). *No health without mental health: A cross-government mental health outcomes strategy for people of all ages.* London: UK Government. Available at: https://assets.publishing.service.gov.uk/media/5a7c348ae5274a25a914129d/dh_124058.pdf.

Department of Health. (2016). *Making every contact count (MECC): Consensus statement.* Available at: https://www.england.nhs.uk/wp-content/uploads/2016/04/making-every-contact-count.pdf.

Department of Health (DH). (2018). *Severe mental illness and physical health in equalities (briefing).* GOV.UK. https://www.gov.uk/government/publications/severe-mental-illness-smi-physical-health-inequalities/severe-mental-illness-and-physical-health-inequalities-briefing.

Emerson, E., & Baines, S. (2011). Health inequalities and people with learning disabilities in the UK. Tizard Learning Disability Review, 16(1), 42–48. https://doi.org/10.5042/tldr.2011.0008.

Engel, G. L. (1977). The need for a new medical model: A challenge for biomedicine. *Science*, *196*, 129–136.

Gil, T. (2020). The therapeutic relationship: Its importance to healing and resiliency. *Psychology Today*. Online at: https://www.psychologytoday.com/intl/blog/breaking-the-silence/202012/the-therapeutic-relationship.

Gamble, C., & Brennan, G. (2023). *Working with serious mental illness: A manual for clinical practice* (3rd ed.). London: Elsevier.

Gates, B., & Mafuba, K. (2016). *Learning disability nursing – Modern day practice.* CRC Press – Taylor and Francis Group.

Grande, D. (2020). Active listening skills: Why active listening is important and how to do it. *Psychology Today*. Online at: https://www.psychologytoday.com/us/blog/in-it-together/202006/active-listening-skills.

Heslop, P., Blair, P., Fleming, R., Houghton, M., Marriot, A., & Russ, L. (2013). Confidential inquiry into the deaths of people with learning disabilities. https://www.bristol.ac.uk/media-library/sites/cipold/migrated/documents/fullfinalreport.pdf.

ICD-11 – International Classification of Diseases 11th Revision: The global standard for diagnostic health information. (2022). https://icd.who.int/en.

Institute of Health Metrics and Evaluation. (2019). *Global Health Data Exchange (GHDx)*. https://vizhub.healthdata.org/gbd-results/.

Javaid, A., Nakata, V., & Michael, D. (2019). Diagnostic overshadowing in learning disability: Think beyond the disability. *Prog. Neurology Psychiatry*, *23*, 8–10. https://doi-org.roe.idm.oclc.org/10.1002/pnp.531.

Laursen, T. M., Nordentoft, M., & Mortensen, P. B. (2014). Excess early mortality in schizophrenia. *Annual Review of Clinical Psychology*, *10*, 425–438.

McLeod, S. (2023). *Carl Rogers humanistic theory and contribution to psychology*. Online at: https://www.simplypsychology.org/carl-rogers.html.

McCormick, F., Marsh, L., Taggart, L., & Brown, M. (2020). Experiences of adults with intellectual disabilities accessing acute hospital services: A systematic review of the international evidence. *Health and Social Care in the Community*, *29*, 1222–1232. https://doi-org.roe.idm.oclc.org/10.1111/hsc.13253.

McMahon, M., & Hatton, C. (2020). A comparison of the prevalence of health problems among adults with and without intellectual disabilities: A total administrative population study. *Journal of Applied Research in Intellectual Disabilities*, *34*, 316–325. https://doi-org.roe.idm.oclc.org/10.1111/jar.12785.

McManus, S., Bebbington, P., Jenkins, R., & Brugha, T. (Eds.). (2016). *Mental health and wellbeing in England: Adult psychiatric morbidity survey 2014*. Leeds: NHS Digital.

Mencap. (2007). *Death by Indifference. 2006. 423 report*. https://www.mencap.org.uk/sites/default/files/2016-07/DBIreport.pdf.

Michael, J. (2008). *Healthcare for all: The Independent Inquiry into access to healthcare for people with LD. Healthcare for all: Report of the Independent Inquiry into access to healthcare for people with learning disabilities*. London: Department of Health.

Mind. (2017). Understanding mental health problems. Available at: https://www.mind.org.uk/media-a/2942/mental-health-problems-introduction-2017.pdf.

Mind. (2020). Mental health information. What are mental health problems? *Mind*.

Musket, C. (2014). Trauma-informed care in inpatient mental health settings: A review of the literature. *International Journal of Mental Health Nursing*, *23*(1), 51–59.

NICE. (2019). *Making every contact count. How NICE resources can support local priorities. Making every contact count for physical activity in musculoskeletal outpatient physiotherapy: A service improvement project to implement NICE public health guidance PH44*. NICE.

NICE. (2020). *Generalised anxiety disorder and panic disorder in adults: Management*. NICE.

NICE. (2021). *Shared decision making*. NICE. https://www.nice.org.uk/guidance/ng197.

NICE. (2022). *Depression in adults: treatment and management*. NICE.

Nicol, J., & Hollowood, l. (2023). *Nursing adults with long term conditions* (4th ed.). UK: SAGE Publications Ltd.

Naylor., C., Parsonage, M., McDaid, D., Knapp, M., Fossey, M., & Galea, A. (2012). *Long-term conditions and mental health: The cost of co-morbidities*. King's Fund.

Northway, R. (1998). Disability and oppression: Some implications for nurses and nursing. *Journal of Advanced Nursing*, *26*, 736–743. https://doi-org.roe.idm.oclc.org/10.1046/j.1365-2648.1997.00727.x.

Nursing and Midwifery Council (NMC). (2018). *Future nurse: Standards of proficiency for registered nurses*. London: NMC.

Office for Health Improvement and Disparities. (2022). *Guidance: Working definition of trauma-informed practice*. Pub: UK Government. Online at: https://www.gov.uk/government/publications/working-definition-of-trauma-informed-practice/working-definition-of-trauma-informed-practice.

Office of National Statistics. (2020). *Home*. ons.gov.uk.

Office of National Statistics (ONS). (2022). Cost of living and depression in adults. *Great Britain: 29th September to 23rd of October. Office for National Statistics*. https://www.ons.gov.uk/peoplepopulationandcommunity/healthandsocialcare/mentalhealth/articles/costoflivinganddepressioninadultsgreatbritain/29septemberto23october2022#:~:text=The%20following%20information%20is%20for,%2Dpandemic%20levels%20(10%25).

O'Leary, L., Cooper, S. A., & Hughes McCormack, L. (2018). Early death and causes of death of people with intellectual disabilities: A systematic review. *Journal of Applied Research in Intellectual Disabilities*, *31*(3), 325–342. https://doi-org.roe.idm.oclc.org/10.1111/jar.12417.

Oliver, M. (2013). The Social Model of Disability: Thirty years on. *Disability & Society*, *28*(7), 1024–1026. https://doi.org/10.1080/09687599.2013.818773.

Peplau, H.E. (1952/1991). Interpersonal relations in nursing. New York: Putnam.

Prochaska, J. O., DiClemente, C. C., Velicer, W. F., & Rossi, J. S. (1993). Standardized, individualized, interactive, and personalized self-help programs for smoking cessation. *Health Psychology*, *12*(5), 399–405. https://doi.org/10.1037/0278-6133.12.

Rogers, C. R. (1957). The necessary and sufficient conditions of therapeutic personality change. *Journal of Consulting Psychology*, *21*(2), 95.

Rogers, M. L., Joiner, T. E., & Golan, S. (2021). Suicidality in chronic illness: an overview of cognitive-affective and interpersonal factors. *Journal of Clinical Psychology in Medical Settings*, *28*(1), 137–148.

Royal College of Nursing. (2018). Literature review: Scoping selected literature on the role of the mental health nursing on improving the physical health care of clients diagnosed with severe mental illness. *Clinical Professional Resource*.

The Equality Act. (2010). *Equality act 2010: guidance. GOV.UK*. https://www.gov.uk/guidance/equality-act-2010-guidance#:~:text=Equality%20Act%20provisions%20which%20came,work%2C%20education%2C%20associations%20and%20transport.

The Mental Capacity Act. (2005). *Mental capacity act 2005*. https://www.legislation.gov.uk/ukpga/2005/9/contents.

Thornicroft, G. (2013). Premature death among people with mental illness. *British Medical Journal (BMJ)*, *346*.

UPIAS. (1976). *Fundamental principles of disability*. London: Union of the Physically Impaired Against Segregation. https://www.google.com/url?sa=t&rct=j&q=&esrc=s&source=web&cd=6&ved=0ahUKEwjumbfclI3QAhXsCcAKHQuKCCoQFgg4MAU&url=https%3A%2F%2Ftonybaldwinson.files.wordpress.com%2F2014%2F06%2F1975-11-22-upias-and-disability-alliance-fundamental-principles-of-disability.pdf&usg=AFQjCNFse9ckEOTWZ2bdoxP_3Fo4b9-1Kw. (Accessed 19 February 2017). [Google Scholar].

University of Bristol Norah Fry Centre for Disability Studies. (2017). *The Learning Disabilities Mortality Review (LeDeR) Programme. Annual report*. London: Healthcare Improvement Quality Partnership.

Willard-Virant, K. (2021). Suicide and chronic illness: Risks, interventions and hope. *Psychology Today*. Online at: https://www.psychologytoday.com/gb/blog/chronically-me/202109/suicide-and-chronic-illness.

Wilson, N. J., & Charnock, D. (2017). Developmental and intellectual disability. In E. Chang, & A. Johnson (Eds.), *Living with chronic illness and disability: Principles of nursing practice* (3rd ed.) (pp. 129–145). Elsevier.

World Health Organization. (1992). The ICD-10 classification of mental and behavioural disorders: Clinical descriptions and diagnostic guidelines. Geneva: World Health Organization.

World Health Organization. (2022). *World mental health report: Transforming mental health for all.* https://www.developmentaid.org/api/frontend/cms/file/2023/07/9789240049338-eng.pdf.

CHAPTER 12

Palliative Care by Community Nurses

Karen Heggs ■ Samantha Rose ■ Vanessa Heaslip

LEARNING OUTCOMES

After reading this chapter you should be able to:

- Have an awareness of palliative care and the role of community nurses
- Understand current policy and practice drivers leading palliative care practice
- Reflect upon personal knowledge and skills in managing people living with and dying of life-limiting illnesses within a multiprofessional team

12.1 Introduction

Palliative care is a holistic approach to care for people who are living with a life-limiting illness. The World Health Organization (WHO, 2023) definition focuses on the importance of quality of life for people with a life-limiting illness and those close to them. They state that palliative care 'prevents and relieves suffering through the early identification, impeccable assessment and treatment of pain and other problems, whether physical, psychosocial, or spiritual'.

In 2004, National Institute for Clinical Excellence (NICE) now called National Institute for Health and Care Excellence identified that general palliative care is the responsibility of all practitioners, in the provision of symptom management and holistic care. Access to specialist palliative care services is essential when the needs of the person and their family are complex and all avenues have been exhausted in general care delivery, assuring a rapid response to the needs of people as their illness progresses (National Palliative and End of Life Care Partnership, 2021). It can be challenging to identify when to recommend palliative care as a care option, due to the variation in trajectories in illness and the possibility of multiple comorbidities. Each illness has its unique and often complex trajectory that can make planning of care challenging. But understanding the general process of illness can be a starting point. Lynn and Adamson (2003) developed an overview of the three main illness processes of decline depicted in Fig. 12.1, which have been used to support the gradual development of tools to support palliative care delivery.

12.2 Personal Choices at End of Life

Meier et al. (2016) conducted a literature review of 36 studies to identify principles of a good death and identified 11 core themes (Table 12.1). It is evident that a good death is

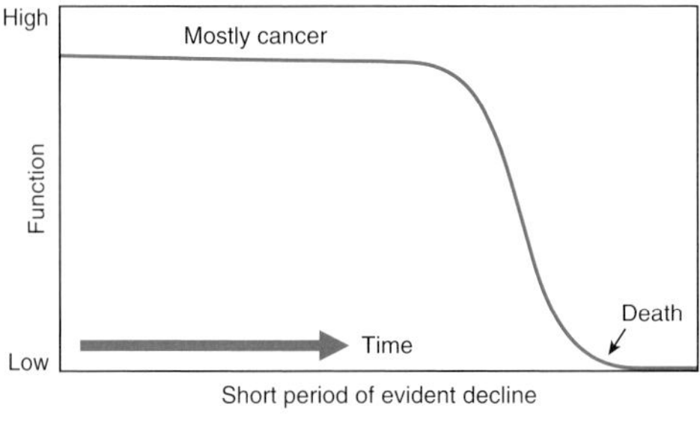

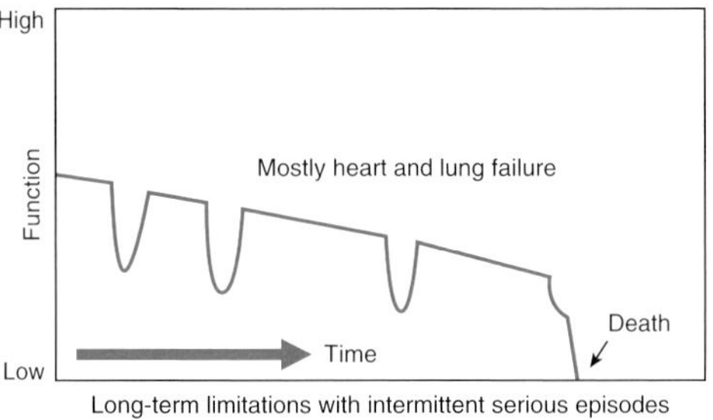

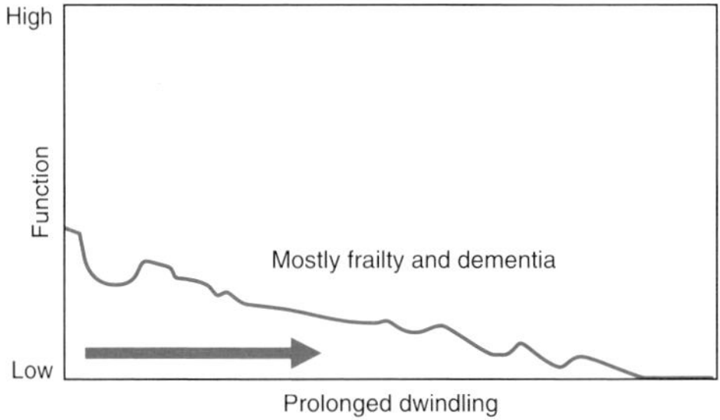

Fig. 12.1 Trajectories of chronic illness. (From Lynn, J., & Adamson, D. M. (2003). Living well at the end of life: Adapting health care to serious chronic illness in old age. https://www.rand.org/content/dam/rand/pubs/white_papers/2005/WP137.pdf.)

a multifaceted process which concerns the past, present and the future. To ensure that a good death is met requires skilled management and oversight and is a large role of the community nurses' caseload (Robinson et al., 2023).

Community nurses do not work in isolation and are supported by general practitioners (GPs) and specialist palliative care services. However, in the UK, it is estimated that over 100,000 people die without access to palliative care services (Hospice UK, 2017, cited in UK Parliament Post, 2022), including deaths in hospitals and community settings. This shortfall is likely to increase with the demand for palliative care services from 25%–47% by 2040 (Etkind et al., 2017) due to an ageing population and increased multimorbidity. Research into community nurses' experiences of managing palliative care at home identified that they find it a rewarding but stressful and demanding aspect of their role (Midlöv & Lindberg, 2020).

TABLE 12.1 **Principles of a Good Death**

Principle	**This Included**
Preferences for the dying process	Preparation, location of death and who was present
Pain free status	Not suffering, pain and symptom management
Emotional well-being	Emotional and psychological support as well as opportunities to discuss death
Family	Family acceptance, preparation for death as well as family support and desire not to be a burden
Dignity	Both respect as an individual as well as retaining independence
Life completion	Chance to say goodbye, accepting one's death and recognition of a good life
Religiosity/spirituality	Opportunities for religious and spiritual comfort
Treatment preference	No prolonging life, control of treatment options, both a belief that all treatments were used but also euthanasia
Quality of life	Living whilst dying and enjoying life
Relationship with healthcare professional	Having trust and professional support, opportunities to discuss fears and beliefs
Other	Cultural sensitivity and importance of touch, pets and costs associated with dying

(Adapted from Meier, E., Gallegos, J., Montross-Thomas, L., Depp, C., Irwin, S., & Jeste, D. (2016). Defining a good death (successful dying): Literature review and a call for research and public dialogue. *American Journal of Psychiatry, 24*(4), 261–271.)

REFLECTION

Please consider the following statements and self-assess your skills and confidence in each of these from 0 (no confidence) to 5 (high confidence)

- Knowledge and skills in planning end-of-life care
- Ability to recognise deterioration in a patient and ability to manage this in the patients' home
- Awareness of wider professional services in your area
- Knowledge of local and national protocols and guidance in palliative care

12.3 Planning and Supporting End-of-Life Care

Death and dying remain a taboo subject for many people, but conversations about death and dying are central to ensuring the principles of a good death, empowering people to plan and make decisions about the end of their lives. The introduction of the Mental Capacity Act (MCA) in 2005 has had a significant impact on developments in how people make decisions about their care. The advent of the Act also assures that people are protected if they are unable to make informed decisions for themselves.

Advance care planning (ACP) is a process that has been identified to provide many benefits to patients and families, including facilitating autonomy, ownership of care

TABLE 12.2 ■ **Universal Principles for Advance Care Planning**

1. The person is central to developing and agreeing their advance care plan including deciding who else should be involved in the process.
2. The person has personalised conversations about their future care, focused on what matters to them and their needs.
3. The person agrees the outcomes of their advance care planning conversation through a shared decision-making process in partnership with relevant professionals.
4. The person has a shareable advance care plan which records what matters to them, and their preferences and decisions about future care and treatment.
5. The person has the opportunity, and is encouraged, to review and revise their advance care plan.
6. Anyone involved in advance care planning is able to speak up if they feel that these universal principles are not being followed.

(From NHS England. (2022). Universal principles for advance care planning (ACP). https://www.england.nhs.uk/wp-content/uploads/2022/03/universal-principles-for-advance-care-planning.pdf.)

and reducing inequalities in access to care (Hall et al., 2019). The publication of the 'Universal Principles for Advance Care Planning' (NHS England, 2022) has sought to provide clarity and consistency in the ACP process, with six universal principles (Table 12.2) at its core, and an awareness of this is vital for community nurses if the principles of a good death are to be met.

The following reflection explores your understanding of the Mental Capacity Act and ACP.

REFLECTION

Consider the five principles of the Mental Capacity Act and six principles of ACP.

- Are you aware of the details of these and do you need to understand more?
- How do you see these enacted in your day-to-day practice?
- What processes and procedures are in place to support you, your patients and their families?

The introduction of the Gold Standards Framework (GSF) promoted opportunity for timely discussion, and to support people and their families to plan for care at the end of life, if they wish to do so. The developed Proactive Identification Guidance (GSF, 2022) supports recognition when a person may be in the last year of life and prompts not only ACP discussion but also coordination of care through multiprofessional team working and communication. Through ACP, patients and their carers can live well and, when the time comes, die well. Equally, families and carers are supported through their bereavement process (NICE, 2015). There are many considerations which should be discussed, including the 'do not attempt cardiopulmonary resuscitation' (DNACPR) and Recommended Summary Plan for Emergency Care and Treatment (ReSPECT) document (Goswami et al., 2020). Documentation and sharing of plans of care will ensure that the patient's dignity is at the forefront of their care (Churchill et al., 2020). Having these discussions with family/carers and healthcare professionals can empower some patients to enable difficult discussion to be undertaken in a structured process (Johnson et al., 2011).

As the patient's care needs increase at home, an application for Continuing Healthcare and National Health Service (NHS)-funded Nursing Care can be considered (NHS, 2018). This national framework uses a decision-making tool to look at the eligibility for care funded by the NHS. Community nurses will be involved in the coordination of care for patients funded in this way and will complete assessments that recognise deteriorating health usually completing a Specialist Health Needs Assessment during reviews and in some cases the need for Fast-Track funded care supporting people at the end of their life (NHS, 2018). Community nurses then coordinate care for adults in the last days of their life. Using guidelines can reduce uncertainty, ensuring people have the right to be involved in their care (Jackson et al., 2022). NICE (2015) recommends that healthcare professionals recognise when a person is approaching the end of their life by assessing for changes using observations, signs and recognition of symptoms associated with end-of-life changes, to support patients through deterioration, ensuring they are symptom-free, creating a good death for the patient, their family and carers.

12.4 Supportive and Palliative Care in Socially Excluded Groups

People's experience of death is also influenced by the groups to which they belong. There is a wealth of evidence noting that people from socially excluded groups have poorer experiences of care, and this is influenced by poor access as well as discrimination. This section explores the impact of poverty as well as a particular group: Gypsy, Roma, Travellers.

12.4.1 POVERTY

Poverty is the single largest determinate of health; poorer people have shorter lives and greater health and well-being challenges (World Health Organization, 2021). In terms of palliative care, a review conducted by Davies et al. (2019) noted that the lower the socio-economic position (i.e. increased poverty) the more likely the individual would die in hospital and the less likely they would be in receipt of specialist palliative care. Rowley et al. (2021) highlight people living in poverty are more likely to experience pain at the end of their life, yet they are less likely to have their pain recognised by health professions and to receive pain relief. Poor quality palliative care at home for people living in poverty is also influenced by wider social issues. Research by Marie Curie and the Queens Nursing Institute (2023) highlighted that 46% of people dying at home are struggling to access food and a further 47% struggled to access heating.

12.4.1.1 Gypsy, Roma, Travellers

Gypsy, Roma, Traveller communities have a strong family-based culture and as such in terms of death and dying it is not uncommon to have large numbers of family members gathering to support the person who is dying (Heaslip, 2015) and this can be challenging for nurses who may feel uncomfortable with such large numbers of people. There is a preference to die at home being cared for by their family and challenges exist linked to poor literacy levels, misunderstanding of medical terminology, and poor cultural awareness by healthcare practitioners (Dixon et al., 2021).

12.5 Working in Multidisciplinary Teams

Understanding the function of the multidisciplinary team is important to provide holistic care (WHO, 2023). Building a robust support network can aid in the management of

CASE STUDY 12.1

Mary is a 57-year-old White female, who has Down syndrome and a recent diagnosis of bowel cancer and has been deteriorating over the past 6 months. Her ability to maintain nutritional intake has been affected and she has lost weight and become quite weak. She has also had four hospital admissions in the last 6 months, with a recent 2-week admission due to dehydration and pneumonia.

Discharge was planned to her home address in an assisted living care facility with carers providing personal care, medication administration and supporting her activities of daily living as they had done previously. Unfortunately, the wider multiprofessional team were not involved or informed of the outcome of the discharge planning meeting, therefore an adequate plan of care was not put into place to support her transition to her preferred place of care and death. Mary was discharged with a DNACPR and statement of intent (SOI), her medications including authorisation for anticipatory medications, and had a completed Continuing Health Care (CHC) fast-track discharge application for support.

After 3 days at home, her carers made contact with the community nursing team to ask when 24-hour nursing care would commence at home as they were not able to manage her increasing needs. She was no longer able to take her medications orally and they required a nurse 24 hours a day to support her. Mary was starting to experience pain and nausea.

Questions for consideration:

- What needs considering in the initial assessment?
- How would you plan and provide ongoing safe care?
- What other members of the multidisciplinary team need to be involved?
- How would you respond to her needs as well as supporting her family and carers?
- Explore the gaps in the communication at discharge, how would you prevent this situation occurring again?

end-of-life care for the patient, family, carers and the community teams, leading to better outcomes (Choi, 2015). Community nurses are the coordinators of end-of-life support (Quinn et al., 2021) and as such need an in-depth knowledge of services available to the person. Developing strong leadership role is imperative and is supported by the Nursing and Midwifery Council (NMC) Standards of proficiency for community nursing specialist practice qualifications (SPQ) (NMC, 2022). These Standards support the knowledge and skills required by community nurses to ensure they can support the person as they navigate deteriorating health and management of increasing needs, signposting to appropriate support (Amo-Setién et al., 2019), whether this be in the person's home, hospice or hospital care (Grindrod, 2020). Community nurses have an advocacy role here, communicating the wishes of the person to the wider team which requires advanced communication skills and the ability to minimise conflict for better outcomes (Taberna et al., 2020). Overall, knowledge, understanding compassion, effective communication and planning ensure the patient's journey at the end of their life is effectively supported (see Case Study 12.1).

12.6 Conclusion

This chapter has covered a range of issues related to the management and provision of palliative care services within community settings and the role of community nurses in delivering these. Throughout the chapter, the profound importance of providing compassionate, holistic care to individuals facing serious illness, advanced disease or end-of-life issues has been explored. The chapter explores fundamental principles, key components and essential practices of palliative care, illuminating its role in enhancing quality of life, relieving suffering and supporting patients and their families through difficult times. Having read this chapter and participated in the activities, you are now invited to complete a reassessment of your confidence and then to develop a personal action plan.

REFLECTION

Reassessment and Personal Action Plan—Please consider the following statements and self-assess your skills and confidence in each of these from 0 (no confidence) to 5 (high confidence).

- Knowledge and skills in planning end-of-life care
- Ability to recognise deterioration in a patient and ability to manage this in the patients' home
- Awareness of wider professional services in your area
- Knowledge of local and national protocols and guidance in palliative care

Following this and where appropriate, develop a list of actions to work on over the next 6 months to further develop your knowledge and skills in palliative and end-of-life care.

References

Amo-Setién, F. J., Abajas-Bustillo, R., Torres-Manrique, B., Martin-Melon, R., Sarabia-Cobo, C., Molina-Mula, J., et al. (2019). Characteristics of nursing interventions that improve the quality of life of people with chronic diseases. A systematic review with meta-analysis. *PLoS One*, *14*(6), e0218903.

Choi, P. P. 2015. Patient advocacy: The role of the nurse. *Nursing Standard (2014+)*, *29*(41), 52.

Churchill, I., Turner, K., Duliban, C., Pullar, V., Priestley, A., Postma, K., et al. (2020). The use of a palliative care screening tool to improve referrals to palliative care services in community-based hospitals: A quality improvement initiative. *Journal of Hospice & Palliative Nursing*, *22*(4), 327–334.

Davies, J., Sleeman, K., Leniz, J., Wilson, R., Higginson, I., Verne, J., et al. (2019). Socioeconomic position and use of healthcare in the last year of life: A systematic review and meta-analysis. *PLOS Med*, *19*(4), e1002782. https://doi.org/10.1371/journal.pmed.1002782

Dixon, K. C., Ferris, R., Kuhn, I., Spathis, A., & Barclay, S. (2021). Gypsy, Traveller and Roma experience, views and needs in palliative and end of life care: A systematic literature review and narrative synthesis. *BMJ Supportive & Palliative Care*. https://doi.org/10.1136/bmjspcare-2020-002676. Published Online First: 22 February 2021.

Etkind, S. N., Bone, A. E., Gomes, B., Lovell, N., Evans, C. J., Higginson, I. J., et al. (2017). 2017. How many people will need palliative care in 2040? Past trends, future projections and implications for services. *BMC Med*, *15*, 102. https://doi.org/10.1186/s12916-017-0860-

Gold Standard Framework. (2022). *How to use the NEW 2022 GSF PIG in your practice [online]*. Available from: goldstandardsframework.org.uk/how-to-use-the-new-2022-gsf-pig-in-your-practice.

Goswami, P., Mistric, M., & Barber, F. D. (2020). Advance care planning: Advanced practice provider—Initiated discussions and their effects on patient-centred end-of-life care. *Clinical Journal of Oncology Nursing*, *24*(1).

Grindrod, A. (2020). Choice depends on options: A public health framework incorporating the social determinants of dying to create options at end of life. *Progress in Palliative Care*, *28*(2), 94–100.

Hall, A., Rowland, C., & Grande, G. (2019). How should end-of-life advance care planning discussions be implemented according to patients and informal carers? A qualitative review of reviews. *Journal of Pain and Symptom Management*, *58*(2), 311–335. https://doi.org/10.1016/j.jpainsymman.2019.04.013

Heaslip, V. (2015). *Experiences of vulnerability from a Gypsy/Traveller perspective: A phenomenological study (PhD)*. Bournemouth: Bournemouth University.

Jackson, J., Maben, J., & Anderson, J. E. (2022). What are nurses' roles in modern healthcare? A qualitative interview study using interpretive description. *Journal of Research in Nursing*, *27*(6), 504–516.

Johnson, C., Girgis, A., Paul, C., Currow, D. C., Adams, J., & Aranda, S. (2011). Australian palliative care providers' perceptions and experiences of the barriers and facilitators to palliative care provision. *Supportive Care in Cancer*, *19*, 343–351.

Lynn, J., & Adamson, D. M. (2003). Living well at the end of life: Adapting health care to serious chronic illness in old age [online]. Available from: www.rand.org/content/dam/rand/pubs/white_papers/2005/WP137.pdf. [Accessed 8.1.24].

Marie Curie & Queens Nursing Institute. (2023). 70 years of end-of-life care in the community. Available from: https://www.mariecurie.org.uk/globalassets/media/documents/policy/policy-publications/2023/1952-report-final.pdf. [Accessed 8.1.24].

Meier, E., Gallegos, J., Montross-Thomas, L., Depp, C., Irwin, S., & Jeste, D. (2016). Defining a good death (successful dying): Literature review and a call for research and public dialogue. *American Journal of Psychiatry*, *24*(4), 261–271.

Mental Capacity Act, 2005. S1. Available at: https://www.legislation.gov.uk/ukpga/2005/9/contents. [Accessed 21.1.24]

Midlöv, E. M., & Lindberg, T. (2020). District nurses' experiences of providing palliative care in the home: An interview study. *Nordic Journal of Nursing Research*, *40*(1), 15–24. https://doi.org/10.1177/2057158519857002.

National Institute for Clinical Excellence. (2004). *Improving supportive and palliative care for adults with cancer (NICE guideline). Guidance on Cancer Services*. National Institute for Health and Clinical Excellence [online]. Available from: www.nice.org.uk/guidance/csg4/resources/imporving-supportive-and-palliative-care-for-adults-with-cancer-pdf-773375005. [Accessed 8.1.24].

National Institute for Clinical Excellence. (2015). *Care of dying adults in the last days of life. NICE guideline*. National Institute for Health and Clinical Excellence [online]. Available from https://www.nice.org.uk/guidance/ng31.

National Palliative and End of Life Care Partnership. (2021). Ambitions for palliative and end of life care: A national framework for local action 2021–2026. Available from https://www.england.nhs.uk/publication/ambitions-for-palliative-and-end-of-life-care-a-national-framework--for-local-action-2021-2026/. [Accessed 21.1.24].

NHS. (2018). *NHS continuing healthcare*. Available from: https://www.nhs.uk/conditions/social-care-and-support-guide/money-work-and-benefits/nhs-continuing-healthcare/. [Accessed 21.1.24].

NHS England. (2022). *Universal principles for advance care planning (ACP) [online]*. Available from: www.englad.nhs.uk/wp-content/uploads/2022/03/universal-principles-for-advance-care-planning.pdf. [Accessed on 21/01/2024].

Nursing and Midwifery Council. (2022). Standards of proficiency for community nursing specialist practice qualification nurses. Available from: nmc_standards_of_proficiency_for_community_nursing_spqs.pdf. [Accessed 26.1.24].

Quinn, K. L., Wegier, P., Stukel, T. A., Huang, A., Bell, C. M., & Tanuseputro, P. (2021). Comparison of palliative care delivery in the last year of life between adults with terminal noncancer illness or cancer. *JAMA Network Open*, *4*(3) e210677-e210677.

Robinson, J., Goodwin, H., Williams, L., Anderson, N., Parr, J., Irwin, R., & Gott, M. (2023). The work of palliative care from the perspectives of district nurses: A qualitative study. *Journal of Advanced Nursing*. https://doi.org/10.1111/jan.16030.

Rowley, J., Richards, N., Carduff, E., & Gott, M. (2021). The impact of poverty and deprivation at the end of life: A critical review. *Palliative Care and Social Practice*, *15*. https://doi-org.salford.idm.oclc.org/10.1177/26323524211033873.

Taberna, M., Gil Moncayo, F., Jané-Salas, E., Antonio, M., Arribas, L., Vilajosana, E., et al. (2020). The multidisciplinary team (MDT) approach and quality of care. *Frontiers in Oncology*, *10*, 85.

UK Parliament Post. (2022). Palliative and end of life care. Available from: https://researchbriefings.files.parliament.uk/documents/POST-PN-0675/POST-PN-0675.pdf. [Accessed 8.1.24].

World Health Organization. (2021). Poverty and social determinates. Available from: https://www.who.int/health-topics/social-determinaffnts-of-health#tab=tab_3. [Accessed 8.1.24].

World Health Organization. (2023). Palliative care [online]. Available from www.who.int/europe/news-room/fact-sheets/item/palliative-care. [Accessed 8.1.24].

CHAPTER 13

Caseload Management

Emma Budd ■ Linda Duggan ■ Michelle McBride ■
Anna Robert ■ Emily Winter

LEARNING OUTCOMES

After reading this chapter you should be able to:

- Understand the complexity of managing district nursing (DN) caseloads
- Comprehend potential facilitators and barriers to implementing skill mix in community nursing services
- Appreciate ways to facilitate smooth and successful transitions for patients from hospital to their homes or other care settings

13.1 Service Planning and Caseload Allocation

13.1.1 INTRODUCTION

Working in the community often involves spontaneous, autonomous decision-making which is difficult to measure or predict (QNI, 2022b). This requires community nursing services to be adaptable and resilient. District nurses (DNs) manage caseloads of patients within their localities and are accountable for the care being delivered by the team they lead. Therefore, DNs are required to review their caseloads regularly to ensure that quality care is being provided (McCrory, 2019). The following information will provide insight into what DN caseloads comprise of and the complexity of managing them in the community setting.

13.1.2 BACKGROUND

The complexity of DN caseloads continues to increase due to the drive of national initiatives and an ageing population living with multiple comorbidities (Horner, 2022). The Five Year Forward View (National Health Service (NHS) England, 2014) highlighted the importance of primary care to the wider healthcare system, and the need for integrated care amongst general practice, community nursing services, specialist nursing and social care to avoid unnecessary hospital admissions and to expedite hospital discharges. Building upon the Five Year Forward view (2014), the Long Term Plan (2019), commits to addressing clinical priorities and focusing on integrated care to meet the needs of the population and increasing the budget for community services (King's Fund, 2022).

As we shift from hospital-based care to care being provided closer to home (NHS, 2019), the pressures on community nursing services across the country are immense (Grundy & Wheeler, 2018). Community nursing services are described by the Queen's

Nursing Institute (QNI, 2016) as sponges, absorbing additional work without a defined number of beds. With a declining DN workforce and an increase in the number of patients on caseloads, it is of high importance that caseloads are effectively managed to ensure safe caseloads are sustained.

13.1.3 CASELOAD MANAGEMENT

The National Quality Board (2017) defines a DN caseload as the care of patients, their families and carers both at an individual and a team level, within a specific locality. DN caseloads can vary in size and complexity and are dependent upon the geographic profile of the population. The QNI (2022a) argues that there is no one definition of a caseload, advising that there is no differentiation between workload and caseload due to the different levels of complexity experienced by community nursing services within their localities.

The QNI (2022a) advises caution with caseloads that exceed 150 patients per whole time equivalent (WTE) DN as this is linked with increased deferred visits. There is no current definition for a deferred visit; however, within some organisations, it is described as a visit that has passed the clinical window of care and requires retriage by a trained clinician. Furthermore, the QNI (2022a) recommends that caseloads be capped at 150 patients as it is deemed as a trigger point for patient visits being deferred or work being left 'undone' such as onward referrals. The report advised that anything above 150 patients should be escalated as a risk. At present, there is no set number of patients on a caseload. The QNI's DN survey (2019) identified the infrequency of DN teams declining referrals. Historically, community nursing services have been defined as 'wards without walls' and a 'Cinderella' service, meaning that care is delivered behind closed doors and is not seen (Green et al., 2020). Community nursing services are often seen as a 'failsafe' option when other services do not have the capacity within themselves to see the patient (QNI, 2022a). However, there are steps in place to raise caseload management concerns with commissioners (see Box 13.1).

McCrory (2019) describes caseload management as a core component of the DN's role and outlines the challenges DNs face when managing effective caseloads. Caseload management is complex and requires confident decision-making skills as well as expert clinical assessment to mitigate risks to patients whilst ensuring the workload of staff is manageable (McCrory, 2019). A DN's caseload that is not effectively managed can lead to poor patient outcomes and restrict a patient's access to timely care (McCrory, 2019). Whilst a DN remains accountable for the quality of nursing care being provided by their teams, the delegation of visits is required to

BOX 13.1 ■ Red Flags for Escalating Concerns in Caseload Management

The QNI (2022a) have identified 'red flags' for when escalation to commissioners of services is required.

1. District nursing services are unable to close caseloads which leads to unmanageable demand.
2. The deferral of routine patient visits every day or most days should be escalated.
3. The deferral of high-priority visits should be escalated as a safety concern.
4. High staff turnover and staff sickness should also be deemed as a red flag for patient safety and system resilience.

ensure that the patient's needs are met. Effective caseload management is therefore imperative in ensuring a high standard of care is delivered, whilst assuring that the right nurse is in the right place with the right skill at the right time, maintaining patient safety (Nursing and Midwifery Council, 2018).

13.1.4 CASELOAD REVIEW

A caseload review ensures that care is planned appropriately to avoid over/undervisiting as well as ensuring visits are prioritised appropriately. This ensures cost-effective, high-quality care is delivered (Gould, 2018). Within some organisations, DNs are assigned management days which can differ between trusts/organisations. The expectation during management time is that the patients on the DN's caseload(s) are reviewed. A caseload review can consist of but is not exhaustive to the following:

- Checking that all patient assessments have been completed
- Checking schedules are in place and not missed
- Checking care plans are in place and appropriate
- Identifying if any onward referrals are required and complete if outstanding
- Identifying when the last DN review took place
- Checking if a patient is being seen by a registered nurse (RN) at least every fourth visit
- Checking if visits remain appropriate
- Reviewing the appropriateness of the frequency of visits and the prioritisation of these. This will ensure that patients are reviewed appropriately and reduce the risk of deferred visits unnecessarily
- Identifying outstanding Dopplers assessments
- Documenting actions taken and any actions required onto software application such as EMIS.

13.1.5 COMPLEXITY OF CASELOADS

Due to the unprecedented demand for community nursing services, DNs are faced with the reality of deferring visits. For this reason, it is essential that new referrals are triaged concisely ensuring that patients are seen in the correct place for them. In most areas, the community nursing services visit patients that are housebound. This means that a patient is unable to leave their home via any mode of transport other than a hospital ambulance. This ensures that the community nursing services are visiting the most vulnerable at home whilst promoting independence for those patients who can attend their general practice nurse (GPN) or other services such as walk-in clinics. This can provoke difficult conversations with patients; however, it is essential to ensure they are receiving care from the correct service in line with their needs.

During the height of the COVID-19 pandemic, patients were often scared of community nursing teams visiting, which prompted self-care at home. Teams utilised technology to review patients at home where appropriate. Moving on from the pandemic, it is important that self-care is promoted where possible to protect community nursing services but also to ensure that patients remain as independent as possible.

Grindle (2021) provides a critical reflection on the use of technology throughout the COVID-19 pandemic, highlighting the positive and negative influences that this had.

13.1.6 SERVICE PLANNING

In order to plan services appropriately, establishments should be based on demand within their specific area. This requires commissioners of services to work alongside their teams to gather and analyse data so that they can estimate demand when determining establishments (QNI, 2022). The Royal College of Nursing (RCN) (2021) workforce standards advise that establishments should include an uplift on the WTE of employees to include leave/unplanned leave and absence. It is important to recognise that if this is not worked out efficiently, staffing requirements will not be met and will ensue over reliance on bank and agency staff as well as compromising patient safety. Recommendations from the QNI (2022a) suggest a skill mix ratio within community nursing services of 60% registered nurses (RNs), 20% newly qualified nurses and 20% nursing support workers (Fig. 13.1). Further recommendations were that an RN should attend every fourth visit of patients to ensure that care is monitored and evaluated appropriately.

Community nursing services are delivered by block contracting which makes it difficult to capture outcomes of care delivered. This is because in the community setting, activity is not measured by each care episode delivered, unlike other NHS services (King's Fund, 2022). Community services receive a lump sum of money to deliver the care so therefore outcomes of care are difficult to capture.

13.1.7 CONCLUSION

Managing a DN caseload is a complex skill to learn and develop. The DN's role is important in sustaining safe caseloads and ensuring that patients are seen by the right nurse, at the right time, in the right place. A DN is accountable for the patients on their

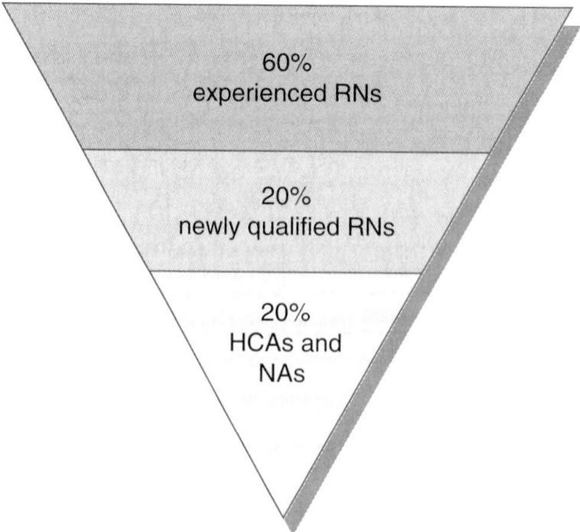

Fig. 13.1 Recommended ratio of RNs and support workers within a community nursing team (QNI, 2022a). *HCA*, Health care assistant; *NA*, nurse associate; *RN*, registered nurse.

caseload and the allocation of patient care needs to be individualised. It is important that commissioners of community nursing services work alongside their teams to develop establishments alongside the demand within their locality.

13.2 Skill Mix in the Community

13.2.1 INTRODUCTION

To use the workforce efficiently and effectively and deliver optimal, safe, patient-centred care it is necessary to establish the right staff, with the right level of skill to deliver it. Definitions of skill mix include the number of and educational experience of nurses working in clinical settings (Kushemererwa et al., 2020; QNI, 2022a; RCN, 2021). The World Health Organisation back in 2000 identified that determining the correct skill mix of health professionals is a longstanding challenge for healthcare organisations and health systems. When analysing skill mix in community nursing, consideration needs to be given to the growing body of evidence that suggests a link between skill mix and mortality (Kushemererwa et al., 2020; RCN 2021). Up until now, the work conducted on skill mix has primarily focused on acute nursing settings. However, due to workload demand exceeding capacity in the district nursing service (QNI, 2022a) and national challenges with staff retention and recruitment and patient safety incidents, there has been a renewed drive to look at skill mix in district nursing.

When discussing skill mix within community nursing services, this goes further than clinical skills competencies and tasks (QNI, 2022a). Focusing on the task alone can be reductionist and minimalist and risks moving away from person-centred holistic assessment and care (Kushemererwa et al., 2020; QNI, 2022a). Maybin et al. (2016) also highlight the importance of continuity of the same DN(s) or community nurse(s) delivering care to a person over a period of time as central in maintaining quality of care.

REFLECTION

- Consider the potential limitations and potential risks of using an allocation tool that, for example, looks at allocating visits by blocks of time.

13.2.2 PROFESSIONAL JUDGEMENT AND SKILL MIX

The National Quality Board (2017) identified that although some tools exist, for example those that measure patient's dependency, frailty or complexity of care, ultimately professional judgement is relied on to identify the skills required to meet patient needs and deliver a high-quality district nursing service; this is supported by Maybin et al. (2016). Using their professional judgement, community nurses and DN team leaders need to consider and interpret the evidence available, utilise evidence-based tools and take account of the local context and the individual patient, family and carer needs. This involves clinical decision-making and is a dynamic process that enables real-time decisions on staffing skill mix in response to the caseload, acuity, dependency, frailty, complexity and activity of the team (Box 13.2). Consideration will

BOX 13.2 ■ Scenario

A referral for a 'routine blood test' is received. The blood test is allocated to a phlebotomist/healthcare assistant and the visit is completed. However, a few days later, another referral is received that the patient has fallen and has a superficial wound to their lower limb. The healthcare assistant visits and dresses the wound to the patient's lower limb. The patient continues to be seen by the healthcare assistant as they are deemed to have a 'simple wound'. The following week the team receives a call to say the patient has been admitted to hospital with acute cellulitis leading to sepsis; they were found unconscious and have been identified as a newly diagnosed diabetic.

1. Consider if there is such a thing as a 'routine' visit or a 'simple wound'.
2. What factors should be taken into consideration when identifying the health professional with the appropriate skill to undertake this visit?
3. How might comprehensive assessment and the identification of potential risk factors have impacted on the outcome for the patient?

also have to be given to geographical factors such as travel and shift patterns as well as the above (QNI, 2022a).

13.2.3 BARRIERS TO IMPLEMENTING SKILL MIX

The biggest barrier to delivering good quality care is the gap between service demand and capacity, given the numbers of staff in post and their levels of skills and experience (QNI, 2016, 2022a). In a recent study carried out by the QNI (2022a), reported high rates of deferred visits and that too much of the complex work was delegated. Likewise, nursing support workers report sometimes feeling uncomfortable with the acuity of the work they were being asked to undertake. With current pressures on recruitment and retention of staff, appropriate skill mix and ensuring staff well-being have the potential benefit of reducing the risk of burnout and staff staying in position and encouraging new staff into the community nursing setting.

The QNI (2022a) suggests that allocation and scheduling of work should not be solely delegated to an online app or electronic schedulers alone; whilst they may be able to guide or advise allocation, they are not supported by sufficient evidence to demonstrate their safety and community work is unpredictable and complex. It can be argued that current approaches to skill mix do not always consider the wider resources and assets available to community nursing services. An understanding of the wider interprofessional team and their skills and roles is essential (Gilbert, 2016). The use of other groups such as private and the voluntary sector should also be considered, for example social prescribing link workers (NHS, 2019). Community nursing and the multidisciplinary team (MDT) with overlapping skills are complex and changing; there are a plethora of different services and roles developing locally and nationally. It is important to be aware of referral criteria and job roles so that they can be utilised to work for the benefit of the patient, but also enable effective and efficient use of healthcare budgets (Gilbert, 2016). DNs and community nurses must have in-depth knowledge and understanding of their local areas through community profiling and the skills as mentioned previously to communicate effectively to form working relationships.

REFLECTION

- What needs to be in place for 'safe' skill mix in community nursing teams?
- Do you know the referral criteria for other members of the primary care team? Is there potential overlap in skill set?

13.2.4 CONCLUSION

This section provides a comprehensive exploration of the deployment and optimisation of diverse skills within the community nursing workforce, emphasising the importance of achieving a balance that enhances overall organisational effectiveness and service delivery as well as ensuring patient safety. Nurses working in the community need to maintain awareness of the wider community assets available to meet patient needs, such as statutory and nonstatutory organisations including patient support groups, nursing homes, residential homes and beyond.

13.3 Effective Hospital Discharge Planning Onto Community Caseloads

13.3.1 INTRODUCTION

Most people wish to return home from a hospital admission, and to support this, they must be discharged effectively and safely when clinically ready. Many patients in hospitals have ongoing care needs requiring input from community nursing services (NHS England, 2019). They may already be known to the team or new to the caseload. Either way, the process to support efficient discharge planning is much the same. The underlying principle is the right place, right time with the right support to maximise the individual's independence for the best possible outcome and prevent readmission or crisis situations (Department of Health and Social Care (DHSS), 2022a).

13.3.2 HOSPITAL DISCHARGE BACK TO THE COMMUNITY

Effective discharge planning begins at the moment of hospital admission or before elective procedures and is reliant upon the MDT working across all sectors with robust communication, documentation and timely action by all (DHSS, 2022b). This process should focus on patient autonomy and include key individuals for the patient such as family, friends, neighbours or the voluntary sector, ensuring consent is obtained to liaise with them. Holistic discharge planning has been recognised in policy, with The Health and Care Act (DHSS, 2022b) introducing a new duty for NHS Trusts and Foundations to include patients and carers (including young carers) in discharge planning when adults continue to need care and support in the community.

Culture plays a significant role in the process of discharging a patient from a hospital. It encompasses a broad range of factors, including the patient's cultural background, beliefs, values and preferences, as well as the cultural competence of healthcare providers. Considering cultural aspects during the discharge process is essential for ensuring effective communication, understanding and adherence to the care plan. By integrating cultural considerations into the discharge planning process, healthcare providers can promote better patient outcomes, enhance patient satisfaction and contribute to a more equitable and patient-centred healthcare system.

Effective discharge planning aims to work towards a safe seamless transfer meeting the individual's needs and expectations in their chosen place of residence with the support they need, ensuring continuity of care (National Institute for Health and Care Excellence (NICE), 2015). It may be necessary to have a case conference if there are complex needs that need to be addressed, and it is important that the district nursing team is included. This might involve rehabilitation for a patient with a spinal injury (NICE, 2022), or degenerative neurological disease requiring ventilated support, as well as end-of-life care, chronic disease management or tissue viability needs. Unfortunately, in practice, this does not always take place (QNI, 2016). It may be necessary for the patient to transfer to a care home rather than return home, or perhaps go and stay with another family member initially (DHSS, 2022b). No matter the circumstances, it is key to ensure that individuals are not coerced into making decisions when they are in crisis (NICE, 2016). There are also occasions when transferring to an intermediate or community hospital is appropriate, when individuals have been clinically optimised, but care is still required (a step down from a specialist or general hospital setting in preparation for discharge home). Reasons for this may include a need for therapy, awaiting an available package of care or for the arrival of specialist equipment/housing adaptations or similar. However, hospital-based services are not always aware of what is available in the community (QNI, 2016).

As soon as possible, a specific date and time of expected discharge are made known to all relevant disciplines and identification of whether the care needs are simple or complex. The clinical care plans and risk assessments should be made available to the district nursing team to ensure the patient will have their clinical care needs met. If required, time needs to be allocated for the district nursing team to be trained in specific clinical skills. This may include the use of chest drains, managing vacuum assisted closure therapy, chemotherapy or learning patient specific moving and handling techniques. Nonclinical aspects must be considered, including home adaptations and equipment. Provisions can be put in place if required, such as a profiling bed or pressure prevention equipment (DHSS, 2022b). If necessary, a social worker can support with other benefits and reviews, as well as support the setting up of a care package for the patient when they return home (DHSS, 2022b). A home visit may be necessary before discharge, in conjunction with family, occupational therapist and physiotherapist to look at specific aspects of ongoing care needs the patient may have, such as moving and transferring.

13.3.3 COMMUNICATION AND INFORMATION SHARING

Documentation of the discharge planning process is vital, including agreed care needs and how they will be met. As the QNI (2016) suggests, effective communication between teams is one of the most imperative factors in an effective discharge to the community. Each member of the coordinating team should understand their responsibilities for specific actions and be proactive in meeting them. If the patient has complex needs, then a named discharge coordinator should have responsibility for this, documenting and informing the rest of the MDT when actions are complete or if there will be a delay, to facilitate safe transition from hospital (DHSS, 2022b; NICE, 2016). This information will form the baseline for ongoing nursing documentation that accompanies the patient throughout their journey on the district nursing caseload. For best practice, the district nursing team must be kept informed of any changes in expected hospital discharges, especially around complex care needs and end-of-life care, to enable forward planning and a safe transition.

13.3.4 HOSPITAL DISCHARGES

It should be noted that hospitals work on a 7-day-a-week discharge criterion, some having a dedicated Discharge Team or Transfer of Care Hub, comprising of professionals from across relevant services, whose job is to coordinate discharges as part of the management of hospital beds, which will vary across the country (NHS Improvement, 2017a). There can often be a need to clear beds in time for weekends or upcoming bank holidays which can add pressure to the district nursing teams, who often operate with minimal staff at these times. This emphasises the need for everything to be in place ahead of the agreed time of discharge; if this is not in place, then there is a risk of harm to the patient. A lack of planning can increase inappropriate hospital readmissions and impact on the patient experience (QNI, 2016).

13.3.5 MENTAL STATUS/CAPACITY

As the DHSS (2022b) states, mental capacity should be assessed on a decision-specific basis. However, where there is no capacity for the patient to make decisions or give consent, they are given rights and obligations under the Mental Capacity Act 2005. A mental capacity assessment may be required if there is cognitive impairment, learning disability or memory problems. If there are capacity concerns, then an MDT '*Best Interests*' decision should be put in place (Mental Capacity Act, 2005). It should be established if there is Lasting Power of Attorney with a family member, friend or other advocate. If there are none, then the existing MDT, family members or friends work together to make a Best Interests decision which should be fully documented and agreed by all. This may include social services or legal representation as there could be a financial element involved for ongoing care needs. At times, it may be appropriate for an independent advocate to support the patient during the discharge planning process and referrals to these services should be made as soon as possible (DHSS, 2022b).

13.3.6 IMMEDIATELY PRIOR TO DISCHARGE

Timely communication is imperative for an effective discharge to take place and therefore the DN should make verbal contact with the ward a few days before the expected discharge; this is particularly relevant for patients with complex needs. This is to establish and confirm everything is in place and that they have received all transfer of care documentation including details of medication regime, wound assessments and care plans, catheterisation details or any other clinical care needs. Often, there is a discrepancy regarding the level of data exchange between inpatient and community settings which presents obstacles to efficient care at this crucial stage (Lino, 2021). Last-minute discussions are often essential for a smooth and safe transition of care. However, according to the QNI (2016), last-minute discussions do not take place as often as needed.

REFLECTION

Think back to when you were involved with a delayed discharge. Were any of the following a contributing factor and what were the potential solutions?

- Lack of available care packages including the provision of meals and personal care
- Environmental factors—relating to property/falls risk/equipment provision
- Patient or family not in agreement with recommended discharge plans
- Lack of medication, specialist equipment or suitable transport
- Lack of specialist training for nursing and care staff
- Communication delays between services

13.3.7 BARRIERS TO DISCHARGE PLANNING

Lino (2021) identified fragmentation in communication and misconceptions surrounding district nursing services as key barriers to the effective transition of care from the hospital to the community. The QNI (2016) added that the lack of care packages and equipment provision, particularly for those in rural areas, often prevents discharges from happening in a timely manner (Box 13.3). A policy-driven approach is key to ensure fundamentals are in place through the discharge planning process, with the inclusion of patient and family being paramount (DHSS, 2022b).

13.4 Discharge Planning

13.4.1 DISCHARGE OF PATIENTS FROM DISTRICT NURSE CASELOAD

District nursing caseloads can often be extremely busy and, without the physical restriction of a defined number of beds, are often seen to accept additional workload (QNI, 2016; NHS Improvement, 2017b). It is therefore expedient for established criteria for discharging patients to be in place, which need to be under continual review. The general principle of these criteria is based in promoting the patient to be independent of the

BOX 13.3 ■ Barriers to Discharge Planning

- A lack of time to adequately involve key people to ensure the plan is appropriate and workable.
- A lack of awareness by hospital teams of both the capability and scope of the district nursing service and also of the challenges in relation to, for example, access to drugs and community health equipment loans.
- Differing information technology (IT) systems in hospitals, general practitioner (GP) surgeries and community providers, which result in duplication of entries and fragmentation of records and frustration for the users.
- Poor communication between hospitals/social services and community-based teams.
- Hurried ineffective discharges due to the pressure on beds in hospitals and a lack of understanding of what is available in the community or 'step-down' services to ensure optimum care of patient and suitable placement.
- A lack of knowledge regarding medication management services within a community team and limited or no rehabilitation in hospital to ensure patients who are capable of self-care regarding medication maintain their independence.

BOX 13.4 ■ Scenario

Lin is a 78-year-old female who has been in hospital for 2 weeks following a fall. She was known to the district nursing service prior to this as she was receiving wound care. During admission, she was diagnosed as having a stroke, which has left her with a severe left-sided weakness. Her mobility has deteriorated and she is going to need a robust care package on discharge. She lives on her own in a fairly run-down property in a rural community. The ward staff have reported that she has been confused at times which is also new for her. You have been asked to attend an MDT meeting to plan discharge home.

- Which other professionals do you expect to be present?
- Which assessments do you feel should take place prior to discharge?
- Do you have any concerns regarding this discharge and why?
- Are there any barriers to a safe discharge here?

service, which may involve teaching them or a family member to continue an element of care. There are, of course, patients who do not want the community nursing services, even if they might still need it.

All discharges of people who use the service must be properly documented whether it be due to death, transferring to a care home, moving to another area or because there is no more need of the service. This documentation must be robust and include the date, time and discharging nurse details. In addition, any transfer of care documentation needs to be forwarded to the relevant service. All team members need to be informed of discharges and transfers to facilitate excellent levels of communication and seamless transition of patient care. Comprehensive discussions need to take place with the patient and their family to ensure they have understood the process and that they know where to access support if it should be needed in the future. Consider the scenario in Box 13.4, which focuses on multidisciplinary working in the community.

13.4.2 CONCLUSION

Effective hospital discharge planning for community caseloads is a multifaceted process that requires a comprehensive set of skills and knowledge from healthcare professionals. The emphasis on cultural competence, legal and ethical considerations and patient and family education underscores the importance of holistic and patient-centred care. Discharges from hospital to community services can often be challenging and patient needs can be complex. The key to maximising safety and promoting patient independence relies on timely preparation and excellent communication between services. A team approach is essential and a mutual appreciation of the barriers from all perspectives will enable a smoother transition.

13.5 Conclusion

In conclusion, this chapter underscores the critical importance of effectively managing caseloads within the district nursing settings providing insights into the key principles and strategies involved in handling caseloads efficiently. Effective caseload management is a multifaceted and dynamic process that requires a combination of organisational skills, interpersonal competence and a dedication to safe evidenced-based nursing care.

References

Department of Health and Social Care. (2022a). Health and Social Care Act. Crown. https://assets.publishing.service.gov.uk/government/uploads/system/uploads/attachment_data/file/1115453/health-and-care-act-2022-summary-and-additional-measures-impact-assessment.pdf.

Department of Health and Social Care. (2022b). Hospital discharge and community support guidance. https://www.gov.uk/government/publications/hospital-discharge-and-community-support-guidance.

Gilbert, H. (2016). *Supporting integration through new roles and working across boundaries*. The King's Fund. https://www.kingsfund.org.uk/sites/default/files/field/field_publication_file/Supporting_integration_web.pdf.

Gould J. (2018). Organisation and management of care, 2nd edn. In: Chilton S, Bain H (eds). London: Routledge.

Green, J., Doyle, C., Hayes, S., Newnham, W., Hill, S. IZeller, I., Graffin, M. and Goddard, G. (2020) COVID-19 and district and community nursing, *British Journal of Community Nursing*, 25:5, pp.213–213.

Grindle, K.R. (2021). Impact of technology on community nursing during the pandemic. *British Journal of Community Nursing*, 26(3), 110–115.

Grundy, C., & Wheeler, H. (2018). The development of a district nursing caseload review tool. *British Journal of Community Nursing*, *23*(6), 220–226. https://doi.org/10.12968/bjcn.2018.23.6.220.

Horner, R.L. (2022). The role of the district nurse in screening and assessment for frailty. *British Journal of Community Nursing*, 27(5), 226–230.

King's Fund. (2022). What are integrated care systems? Available at: https://www.kingsfund.org.uk/insight-and-analysis/long-reads/integrated-care-systems-explained.

Kushemererwa, D., Davis, J., Nompilo, M., Gilbert, S., & Gray, R. (2020). The association between nursing skill mix and mortality for adult medical and surgical patients: Protocol for systematic review. *International Journal of Environmental Research and Public Health*, *17*, 8604. https://doi.org/10.3390/ijerph17228604.

Lino, P. (2021). Challenges and complexities of discharge planning from a district nursing perspective. *British Journal of Community Nursing*, *26*(4).

Maybin, J., Charles, A., & Honeyman, M. (2016). *Understanding quality in district nursing services*. The King's Fund.

McCrory, V. (2019). Caseload management: A district nursing challenge. *British Journal of Community Nursing*, *24*(4), 186–190. https://doi.org/10.12968/bjcn.2019.24.4.186.

Meeley, N.G. (2021). Undergraduate student nurses' experiences of their community placements. *Nurse Education Today*, 106. https://doi.org/10.1016/j.nedt.2021.105054.

Mental Capacity Act. (2005) [monograph on the Internet]. Crown copyright; 2005 [cited 2011 Feb 16]. Available from: http://www.legislation.gov.uk/ukpga/2005/9/pdfs/ukpga_20050009_en.pdf.

National Quality Board. (2017). Safe, sustainable and productive staffing, An improvement resource for the district nursing service. Available at: https://www.england.nhs.uk/wp-content/uploads/2022/03/improvement-resource-for-district-nursing-service.pdf.

NHS. (2019). Long-Term Plan. https://www.longtermplan.nhs.uk/.

NHS England. (2014). NHS five year forward view. Available at: https://www.england.nhs.uk/publication/nhs-five-year-forward-view/.

NHS England. (2019). The Long Term Plan. https://www.longtermplan.nhs.uk/wp-content/uploads/2019/08/nhs-long-term-plan-version-1.2.pdf.

NHS Improvement. (2017a). Equality for all – Delivering safe care-seven days a week. https://www.england.nhs.uk/improvement-hub/wp-content/uploads/sites/44/2017/11/Equality-for-all-Delivering-safe-care-seven-days-a-week.pdf.

NHS Improvement. (2017b). Safe, sustainable and productive staffing. An improvement resource for the district nursing service. https://www.england.nhs.uk/wp-content/uploads/2022/03/improvement-resource-for-district-nursing-service.pdf.

NICE. (2015). Transition between inpatient hospital settings and community or care home settings for adults with social care needs. Available at: https://www.nice.org.uk/guidance/ng27.

NICE. (2016). Transition between inpatient hospital settings and community or care home settings for adults with social care needs. *NICE Quality Standard*. https://www.nice.org.uk/guidance/qs136.

NICE. (2022). Rehabilitation after traumatic injury: NICE guideline. https://www.nice.org.uk/guidance/ng211.

Nursing and Midwifery Council. (2018). The code: Professional standards of practice and behaviour for nurses, *midwives and nursing associates*. London: NMC.

Queen's Nursing Institute. (2016). Discharge planning. *Best Practice in Transitions of Care*. https://qni.org.uk/wp-content/uploads/2016/09/discharge_planning_report_2015.pdf.

QNI. (2022a). Workforce standards for the district nursing service. ICNO [on-line] https://qni.org.uk/wp-content/uploads/2022/02/Workforce-Standards-for-the-District-Nursing-Service.pdf. (Accessed 13/07/23).

QNI. (2022b). Field Specific Standards of Education and Practice for Community Specialist Practitioner Qualifications Raising the Standards for People being Cared for in the Community. Available at: https://qni.org.uk/wp-content/uploads/2023/04/Background-to-QNIs-Field-Specific-Standards-for-Education-and-Practice.pdf.

Royal College of Nursing. (2021). *Nursing workforce standards. Supporting a safe and effective nursing workforce* [online]. https://www.rcn.org.uk/professional-development/publications/rcn-workforce-standards-uk-pub-009681. (Accessed 13/07/23).

CHAPTER 14

Leadership and Career Progression

Caroline Ogunsola Anthea Thorpe Hayley Thrumble Fiona Kaye

LEARNING OUTCOMES

After reading this chapter you should be able to:

- Understand the importance of leadership within community nursing
- Appreciate different leadership theories applicable to community nursing
- Explore ways in which to network via social media

14.1 Introduction

Community nursing plays a vital role in delivering healthcare services to individuals, families and communities within their own homes and community settings. Effective leadership is essential in community nursing to ensure high-quality care, optimise patient outcomes and drive positive change. This chapter explores the concept of leadership in community nursing and delves into the various aspects of career progression within the field in the United Kingdom.

14.2 Definition and Importance of Leadership in Community Nursing

Defining leadership and its importance in community nursing involves understanding the multifaceted role of a nurse leader and the impact they have on healthcare outcomes (QNI, 2016). Leadership in nursing extends beyond positional authority and encompasses the ability to inspire, guide and influence others towards a shared vision of providing excellent patient care. It involves taking responsibility, making decisions and facilitating change to improve healthcare delivery and patient outcomes (NMC, 2024).

Nursing leadership involves mobilising and empowering the nursing team to work collaboratively, efficiently and effectively. It requires a combination of skills, knowledge and qualities that enable nurses to navigate complex healthcare systems, manage resources and advocate for patients and the nursing profession. Leadership in nursing is not confined to those in formal managerial positions but can be demonstrated at all levels of nursing practice (Ellis, 2021).

14.3 Leadership Theories and Models

Leadership theories in nursing encompass various models and frameworks that inform leadership practices within healthcare settings. Leadership theories provide valuable frameworks for understanding leadership dynamics in nursing and guiding leadership development efforts to promote effective, ethical and compassionate leadership practices within healthcare organisations.

Compassionate leadership is the current ambition for the future of NHS leadership (NHS England, 2021), and is thought to be the optimum leadership model for producing high-quality, inclusive care by promoting an empathetic culture in which colleagues feel respected, supported and listened to (Bailey and West, 2022). Due to the autonomous nature of the role, community nurses require encouraging and considerate teamwork to promote shared decision-making and uphold staff wellbeing, thus highlighting the importance of a compassionate leader within this environment to foster and develop an engaged and supported workforce (Ali and Terry, 2017).

Democratic leadership is also well suited to community nursing due to its significant impact on team empowerment, the basis of which utilises team inclusion within decision-making and delegation. This approach extrinsically motivates colleagues by utilising individual skill sets, promoting a collective purpose and facilitating collaborative working (Al Junaid and Al Samman, 2021; Herzer and Pronovost, 2013). Like compassionate leadership, this collective purpose enables an open and honest culture, which Francis (2013) identified as crucial for enhancing patient safety and quality. Staff are encouraged to speak up, and the process of raising concerns is normalised, promoting learning through reflection. Although this leadership model requires team effort and contribution, in community nursing a District Nurse following the democratic leadership style may lead these group discussions, such as within handover and listen to the viewpoints of all involved before utilising the feedback gained through open discussion to make a final decision.

The theory behind participative leadership complements the above leadership models well, as it suggests equal and shared responsibility or power to achieve the set targets and goals, with all team members capable of providing input (Likert, 1961). Whilst it is more commonly linked to democratic leadership as it could be considered a sub-type of this (Wang, Hou and Li, 2022), elements of compassionate leadership such as empathy and understanding, can be shown through active listening and providing both clinical and managerial support to other colleagues. This enhanced support for employee wellbeing also results in higher motivation (West, 2021), which increases inspiration and engagement among the team and subsequently promoting higher levels of participation and performance. Within community nursing, there is a significant need to work closely with members of the multidisciplinary team to promote person-centred care, yet it is important that these interactions involve detailed discussions and debates rather than being task orientated (QNI, 2017). Therefore, this theory is well-suited to leadership within the community, as it enhances the ability to build professional relationships and improve levels of organisational collaboration and commitment (Xu, 2017).

Leadership within community nursing requires the ability to empower others. With an increasingly more complex caseload of patients, team members must feel empowered and supported to uphold high standards of patient care (Maybin, Charles and Honeyman, 2016). Similarly, complex developments in patient needs can require flexibility and adaptation to change. Utilisation of the situational leadership theory promotes the adaptation of the leader to suit the team they are attempting to lead (Hersey and Blanchard, 1969), therefore encouraging a balanced approach to leading unfamiliar or complex situations. Whilst the leader's chosen approach may depend on factors affecting the team's competence and readiness such as experience, motivation and confidence (Henkel and Bourdeau, 2018), this theoretical flexibility promotes the sharing of experience, to educate and empower others within the team to develop the skills required to meet the increasing complex needs of service users in the community.

As clearly highlighted, educating, enabling and empowering those we lead is a significant part of leadership within community nursing. This provides the opportunity for growth and development and supports employee wellbeing. However, these opportunities may also be used to promote empowerment and engagement among team members. Kanter's (1993) theory of structural empowerment supports this, suggesting empowerment among employees can be promoted through providing the opportunities required to develop, alongside access to suitable information, support and resources. This provision of support and resources may include protected time, feedback and encouragement. Application of Kanter's (1993) theory to practice produces nursing leaders who are present and available to help others, offering supportive relationships among the team, promoting a safe and empowered group structure, and increasing the effectiveness of teamwork as nurses have timely access to information, increasing their ability to complete tasks and trust in their leader to ensure they have the support they need to complete their role to a high standard (Lundin et al., 2021). Similarly, a greater perception of empowerment through the application of Kanter's (1993) theory is directly correlated with reduced levels of burnout and increased work satisfaction (Valdez et al., 2019).

14.4 Essential Leadership Qualities in Community Nursing

Leaders in community nursing need to be authentic, visionary and proactive to meet challenging demands and changes within the healthcare setting. This is the reason that many nurses have chosen the community setting as a place to work. Table 14.1 presents the characteristics of effective nursing leadership

14.5 Professional Development and Continuous Learning

Community nursing is changing in response to a shift in care from hospital to home, brought about by increasing costs to care because of an ageing population and increasing need for acute care at home (QNI, 2016). Until now, community nursing positions and scope of practice have been dependent on service focus and location, which has led to the role being unclearly defined. Lack of appeal for a career in community practice and a looming workforce shortage necessitate a review of how community nursing transition to practice is supported. Because of the autonomous way in which community nurses practice, regular supervision is central to their clinical practice.

Leadership and career progression within community nursing offer numerous opportunities for professional growth and advancement. Indeed, community nurses are placed in a privileged position to be able to progress career-wise because of the varieties of specialties and pathways available in the area, and the growing complexity of care delivered at home. Working as a community nurse has a different challenge to working in a ward environment and one that involves a great deal of autonomy, but it can be incredibly rewarding (West et al., 2015). It is advised that working in the community as a newly qualified nurse is better as it enables the nurse to develop and grow with the knowledge acquired during training, enlarging these and embedding the skills and abilities (West et al., 2015). When starting a career as a community nurse, it is important to choose an employer who reflects

TABLE 14.1 ■ **Characteristics of Effective Nursing Leadership**

Vision and strategic thinking	Nurse leaders have a clear vision of the desired future state of nursing practice and healthcare delivery. They strategically plan and set goals to achieve this vision, considering factors such as patient needs, organisational objectives and industry trends.
Communication and collaboration	Effective leaders in nursing possess strong communication skills and actively engage in open and transparent communication with patients, interdisciplinary teams and stakeholders. They foster collaboration and build relationships based on trust and respect.
Clinical competence	Nurse leaders are clinically competent and stay abreast of current evidence-based practices. They demonstrate expertise in their area of specialisation, providing guidance and support to the nursing team and ensuring safe and high-quality care.
Emotional intelligence	Leadership in nursing requires emotional intelligence, including self-awareness, empathy and the ability to manage emotions effectively. Nurse leaders understand and respond to the emotional needs of patients, families and colleagues, promoting a positive and supportive work environment.
Critical thinking and decision-making	Nurse leaders possess strong critical thinking and problem-solving skills. They analyse complex situations, gather relevant information and make informed decisions that promote optimal patient outcomes and nursing practice.
Advocacy and ethics	Nurse leaders act as advocates for patients, ensuring their rights, needs and preferences are respected. They also advocate for the nursing profession, promoting ethical practice and ensuring nursing standards and regulations are upheld.
Change management	Effective nursing leaders are adaptable and skilled in managing change. They recognise the need for innovation and improvement, facilitate change processes and support the nursing team in embracing and adapting to change.
Mentorship and development	Nurse leaders are committed to fostering the professional growth and development of their team members. They serve as mentors, providing guidance, feedback and opportunities for learning and advancement.

personal values and provides them with a sustainable career. Fig. 14.1 gives an idea of what is needed in each area for personal and professional development.

14.5.1 DISTRICT NURSE

To be a district nurse (DN), you need to already be a qualified nurse and be willing to undertake further training. DN training is a specialist practitioner programme and usually takes not less than one academic year to complete (QNI, 2016). Training can be privately funded with a sponsor, provided on a secondment from an NHS trust, or by sponsorship on the Apprenticeship route. However, to be successful as a DN, a nurse must be autonomous, resourceful, organised, confident and able to handle complex and challenging situations (QNI, 2016). The DN advanced specialist role sees them promoting care for all and supporting the family from cradle to grave.

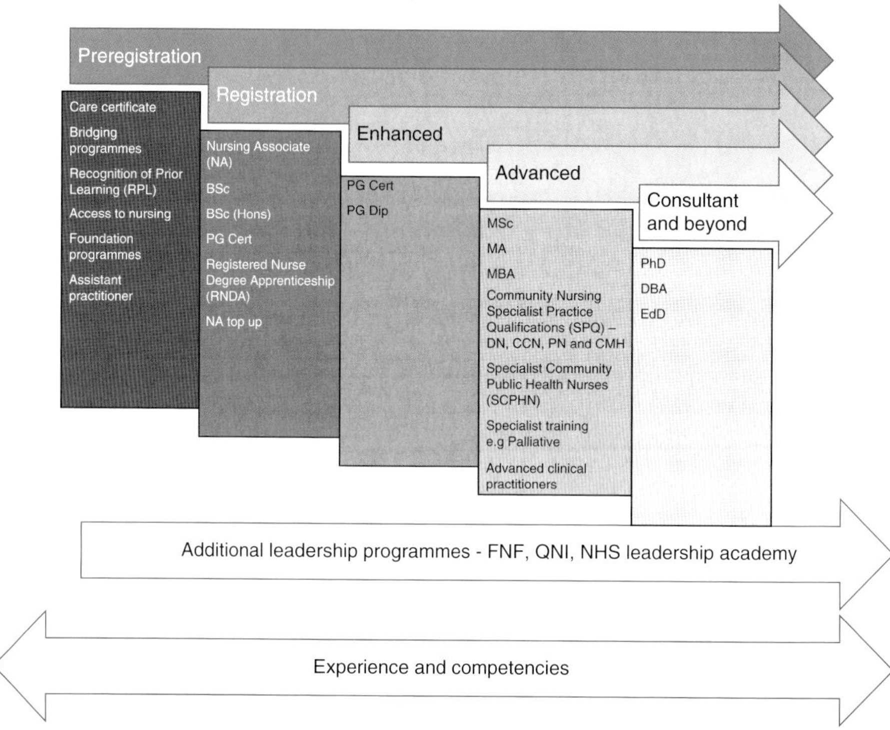

Fig. 14.1 Personal and professional development.

The district nurse is the lynchpin of community care services for adults in the community (QNI, 2016). The district nurse title is used by nurses who have undergone the Community Nursing Specialist Practice Qualifications (District Nursing) training which is a postgraduate programme in any of the Nursing and Midwifery Council (NMC) accredited universities in the UK. The qualification is recordable on the Nursing and Midwifery register and renewed annually but revalidated every 3 years in line with the NMC (2022). The primary role of the district nurse is to visit patients in their own homes to provide nursing care and support the family directly involved in looking after the individual (QNI, 2016). District nurses are professionally responsible for arranging and monitoring the care provided, and in conjunction, they also teach family members and sometimes the patient to care for themselves. Ongoing assessments are a key part of the working practice of a district nurse, and there are a variety of conditions to manage in the caseload (NMC, 2022). Some patients will be elderly, others living with dementia, learning disabilities or physical disabilities, all of whom require individual care plans to be organised by a district nurse.

Engaging in continuous professional development (CPD) is essential for career progression and clinical currency; therefore, community nursing provides the opportunity to grow in this way (Harvey et al., 2019). CPD activity could involve attending relevant conferences, workshops and courses to enhance knowledge and skills. Being a clinical champion in an area of nursing helps to boost interest in the said area. For example, being a tissue viability clinical champion in a team could potentially lead to the nurse becoming a tissue viability specialist by gaining additional qualifications, such as a Master's degree in a related field which can also strengthen leadership prospects.

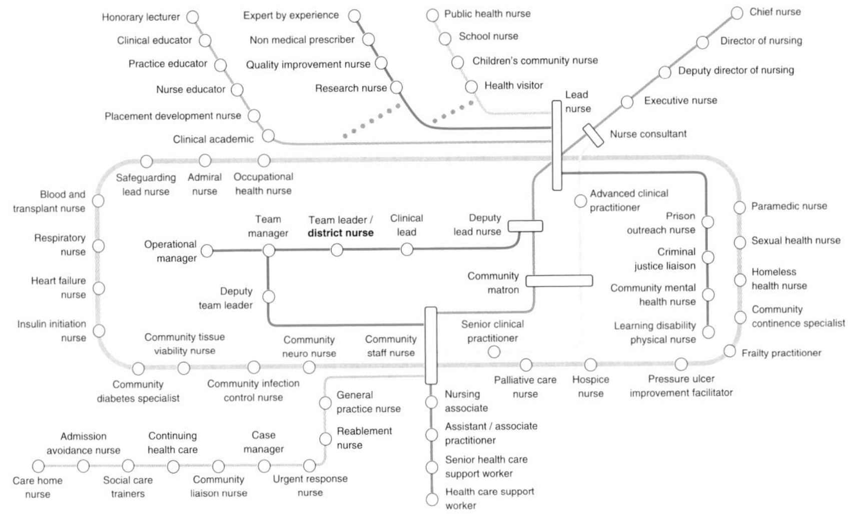

Fig. 14.2 Diverse career paths in community nursing.

14.5.2 LEADERSHIP COURSES AND PROGRAMMES

Appraisals are crucial in identifying talents and gaps in knowledge and what to do to bridge the gap (Berridge et al., 2007). Taking advantage of leadership courses and programmes specific to community nursing can provide valuable insights into leadership theories, skills and strategies. These programmes often cover topics like effective leadership styles, change management, project management and strategic planning which can help develop a nurse's career.

14.5.3 LEADERSHIP ROLES

Community nursing provides various opportunities to develop a specialisation in many areas other than district nursing which can include health visiting, school nursing and palliative care nursing. Pursuing advanced practice roles within these specialisations, such as nurse practitioner or advanced nurse practitioner is also an option (Fig. 14.2).

14.5.4 CLINICAL LEADERSHIP ROLES

Community nursing offers various clinical leadership roles that denote the individual's clinical credibility and ability (Harvey et al., 2019). The district nurse role as well as other roles, such as community matron, clinical nurse specialist, team leader and advanced practitioners, give deserved recognition to highly skilled clinicians who enable positive outcomes for their patients at all times. These roles involve overseeing a team of nurses, coordinating care and ensuring the delivery of high-quality services within the community.

14.5.5 MANAGEMENT POSITIONS

An experienced community nurse in the health service may choose a career in management (Ogunsola & Thorpe, 2023). It is preferred that community nurses manage their discipline because they will have a better in-depth understanding of clinical issues and supervision to promote greater model of service delivery and better outcomes for service users. Advancing into management positions within community nursing organisations is another avenue for career progression. These positions include roles like clinical service manager, operations manager, team lead and service lead. They involve broader responsibilities related to managing budgets, managing resources, managing service-related projects and strategic planning (HEE, 2015).

14.5.6 RESEARCH AND EDUCATION

Research development is an area of career progression that is currently being promoted and encouraged in community nursing through the Clinical Academic route. Engaging in research and education is a viable pathway to leadership within community nursing and is a core component of the nurse consultant route. Conducting research, publishing articles and participating in educational initiatives can establish expertise and pave the way for leadership roles in academia, research institutions or educational organisations. Some of the subjects accessed for research trials are community-based patients and the knowledge of community nurses in enabling the right environment for research is very essential.

14.5.7 PROFESSIONAL NETWORKS AND ASSOCIATIONS

There are key professional networks and organisations that promote the work of community nursing. Some are disciplined focussed, e.g., National District Nursing Network (NDNN) and Association of District Nurse and Community Nurse Educators (ADNE), while others support community nursing such as the Queen's Nursing Institute. The work of each of these organisations has been helpful in enabling community nursing to develop and for the voice of the community nurses be heard and acted upon. The Queen's Nursing Institute, Royal College of Nursing or local nursing fora provides opportunities to connect with like-minded professionals, access mentorship and gain exposure to leadership opportunities and resources.

14.5.8 CONTINUOUS SELF-ASSESSMENT AND REFLECTION

Regularly assessing strengths, weaknesses and areas for improvement is essential for career progression (QNI, 2016). Engaging in self-reflection, seeking feedback from peers and supervisors and actively working on personal and professional development goals can contribute to leadership growth. It is important to note that career progression may vary based on individual goals, aspirations and opportunities within specific organisations (Harvey et al., 2019). Building a strong foundation of clinical experience, developing leadership skills and actively seeking growth opportunities are key to advancing in community nursing leadership roles in the UK.

14.5.9 MENTORING

Seeking mentorship and participating in preceptorship programmes can provide guidance and support in career progression (HEE, 2015). Experienced leaders within the community nursing field can offer insights, share their experiences and provide advice on navigating the path to leadership. Some organisations have senior nurses in positions that support career development and career progression as part of a retention strategy.

Shadowing is also encouraged to allow community nurses to have a taste of their career choice (HEE, 2015). Shadowing also provides the opportunity to discuss the role with the expert and understand the challenges and dynamics of the role. It allows exposure to decision-making processes, collaboration with diverse stakeholders and visibility within the community nursing sector (HEE, 2015). It can also help to broaden professional networks and develop leadership skills. These forms of practice learning are valued and seen as central to advancing the skills of community nurses.

14.6 The Role of Social Media and Building a Professional Network

With hundreds of social media platforms in the world, the internet is the backbone of our society (Gamor et al., 2023). Consequently, using social media to network can be a beneficial starting point. More than half of the world's population is already using social media to interact with friends, family and colleagues, meet new people and share interests. Some of the most widely recognised social media sites include Facebook, WhatsApp, Twitter, Instagram, Telegram, Snapchat, YouTube and Google+ (Gamor et al., 2023). As a result of social media saturation worldwide, user bases have become more reflective of the general population, and healthcare professionals are frequently adopting social media to engage in health promotion, patient education, professional development and networking (Gamor et al., 2023). There are a variety of platforms that target different audiences, and this diversity enables users to choose tools that support their individual needs.

14.6.1 CREATING A PROFESSIONAL NETWORK USING SOCIAL MEDIA

Healthcare professionals are empowered by social communities as they can increase engagement and insight into healthcare information and subsequent changes and trends in the professions, along with providing better opportunities for career advancement and developing a sense of belonging (Meiring, 2018). In recent years, there has been a transformation in how nurses build professional networks, and social media has been described as one of the most powerful tools to achieve this (Thrumble & Oozageer Gunowa, 2022).

Many people claim that they have more online than real-world connections, highlighting new opportunities to create and share information and connect with healthcare professionals worldwide (Donelan, 2014). LinkedIn is commonly used to strategically build and maintain networks by allowing members to demonstrate their expertise and achievements and providing professional opportunities for employment and development (Tower et al., 2014). However, strong professional networks take time and effort to build, traditionally requiring nurses to participate in societies and events to increase visibility and reputation (Meiring, 2018). Knowledge gained from these events ripples out, influencing communities, helping others to learn and benefit from personal growth, fostering a professional and collaborative culture in nursing (Donelan, 2014). However, some nursing groups, like community nursing teams, can become marginalised from face-to-face networking events due to the incompatibility of roles and locations and nurses often find networking opportunities particularly difficult due to a lack of confidence (Meiring, 2018). The relative anonymity of social networking can reduce these barriers with increased access to information, and an inclusive environment that allows previously passive observers to actively participate in discussions and debates (Thrumble & Oozageer Gunowa, 2022).

Ninety-two percent of nurses feel that social networking provides an inclusive, respectful environment and presents an innovative learning platform, allowing nurses to explore different opinions and enhance autonomy in learning (Tower et al., 2014). However, the value of this way of networking is not effectively promoted among nurses (Donelan, 2014). Furthermore, 89.8% of nursing students report that professional social media networking increased their knowledge and understanding of subject content, and the dissemination of research via online platforms has been shown to increase downloads of published articles and subsequent citations in further literature (Tower et al., 2014). This has been identified as a mission statement for a widely used social media platform—Twitter (X)—with this platform aiming to provide the ability to share ideas instantly with limited barriers (Power, 2015).

Social media networking has its disadvantages. Twitter and Facebook demonstrate minimal content regulation, which raises concerns regarding compatibility within a profession that values privacy, confidentiality and face-to-face relationship building (NMC, 2023). Utilisation of social media professionally can be an intimidating prospect, due to fears regarding professionalism which have been instilled from undergraduate education (NMC, 2023). Concerns regarding security, privacy and inappropriate content present potential for violation of the nursing Code of Conduct (NMC, 2018) if personal and professional social media accounts are combined (Thrumble & Oozageer Gunowa, 2022). In contrast to traditional networking where professionals have been able to apply distinct personal and professional boundaries, social media accounts provide nonrestrictive access to information, meaning participation in networking events can be accessed from the comfort of an individual's home (Tower et al., 2014). This provides an illusion of privacy which could lead to violations including posts which include breaches of Information Governance and patient confidentiality (Data Protection Act, 2018). However, Power (2015) states that social media can be used in accordance with the NMC Code of Conduct (2018) when appropriate privacy settings and separation of personal and professional accounts are used. Through this, nurses can safely participate while maintaining professionalism and preventing repercussions on professional reputations (Thrumble & Oozageer Gunowa, 2022).

TIPS TO CREATE AND EXPAND A PROFESSIONAL SOCIAL MEDIA NETWORK

Commenting and engaging: build links to your profile so people can follow and engage with you and your work; provide feedback on posts of interest which helps others by sharing your knowledge.

Uploading content you have created: build a support network and post useful resources such as research articles that ensure you share your knowledge and experience; increase your visibility and build your reputation.

14.7 Conclusion

In conclusion, leadership and career progression in community nursing are closely intertwined, providing opportunities for unlimited advancement. As community nurses grow in their roles, they take on greater responsibilities, including leading and influencing teams, driving change, managing projects, and continuously improving the quality of care. These efforts contribute to shaping the delivery of community healthcare services. Additionally, the use of various social media platforms plays a crucial role in building connections across professional networks, enabling easy access to research leaders and colleagues on local, regional, national, and global levels.

References

Ali, S., & Terry, L. (2017). Exploring senior nurses' understanding of compassionate leadership in the community. *British Journal of Community Nursing*, *22*(2), 77–87. https://doi.org/10.12968/bjcn.2017.22.2.77

Al Junaid, A. I., & Al Samman, A. (2021). How employee empowerment is affected by the exercised leadership style. *International Journal of Economics, Commerce and Management*, *4*(9), 295–312. Available at: https://www.researchgate.net/profile/Adel-Al-Samman/publication/354948748_HOW_EMPLOYEE_EMPOWERMENT_IS_AFFECTED_BY_THE_EXERCISED_LEADERSHIP_STYLE/links/61558574eabde032acb93369/HOW-EMPLOYEE-EMPOWERMENT-IS-AFFECTED-BY-THE-EXERCISED-LEADERSHIP-STYLE.pdf?origin=journalDetail&_tp=eyJwYWdlIjoiam91cm5hbERldGFpbCJ9. [Accessed 8 June 2024].

Bailey, S., & West, M. (2022). *What is compassionate leadership?* Available at: https://www.kingsfund.org.uk/insight-and-analysis/long-reads/what-is-compassionate-leadership#:~:text=Compassionate%20leadership%20involves%20a%20focus. [Accessed 8 June 2024].

Bass, B.M. (1995). Comment: Transformational leadership: Looking at other possible antecedents and consequences. *Journal of Management Inquiry*, *4*(3), 293–297. https://doi.org/10.1177/105649269543010.

Berridge, E.-J., Kelly, D., & Gould, S. (2007). Staff appraisal and continuing professional development: Exploring the relationships in acute and community health settings. *Journal of Research in Nursing*, *12*(1).

Data Protection Act. (2018). Available online: www.gov.uk/data-protection. [Accessed 14 November 2023].

Donelan, H. (2014). Social media for professional development and networking opportunities in academia. *J Further Higher Education*, *40*(5), 706–729.

Ellis, P. (2021). Leadership, management and team working in nursing (4th ed.). Learning Matters.

Francis, R. (2013). *Report of the mid staffordshire NHS foundation trust public inquiry: executive summary.* (HC 947). London: The Stationary Office.

Gamor, N., Dzansi, G., Konlan, K.D., & Abdulai, E. (2023). Exploring social media adoption by nurses for nursing practice in rural Volta, Ghana. *Nursing Open*, *10*(7), 4432–4441. https://doi.org/10.1002/nop2.1685. Epub 2023 Feb 25. PMID: 36840611; PMCID: PMC10277433. https://www.ncbi.nlm.nih.gov/pmc/articles/PMC10277433/.

Harvey, C., Hegney, D., Sobolewska, A., Chamberlain, D., Wood, W., Wirihana, L., et al. (2019). Developing a community based nursing and midwifery career pathway – A narrative systematic review. *PLOS One*, *14*(3).

Health Education England [HEE]. (2015). *Health careers: District nursing and general practice education and career framework*. London: HEE.

Henkel, T., & Bourdeau, D. (2018). A field study: An examination of managers' situational leadership styles. *Journal of Diversity Management (JDM)*, *13*(2), 7–14. https://doi.org/10.19030/jdm.v13i2.10218

Herzer, K. R., & Pronovost, P. J. (2013). Motivating physicians to improve quality: Light the intrinsic fire. *American Journal of Medical Quality*, *29*(5), 451–453. https://doi.org/10.1177/1062860613510201

Kanter, R. M. (1993). *Men and women of the corporation* (2nd ed.). New York: Basic Books.

Likert, R. (1961). *New patterns of management*. New York: McGraw-Hill.

Lundin, K., Silén, M., Strömberg, A., Engström, M., & Skytt, B. (2021). Staff structural empowerment—observations of first–line managers and interviews with managers and staff. *Journal of Nursing Management*, *30*(2), 403–412. https://doi.org/10.1111/jonm.13513

Maybin, J., Charles, A., & Honeyman, M. (2016). *Understanding quality in district nursing services*. Available at: https://www.kingsfund.org.uk/insight-and-analysis/reports/understanding-quality-district-nursing-services. [Accessed 10 August 2024].

Meiring, A. (2018). The value of networking for professional nurses. *Prof Nurs Today, 22*(3), 2.

NHS England. (2021). *NHS England» our shared ambition for compassionate, inclusive leadership*. Available at: https://www.england.nhs.uk/ourwork/part-rel/nqb/our-shared-ambition-for-compassionate-inclusive-leadership/. [Accessed 10 August 2024].

Nursing and Midwifery Council. (2018). *The code: Professional standards of practice and behaviour for nurses, midwives and nursing associates*. Available at: https://www.nmc.org.uk/globalassets/sitedocuments/nmc-publications/nmc-code.pdf. [Accessed 28 February 2024].

Nursing and Midwifery Council UK. (2022). *Standards of proficiency for community nursing specialist practice qualifications*. NMC.

Nursing and Midwifery Council. (2023). *Social media guidance*. Available from: https://www.nmc.org.uk/standards/guidance/social-media-guidance/.

Nursing and Midwifery Council. (2024). *Good leadership means better care*. Available from: https://www.nmc.org.uk/standards/guidance/good-leadership-means-better-care/.

Ogunsola, C., & Thorpe, A. (2023). Diverse career pathways in community nursing, an infographic of variety of careers available in community nursing. *COAT – NHSE Clinical Fellow 2022*.

Power, A. (2015). Twitter's potential to enhance professional networking. *BMJ, 23*(1), 65–67.

QNI. (2016). Transition into District Nursing. Accessed at https://qni.org.uk/resources/transition-district-nursing/.

Sfantou, D.F., Laliotis, A., Patelarou, A.E., Sifaki-Pistolla, D., Matalliotakis, M., & Patelarou, E. (2017). Importance of leadership style towards quality of care measures in healthcare settings: A systematic review. *Healthcare (Basel, Switzerland)*, 5(*4*), 73. https://doi.org/10.3390/healthcare5040073.

The Queen's Nursing Institute. (2017). *Transition to district nursing service*. Available at: https://www.qni.org.uk/wp-content/uploads/2017/01/2-Transition-to-District-Nursing-CHAPTER-2.pdf. [Accessed 7 June 2024].

Thrumble, H., & Oozageer Gunowa, N. (2022). Using social media to enhance nursing practice and patient safety. *Journal of General Practice Nursing*, 20–21.

Tower, M., Latimer, S., & Hewitt, J. (2014). Social networking as a learning tool: nursing students' perception of efficacy. *Nurse Education Today, 34*(6), 1012–1017.

Valdez, G. F. D., Cayaban, A. R., Mathews, S., & Doloolat, Z. A. (2019). Workplace empowerment, burnout, and job satisfaction among nursing faculty members: Testing Kanter's theory. *Nursing and Palliative Care International Journal, 2*(1), 29–35. https://doi.org/10.30881/npcij.00012

Wang, Q., Hou, H., & Li, Z. (2022). Participative leadership: A literature review and prospects for future research. *Frontiers in Psychology, 13*(1), 1–12. https://doi.org/10.3389/fpsyg.2022.924357

West, M. A. (2021). *Compassionate leadership: Sustaining wisdom, humanity and presence in health and social care*. London: The Swirling Leaf Press.

West, M.A., Armit, K., Loewenthal, L., Eckert, R., West, T., & Lee, A. (2015) Leadership and Leadership Development in Health Care (Accessed on 6th Feb 2024. https://www.kingsfund.org.uk/insight-and-analysis/reports/leadership-development-health-care.

Wong, C.A., Cummings, G.G., & Ducharme, L. (2013). The relationship between nursing leadership and patient outcomes: A systematic review update. *Journal of Nursing Management,* 21(*5*), 709–724. https://doi.org/10.1111/jonm.12116.

Xu, J.-H. (2017). Leadership theory in clinical practice. *Chinese Nursing Research, 4*(4), 155–157. https://doi.org/10.1016/j.cnre.2017.10.001

CHAPTER 15

Quality and Safety in the Community

Katie Baichoo ■ Hannah Little ■ Paulette Ragan ■
Kendra Schneller ■ Jonathan Taylor

LEARNING OUTCOMES

After reading this chapter you should be able to:

- Understand the fundamentals of measuring quality and patient outcomes in the community
- Contribute to the delivery of safe, high-quality care and protect the well-being of patients in the community
- Appreciate the impact that documentation has on patients and colleagues
- Comprehend how medicines are managed in the community and the role of nurse prescribing

15.1 Patient Safety

15.1.1 INTRODUCTION

Patient safety can be defined as 'the absence of preventable harm to a patient and reduction of risk of unnecessary harm associated with health care to an acceptable minimum' (World Health Organization (WHO), 2023), or 'the avoidance of unintended or unexpected harm to people during the provision of health care' (NHS, 2023). Within the context of a health system, patient safety can be defined as 'a framework of organized activities that creates cultures, processes, procedures, behaviours, technologies and environments in health care that consistently and sustainably lower risks, reduce the occurrence of avoidable harm, make error less likely and reduce impact of harm when it does occur' (WHO, 2023).

Approximately 1 in 10 patients are harmed in healthcare, and unsafe care results in over 3 million deaths each year, more than half of these being preventable (WHO, 2023). Some of the most common causes of patient safety incidents are communication errors and human factors (Chaneliere et al., 2018), trips and falls, infection and sepsis, pressure injuries, medication errors, surgical errors, diagnostic errors and venous thromboembolism (WHO, 2023).

Healthcare organisations have a responsibility to protect patients from avoidable harm. Where harm does occur, there is often an opportunity to learn lessons to drive improvements in safety and quality. Patients and families deserve to know that when something goes wrong, the organisation will learn and prevent anything similar from happening to anyone else.

This section of the chapter will provide an introduction to key matters relating to patient safety, giving an insight into how healthcare systems strive to improve safety for patients.

15.1.2 BACKGROUND

A King's Fund report published in 2023 suggested that comparing the healthcare systems of different countries can help politicians and policymakers understand how the UK is performing, as well as how it could improve (Anandaciva, 2023). According to this report, which reviewed academic literature, analysed quantitative data and interviewed experts in the field, people receiving healthcare in the UK generally experience low levels of total harm compared to other countries. This is an impressive achievement given that, for many years, the UK's spending on healthcare has been below average compared to peer countries (Papanicolas et al., 2019). To explain this, it is important to consider that the UK has relatively high levels of reported harm (Anandaciva, 2023); harm levels are fairly low, but the harm that does occur is reported with good frequency. It might be inferred that the high level of reportage contributes to the safety of the UK's health system. Reporting harm enables organisations to learn and prevent harm from proliferating.

Crucially, reporting harm allows for the development of comparative data on which clinicians and policymakers can draw when considering where to focus improvement efforts. For example, from such data, it is known that rates of postoperative sepsis after abdominal surgery used to be higher in the UK than in peer countries (Papanicolas et al., 2019). Such insight has motivated clinicians and organisations to improve in this area. The Preventing Surgical Site Infection (PreciSSIon) project, for instance, trialled a bundle of evidence-based interventions known to reduce infection in one hospital, before rolling it out across a region via the local Health Innovation Networks (Clayphan et al., 2022). The bundle of interventions was so successful that it was included in in the 2016 WHO global guidelines on the prevention of surgical site infection and in the 2019 update to the National Institute for Health and Clinical Excellence (NICE) guidance (Health Innovation Network West of England, n.d.).

REFLECTION

Improvements made in one part of the healthcare system can have far-reaching benefits.

- Ask some of your most experienced colleagues if they have noticed a reduction in wound infections following abdominal surgery in recent years.
- What advice can you give patients to reduce their risk of pressure injury?
- What do you think could be the next patient safety improvement drive in the community?
- Is there anything you can do now to improve safety for your patients?

Similarly, a project mobilised through the NHS Patient Safety Collaboratives utilised national sepsis data to indicate that using the National Early Warning Score (NEWS) in community and primary care settings can reduce mortality (Pullyblank et al., 2020). If a patient with suspicion of sepsis has a NEWS of 3 in the community, 4 in the ambulance and 5 when they arrive at the hospital, the receiving team can easily see that this person is deteriorating and prioritise them above others who may be stable with similar observations. When there are hundreds of people needing care in a busy emergency department, this kind of insight can save lives.

Data also show that around half a million people in the UK develop at least one pressure ulcer each year (Health Foundation, 2020). A project involving collaboration from different healthcare and academic organisations notes that: 'Many of these occur in the community setting and become long-term, nonhealing wounds, leading to significant discomfort' (Health Foundation, 2020). The project introduced the use of chair and mattress sensors in patients' homes, training up three tissue viability teams and one District nurse team in Southwest England to support patients. This achieved a reduction in the number of pressure ulcers and resulted in significant (57%) ulcer healing rates (Health Foundation, 2020).

15.1.3 SAFER CULTURE AND SAFER SYSTEMS

The recent NHS Patient Safety Strategy (NHS England, 2019a) acknowledges that there is still much to do to optimise safety in the NHS. It proposes that if patients and staff are empowered with the skills, confidence and mechanisms to improve safety, it could be possible to save almost 1000 extra lives and £100 million in care costs each year. The Strategy outlines how the NHS might continuously improve patient safety, building on the following two foundations:

1. Patient safety culture
2. Patient safety systems

Safety culture is inextricably linked to safety systems (NHS England, 2019a). Safety systems include things such as mechanisms to report and learn from incidents. An organisation could have the best safety systems possible, but without a culture that prioritises patient safety, these would likely be used ineffectively (Fig. 15.1).

Incident reporting systems rely on staff reporting incidents, and the effectiveness of this can depend upon the culture. The NHS Patient Safety Strategy (NHS England, 2019a) outlines several key features of a patient safety culture, including 'staff who feel psychologically safe; valuing and respecting diversity; a compelling vision; good leadership at all levels; a sense of teamwork; openness and support for learning'.

If this is applied to an organisation's response to incidents, one could expect to find a culture where staff feel free to raise and report incidents and concerns of all kinds, and that they can trust that their organisation will learn from these. They might expect to be treated fairly when something goes wrong, confident that they will not be unfairly blamed, in accordance with the NHS's Just Culture Guide, which supports organisations

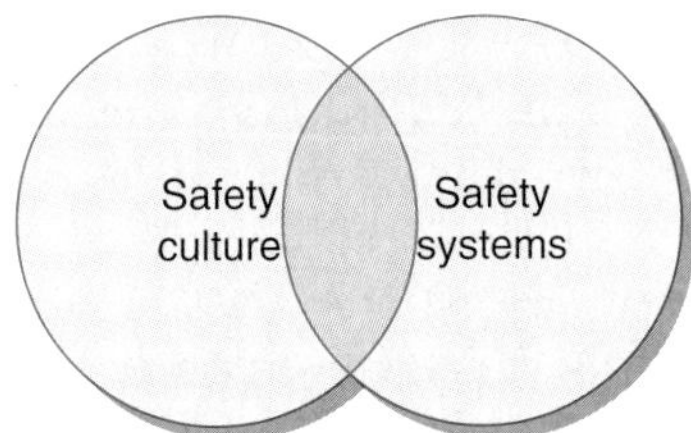

Fig. 15.1 Safety culture and safety systems are inextricably linked.

to treat staff involved in a patient safety incident in a consistent, constructive and fair way (NHS England, 2021).

Blame is a natural and easy response to error and it allows the cause of mistakes to be boiled down to individual incompetence, carelessness or recklessness (NHS England, 2021). However, healthcare staff operate within highly complex systems where multiple factors tend to play a role when something goes wrong. These may include the quality of training provided, clarity of guidelines and volume of tasks assigned to those involved. In a just culture which values a 'systems approach' to learning, all of the relevant factors would be considered and addressed proportionately. Until recently, it was fairly common for managers to conduct a simple root cause analysis (RCA) when something went wrong, which tended to encourage finding a single 'root cause' for a complex problem. Now, it is expected that various relevant factors will be explored for opportunities to learn. RCA can still be a useful tool but should ideally be used alongside other tools. It is also important to acknowledge that incidents may have multiple root causes. Incidents rarely have a single, straightforward cause, and responses to them need to reflect this.

The recent release of the NHS Patient Safety Incident Response Framework (PSIRF), replacing the Serious Incident Framework (SIF) of 2015, is also illustrative of the NHS's shift towards learning from complexity. With the 2015 SIF, all incidents deemed to be serious enough in nature had to be fully investigated using a prescriptive bureaucratic process. PSIRF aims to ensure resources allocated to learning are balanced with those needed to actually deliver improvement (NHS England, 2022a, 2022b). It also places a strong emphasis on compassionate engagement with those affected by patient safety incidents—patients and families—and provides various system-based toolkits and guides to support the embedding of learning in practice (NHS England, 2023b). Many of these resources are designed around the fact that ultimately healthcare is run by humans, with their inevitable flaws and resultant opportunities to learn and improve. Acknowledging this is essential for promoting both a safer culture, where people feel empowered to speak up when things go wrong, as well as safer systems which are primed to learn and progress.

In recent years, key developments in several areas have allowed for the development of both a safer culture and safer systems. These include:

- The study of human factors
- Learning from excellence
- Learning from harm

15.1.4 THE STUDY OF HUMAN FACTORS

The study of human factors in patient safety has made great headway in healthcare systems around the world, including the NHS (NHS England, 2013). Human factors focus on 'optimising human performance through better understanding the behaviour of individuals, their interactions with each other and with their environment. By acknowledging human limitations, Human Factors offer ways to minimise and mitigate human frailties, so reducing medical error and its consequences' (NHS England, 2013).

Hollnagel et al. (2013) described healthcare as 'a complex adaptive system', with emergent properties resulting from a labyrinth of interactions, making it nonlinear and dynamic. As such, learning from patient safety incidents can be hugely complex and require great skill and resources. It can also be extremely interesting, as well as beneficial to both safety systems and culture, if adequate time is given to fully investigate, meaningfully involving those affected and demonstrating learning in action to them and the wider team, organisation and system.

A seminal 2015 white paper by Hollnagel et al. (2015) outlined that learning can be accelerated if healthcare moves from ensuring that 'as few things as possible go wrong' to ensuring that 'as many things as possible go right'. This is known as a Safety-II approach and has been extremely influential in shaping how we learn to improve.

15.1.5 LEARNING FROM EXCELLENCE

A 'systems' approach to patient safety considers all relevant factors which means that the pursuit of safety focuses on strategies that maximise the frequency of things going right, as well as minimising things that go wrong (NHS England, 2019a). Many organisations have set up or adopted systems for excellence reporting alongside incident reporting, which can not only provide rich sources of insight for learning, but they can also provide a welcome morale boost for staff and promote a positive safety culture. Systems include 'GREAT-ix', 'PIMS' (Positive Incident Management System) and Learning from Excellence (LfE) Reporting, which is open to anyone working in healthcare via https://learningfromexcellence.com/open-reporting/

15.1.6 LEARNING FROM HARM

15.1.6.1 The Role of the Community Nurse

The single biggest thing every community nurse can do to contribute to patient safety systems and culture is to complete an incident report when something goes wrong or had the potential to go wrong, often referred to as a 'near miss'. This not only gives local teams the chance to respond but ensures that the duty of candour is appropriately applied, and steps taken to prevent local reoccurrence; it also enables regional, national and international patient safety experts to identify and respond to themes. The duty of candour is defined as 'a professional responsibility to be honest when things go wrong' (Nursing and Midwifery Council (NMC), 2022). There is a difference between the professional duty of candour, as described and required by the NMC Code (2018a), and a statutory duty of candour. Whilst both have similar aims, to ensure that healthcare services are open and transparent when something goes wrong, the statutory duty of candour refers to the requirements outlined in Regulation 20 of the Health and Social Care Act. This regulation requires all health and social care providers registered with the CQC to 'act in an open and transparent way with people receiving care or treatment from them' (Care Quality Commission (CQC), 2022), and defines 'Notifiable Safety Incidents' and what must occur in such cases.

REFLECTION

- Is there anything you can do to encourage excellence reporting in your clinical area?
- Is there an established mechanism for this? If not, how would you feel about asking your organisation's Patient Safety team to either set this up or promote free available options such as: https://learningfromexcellence.com/open-reporting/.
- How can you ensure learning occurs when things go wrong?

15.1.7 RISK

REFLECTION

- How do you assess risk in everyday clinical practice?

15.1.7.1 Managing Risk

Healthcare professionals dynamically assess risk all the time. From the simplest of tasks, such as making a hot drink for a patient, to the most complex of clinical tasks, healthcare professionals are continually considering potential hazards and ensuring control measures are in place to reduce the risk of harm. This is a dynamic risk assessment. It can be documented in a patient's clinical record where appropriate, either as free text or according to local protocol.

Formal risk assessment tends to involve scoring a risk to show how likely it is to cause harm and how severe the harm could be, both before and after steps to mitigate (reduce) the risk have been put in place. Most organisations have a risk assessment matrix, similar to Fig. 15.2.

Formally assessed risks tend to be captured on risk registers, where actions to address and mitigate the risk can be viewed by different leaders and managers to ensure the organisation has adequate measures in place to reduce the risk of harm to patients. Large organisations often have different levels of risk registers. For example, there might be departmental risk registers that inform wider organisational ones, capturing risks which are outside of the control of local departments. Integrated care boards also hold risk registers containing risks outside of the control of individual organisations. See Table 15.1.

Risk assessment matrix example		Severity (Consequences)				
		1 Insignificant	2 Minor	3 Moderate	4 Severe	5 Catastrophic
Likelihood (frequency)	1 Rare	1 Low	2 Low	3 Low	4 Medium	5 Medium
	2 Unlikely	2 Low	4 Medium	6 Medium	8 High	10 High
	3 Possible	3 Low	6 Medium	9 High	12 High	15 Very high
	4 Likely	4 Medium	8 High	12 High	16 Very high	20 Very high
	5 Almost certain	5 Medium	10 High	15 Very high	20 Very high	25 Very high

Fig. 15.2 Risk assessment matrix. The score is determined by multiplying the severity × likelihood. The matrices can vary slightly between organisations. Often the scores are referred to as 'RAG (red, amber, green) ratings'.

TABLE 15.1 ■ **Examples of Risks Captured on Different Levels of Risk Register**

Type of Risk Register	Example of Risk Held Here
Departmental	Risk of delays to patient care due to high staff vacancy.
Organisational	Risk to future service provision as 52% of the nursing workforce are due to retire within the next 5 years.
Integrated care board	Risk to recruitment regionally as the local university plans to stop providing nursing degrees within the next 3 years (this kind of risk might also be captured at organisational level).

BOX 15.1 ■ Future Considerations

- Seek opportunities to report incidents using your local reporting system and encourage others to do the same.
- Communicate with colleagues that learning from incidents is about enabling safer systems for patients. It is not about blame (A Just Culture Guide can help with this).
- Look for opportunities to reduce risk and support learning from both success and harm in your team. Whether this involves making small changes or leading a quality improvement project, share your findings openly and honestly with anyone else who could learn. This could be verbally, via publication, presenting posters, writing blogs or case studies or any other means of spreading learning to make our healthcare systems as safe as possible for patients.
- Be an ambassador for patient safety in the community and beyond, advocating for safer culture and safer systems.

Healthcare organisations can be asked to demonstrate their oversight of risk to commissioners and regulators, such as the CQC. The CQC will expect to see robust action plans in place to mitigate such risks and will want to know that the organisation's leaders are actively engaged in overseeing these action plans.

REFLECTION

- What is the difference between dynamic and formal risk assessment?
- Why do you think it is important that an organisation's leaders, such as their chief nurse and chief executive, have oversight of major risks?

Challenge: Why not ask your team leader if you can view any risk registers they have access to? Awareness of risks might help you to play a role in reducing them in your clinical practice. It may also give you ideas for QI projects which could improve patient safety.

15.1.8 CONCLUSION

Preventing harm by managing risk and learning when something goes wrong is fundamental to patient safety, and can support individual, team and organisational learning. The NHS also has systems in place to facilitate learning regionally and nationally, by analysing and responding to new and emerging themes and trends which show risks to—or adverse effects on—patient safety. Such data are analysed internationally by organisations such as the WHO and translated into intelligence to help healthcare organisations and policymakers ensure that their systems are as safe as can be. The UK, despite having a lower-than-average spend per person on healthcare, repeatedly scores higher than average in various safety measures. It could be suggested that this is due to a culture of open and transparent reporting and subsequent systematic learning. This depends on healthcare professionals reporting incidents and near misses, and on leaders both applying learning locally and sharing learning more widely. Box 15.1 lists other points to consider.

15.2 Patient Documentation

15.2.1 INTRODUCTION

The growing number of people living with comorbidities, noncommunicable diseases and complex care pathways means that providing a person-centred approach that is both tailored to the patient and clinician needs is difficult (Ajibade, 2021). Therefore, effective nursing practice requires comprehensive, accurate and timely completion of records. The benefit of this is not only to the patient and other healthcare professionals involved in the individuals' care, but to ensure safe practice of the nurse in line with NMC regulations (NMC, 2018b).

With effective documentation using objective assessment tools, accurate history taking and subjective patient reports, care can be optimised, and any treatments evaluated for effectiveness. Robust documentation will enable clinicians to flag both deterioration and improvement in health; and multidisciplinary teams can review trends and identify underlying illness that may not have been diagnosed or recognised with inadequate documentation (Williams, 2022).

15.2.2 THE LEGAL ASPECT OF DOCUMENTATION

A patient record is a professional and legal document (NMC, 2018b). Effective record keeping is an essential element of the nurse's role and supports the provision of safe, high-quality patient care (Brooks, 2021). It provides evidence that safe practice has been exercised, allows complaints and concerns to be investigated and facilitates opportunity for reflections (NMC, 2018b). Effective documentation reduces margins of error and maximises patient experience and is evidence that an event happened, what happened during the event and planned next steps after the event. The clarity and accuracy of information documented in chronological order demonstrate response to treatment, thus allowing continuity of care to flow (Brown, 2022).

By taking the time to assess patient need, review previous care and document fully, openness and honesty are promoted (NMC, 2022), which in turn creates safer practice and improves communication between the multidisciplinary workforce. According to the NMC (2022), reporting adverse incidents or near misses encourages a learning culture amongst the wider network of healthcare professionals. This in turn improves the overall patient experience, so it is vitally important that all elements of documentation are completed according to trust frameworks, legal frameworks and the NMC Code (2018a).

Jargon and speculation should be avoided (Royal College of Nursing (RCN), 2023) as it could be argued that it only serves to confuse; many disciplines have abbreviations that can mean different things depending on the area of practice.

REFLECTION

- Consider some abbreviations that you have seen used in your clinical area that could mean something else in a different environment and what risk this may present to the patient.

15.2.3 EFFECTIVE RECORD KEEPING

Nurses often say, 'If it isn't written down it didn't happen'. Documentation provides evidence of your clinical rationale for giving care and protects you from liability (NMC, 2018b). It should be clear and free from jargon or unapproved abbreviations (RCN, 2023). All employers will provide training for their clinicians to maximise the potential use of available systems. Nurses are then responsible after this initial training to familiarise themselves with the systems to manage their potential and ensure the accuracy of their record keeping is maximised.

BOX 15.2 ■ Specific Information Regarding Community Nursing Notes

- Records should be completed at the time of care or as soon as possible after the event.
- All records must be signed, timed and dated if handwritten. If digital, they must be traceable to the person who provided the care that is being documented, using electronic identification cards or similar.
- Ensure that you are proficient in the use of electronic systems in your place of work, including security, confidentiality and appropriate usage, accessing system-specific training as required.
- Records must be completed accurately and without any falsification.
- Jargon and speculation should be avoided; the aim is to be as objective as possible when writing from a clinical viewpoint. The patient's subjective view can be documented in their own words within the body of the text and clearly attributed to them.
- When possible, the person in your care should be involved in the record keeping and should be able to understand what the records say. Remember patients can request access to their records.
- Records should be readable when photocopied or scanned and written in black pen.
- In the rare case of needing to alter a record, the original entry must remain visible (draw a single line through the record) and the new entry must be signed, timed and dated. For electronic records, the 'mark in error' process must be followed and the reason for adjusting an entry clearly documented.
- Records must be stored securely and should only be destroyed following your local policy and Information Governance requirements.

(From RCN (2023) Record Keeping: The Facts. https://www.rcn.org.uk/Professional-Development/publications/rcn-record-keeping-uk-pub-011-016. With permission from Royal College of Nursing.)

Sharing of information with the wider network of care promotes seamless communication. This minimises risks, thus providing an integral record of care given, ensuring safety in care giving is enhanced as patients move between different services within the NHS (NHS England, 2023b). This promotes transparency about the purpose of record keeping which is an integral consideration from a legal perspective and supports good practice, demonstrates accountability and due diligence and is as important as the duty to protect confidentiality. Unmet needs and readmissions are avoided if follow-up care is planned; this can only be successful if there are clear notes on changes from baseline data and concise involvement from patients and carers (NHS England, 2023b). Sharing data aims to improve direct care for individual patients and underpins effective system management. Box 15.2 provides specific information regarding community nursing notes.

REFLECTION

- Have you been involved in a Clinical Record Keeping Audit?
- Did you identify any areas of concern?
- Did you find areas of good practice that can be shared with other services?

15.2.4 INVOLVING PATIENTS IN RECORD KEEPING

Patients have a right to be involved in their care (NICE, 2023); documenting patient experience alongside critical thinking is essential. In addition, documenting the involvement of patients and carers in their health journey creates and maintains respectful and trusting relationships that will enable healthcare professionals to build shared goals with patients and other relevant care givers to optimise positive health outcomes. Good experience of care, treatment and support is increasingly seen as an essential part of an excellent health and social care service, alongside clinical effectiveness and safety, and starts from the very first contact with the system through to the last, which can include end-of-life care (NHS Improvement, 2018).

It is important to consider consultation style to ensure that care is person centred and documented accordingly (Ajibade, 2021). This is significant because nursing documentation represents much more than simply a record of the continuity of care. When patients have a good understanding of the benefits, harms and possible outcomes of their care, improvement in engagement and better management of long-term conditions can be achieved (NICE, 2023).

NHS Improvement (2018) reminds all clinicians that the patient experience is positive when they are involved in the decision-making of their care; documenting patients' understanding of this and any wishes or concerns enables other healthcare professionals who may subsequently be involved to tailor the care given to include this information.

15.2.5 INFORMATION TECHNOLOGY AND BARRIERS TO EFFECTIVE RECORD KEEPING

Community nursing trusts invest widely in mobile working facilities, but if clinicians continue to handwrite notes and then transpose them later, vital information can be overlooked and failure to record substantially results in incomplete data sourcing. Best (2023) reported that paper notes are less safe and efficient.

The Safer Nursing Care Tool Data (The Shelford Group, 2019) report that up to 15% of time is spent documenting care and 10% looking for information. NHS Improvement (2018) suggests that use of technology encourages nursing teams to work in a streamlined fashion. However, the Queen's Nursing Institute (QNI 2023) reports poor connectivity when seeing patients and limited battery life of mobile devices were amongst the highest challenges faced by community nurses when documenting in patients' homes or out in practice, which may account for the number of handwritten notes still being made and transposed later. It has been reported by nurses that leaving documentation to the end of the day is disproportionately time-consuming and a chore rather than central to the act of caring being at the forefront; therefore, it is important to use the clinical systems available contemporaneously, to deliver optimum patient care (Williams, 2022). In a recent survey, none of the investigated patient records at audit fulfilled standards for recommended nursing documentation practice (Moldskred et al., 2021) which indicates that documentation training may be inadequate, or that the barriers identified earlier are continuing to significantly contribute to completing contemporaneous record keeping.

Increasing patient caseloads allow less time for record completion (QNI, 2023). Harper-McDonald (2020) reports that it is vital to maintain contemporaneous and concise, relevant documentation to enable effective remote reviews and effective caseload management. Reduced staffing levels impact the quality and consistency of documentation. Staff shortages have a negative impact on record keeping due to increased workload with lack of time to complete records (Mutshatshi et al., 2018). Nurses must view documentation as a key element of their provision of care.

REFLECTION

- Consider barriers within your scope of practice.
- When staffing levels are compromised, how effectively are records kept?
- Are there obvious omissions of information?
- How easy is it to manage ongoing care from entries made previously?

15.2.6 CONCLUSION

Record keeping is defined and underpinned by legal requirements that have competence and compassion at the core. Records should provide clear evidence of opportunity for fair and transparent communication and demonstrate an understanding of patient need.

Poor documentation leads to legal claims, breakdown in communication and inadequate care provision. Risk of harm is increased, and positive patient outcomes are reduced, with potential for delays in treatment, unnecessary hospitalisation and subsequent recovery. Documentation and care planning should involve the patient and other relevant care providers to optimise recovery and management of long-term conditions by increasing engagement with the clinician and wider team.

Nurses are accountable for the clinical decisions they make and are required to document the rationale behind those decisions and mitigate risks around the recognised barriers to effective communication. Appropriate evidence should be recorded electronically in clear, detailed and appropriate language. Records should indicate collaboration with patients, carers, advocates and other healthcare professionals in care giving and planning.

15.3 Measuring Quality and Patient Outcomes in the Community

15.3.1 INTRODUCTION

The 2008 Darzi report helped to establish the landscape and define the language we use to describe quality within healthcare today. The Darzi report and similar studies' references into quality provided the blueprint to adopt a holistic national quality system, summarising, as part of its findings, the requirement for a quality measurement framework at all levels, and the need to measure service delivery and outcomes before being able to define, understand and improve quality (NHS, 2008).

The Darzi reports findings helped to develop the National Quality Board (NQB) in 2009. The NQB provides advice, recommendations and endorsement on matters relating to quality, and acts as a collective to influence, drive and ensure system alignment of quality programmes, management systems and initiatives (NHS England, 2023a).

Measuring quality and patient outcomes in the community requires a joined-up approach from multiple teams and organisations, focusing on aligned goals and understanding data/outcomes with a unified aim of driving up quality in services (NHS Oversight Framework, 2022).

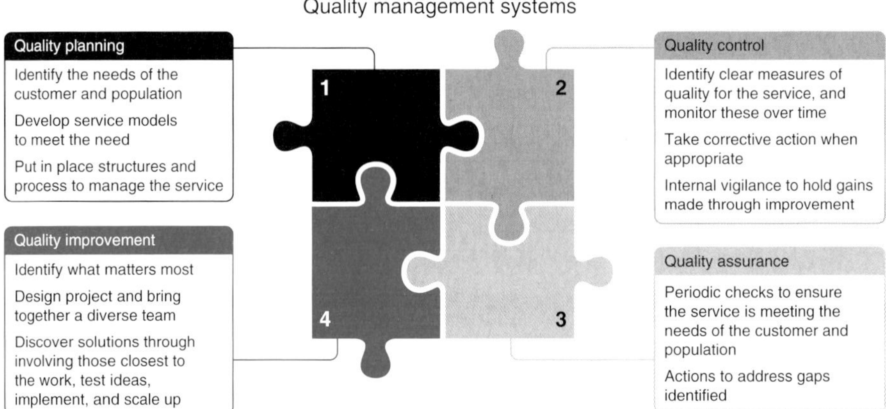

Fig. 15.3 The four aspects of a quality management system: planning, control, assurance, and improvement (From Shah, A. (2020). How to move beyond quality improvement projects. *BMJ (Clinical research ed.)*, *370*, m2319. https://doi.org/10.1136/bmj.m2319).

15.3.2 QUALITY MANAGEMENT SYSTEM

The term 'quality management system' often refers to the cycle of planning, control, assurance and improvement, which takes place in any healthcare system (Rose, 2023). Each facet relies on data and evidence rather than ideology to drive reforms and advancements in quality at all levels, nationally, regionally and locally (Leatherman & Sutherland, 2008). This process requires all areas to embed approaches to planning, control, assurance and improvement, and align actions and directives to meet patient, policy and regulatory requirements (Hon & Hewitt, 2023). This commitment to collaborative improvement-led delivery demands all services to support and engage with constant ongoing developments and support relative components of the quality management system, to increase productivity and deliver better health outcomes for patients and communities through evidence-based learning (Eden, 2023). In Fig. 15.3, quality management systems are explained in more detail, and in Fig. 15.4, the applicability to community nursing is showcased.

15.3.3 USING DATA DAY TO DAY

This advancement in understanding outcomes via the quality management system can only be achieved through capturing, understanding and utilising data. This science of improvement is fundamental to the development of quality and aligning goals for improving patient-reported outcome measures (PROMs) and patient-reported experience measures (PREMs). Useful tools such as statistical process control charts (SPCs) help map outcomes and service delivery and create a visual overview of performance, supporting and planning, key performance indicators (KPIs), trajectories and targets, as well as provide valuable data on PROMs and PREMs (Sewell-Jones, 2019).

The landscape of healthcare in the United Kingdom is changing; the introduction of integrated care boards (ICBs) creates a dependency on healthcare organisations and hospital-based trusts to align the data they collect and, when appropriate, the systems that they use to the benefit of patient care.

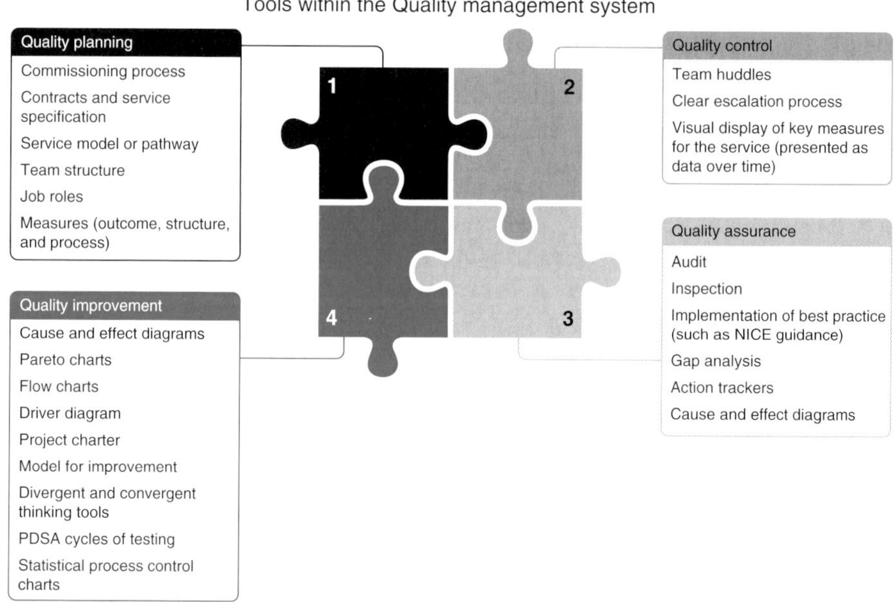

Fig. 15.4 Examples of tools that might be used within each of the four aspects of a quality management system (From Shah, A. (2020). How to move beyond quality improvement projects. *BMJ (Clinical research ed.)*, *370*, m2319. https://doi.org/10.1136/bmj.m2319).

15.3.4 APPLICATION TO PRACTICE

Improving community performance requires services to think wider about how their data are reported and used, and how this translates to measurable patient outcomes and national directives. For example, measuring the clinical outcomes of a patient with type 1 diabetes in the community (quality control) could drive an audit to assess the care received against national/local policy standards (quality assurance). Data collected could feed an improvement project (East London NHS Foundation Trust, n.d.) to transform highlighted aspects of care. Outcomes can then be fed into ICBs/community forums, which help provide a greater picture of diabetes care in the community and provide the evidence to drive meaningful change and reforms.

The application of quality management systems in practice provides assurance and evidence to stakeholders that all aspects surrounding 'quality' are managed, monitored and supported. This assurance is based on the analysis and assessment of data/PROMs/PREMs against national regional and local metrics/standards/criteria (Sewell-Jones, 2019). Without this ability to plan, review, reflect and improve on collected data, community services would be unable to provide effective care plans, plan the daily running of services or plan and deliver transformational change (Rose, 2023).

15.3.5 THE FOUR Qs: FUNDAMENTAL COMPONENTS OF QUALITY MANAGEMENT

The four aspects that create a quality management system rely on each component working in unison to deliver measurable outcomes for staff and patients in all working areas building a working quality management system (QMS) relies on each aspect working with another (The Health Foundation, 2020).

15.3.5.1 Quality Planning

Quality planning requires the service/team/trust/organisation to:

- Understand the population's needs and requirements.
  Example: How many pressure ulcers are on the community caseload?
- Establish KPIs in line with trust/organisation strategic vision and strategy.
  Example: Reduce the number of community-developed pressure ulcers by 10%.
- Design structure and processes to meet the required need for services.
  Example: Establish mandatory pressure ulcer checks for all patients on every visit.

15.3.5.2 Quality Control

Quality control is ensuring systems are in place to react to and record daily occurrences, this involves:

- Real-time reporting.
  Example: Incident reporting or handover of pressure ulcers.
- Utilising collected data effectively.
  Example: Foot ulcer screening for known diabetic patients.
- Embedded mechanisms into teams so they can own and react to their data.
  Example: Reacting to identified training needs of staff from raised reporting when caring for patients with pressure ulcers.
- Identify and/or establish reporting and escalation processes and protocols.
  Example: Monitor number of recorded pressure ulcer checks in handover.

15.3.5.3 Quality Assurance

Quality assurance requires independently checking the quality-of-service delivery against preestablished standards/guidance through:

- Internal and external processes to check the quality.
  Example: Audit/deep dive, into pressure ulcer care.
- Ensuring we are meeting and exceeding the set standards of care, identifying gaps and rechecking for compliance.
  Example: Regularly monitoring policies and standard operating procedures (SOPs) mapped against national and local guidelines and standards for pressure ulcer care.

15.3.5.4 Quality Improvement

- Ensure staff have the capacity and capability to improve what is in their control and escalate those that are not.
  Example: Create a quality improvement (QI) group to review pressure ulcer care and improvements centred around reported incidents or inherited risks.
- Systems and culture to allow test and learn improvement cycles—plan, do, study, act (PDSA).
  Example: Review established measures around pressure ulcer care and utilise QI tools and techniques to establish meaningful change against mapped data and assurances.

- Systems for spreading learning that enables adaptation for local context.
- Triage the right methodology to deliver the change, e.g., 'Just do it' actions, iterative improvements (QI) or fundamental transformation.

15.3.6 CONCLUSION

By implementing a comprehensive approach to measuring quality and patient outcomes in the community healthcare setting, organisations can identify areas for improvement, track progress over time and ultimately enhance the delivery of care to individuals and communities. Effective measurement and evaluation processes are fundamental to driving continuous improvement and achieving better health outcomes for all.

15.4 Medicines Optimisation and Nurse Prescribing in the Community

15.4.1 INTRODUCTION

The UK has an increasingly ageing population, with hospital avoidance and effective person-centred community care becoming increasingly prevalent and essential in the management of long-term conditions (NHS England, 2019b). Ensuring that patients remain outside of the hospital environment is not only appropriate but highly beneficial to outcomes in general health and well-being (Sanderson, 2023). Community-based nurse prescribing, medicine management and medicines optimisation play significant roles in influencing policies, procedures and protocols.

Since the inception of Integrated Care Trusts throughout the UK, hospital and community care providers share policies and procedures relating to prescribing, but the community sector continues to play a more extended role, with the aim of providing a seamless sharing of care for the patient (NHS South West London, 2022). The administration of medicines is an important aspect of nursing professional practice (NMC, 2018b). Community nurses work alongside other members of the multidisciplinary team (MDT) to achieve the best outcomes for their patients and these relationships require advanced communication skills, utilising more joined-up thinking such as electronic documentation systems and regular MDT meetings.

DEFINITIONS

Medicines management is defined as a system of processes and behaviours that determines how medicines are used by the NHS and patients (National Prescribing Centre, 2002 cited in NICE, 2015). For good medicine management to occur, there are elements relating to autonomy, immediate and remote teamwork and lone working that nurses need to be consistently aware of.

Medicines optimisation is defined as 'a person-centred approach to safe and effective medicines use, to ensure people obtain the best possible outcomes from their medicines. Medicines optimisation applies to people who may or may not take their medicines effectively. Shared decision-making is an essential part of evidence-based medicine, seeking to use the best available evidence to guide decisions about the care of the individual patient, taking into account their needs, preferences and values' (Greenhalgh et al., 2014).

15.4.2 MEDICINES ADMINISTRATION IN THE COMMUNITY

It is important to note that most individuals live in their own homes; however, there are many people who take up residence in care homes, nursing homes, sheltered accommodation, temporary housing and hostels. It is worth noting that in each of these settings, there may be different protocols and procedures for medication administration and these need to be considered individually (NICE, 2017). For this section of the chapter, the word 'home' is used to describe the place where the patient normally resides.

15.4.3 MEDICATION IN THE PATIENT'S HOME

The control of medicines in the UK is primarily governed by the Medicines Act (1968) and associated European legislation. Medications are prescribed by medical staff in hospitals, at general practice (GP) surgeries and multiple other clinical areas by other healthcare professionals including nurses, physiotherapists, pharmacists and health visitors. The NMC (2018b) recognises that medication administration is not a mechanistic task to be performed in strict compliance with the instructions of the prescriber but requires thought and expertise with professional judgment.

For patients being seen by community nurses, a prescription is most often completed by the prescriber such as a District nurse, advanced care practitioner or GP, then transferred to a community pharmacy. The prescribed medication is then dispensed and delivered to the patient's home. This systematic process ensures that the patient has the correct medication at their disposal as it is prescribed and therefore intended for use. Alternatively, the patient who has recently had their care transferred from a hospital setting and is returning home will have been prescribed medications known as Tablets to Take Away (TTAs) or Tablets to Take Out (TTOs). These medications are most commonly the drugs used by the patient whilst they were residing in the hospital and may include newly prescribed medications as well as those previously prescribed. These medications are dispensed from the hospital pharmacy and usually enough medication is supplied to cover the patients' needs for 2 weeks. This means that the patient has enough medication to take until they can contact the GP and gain further supplies. In the community, the GP takes up the responsibility of prescribing and supplying further medication. In complex cases when the transfer of care from hospital to home has taken place a member of the local community nursing team may visit the patient and will review and check the dispensed medications. Additionally, the GP will have been informed of the need for more prescribed medication via the patients' hospital discharge summary which is sent electronically.

If medicine supplies are inadequate in the community, all reasonable steps should be taken to ensure they are obtained, and all the actions taken documented in the patient's records to ensure good communication and continuity of care. If a medicine is not available and the patient does not receive the prescribed medication, the prescriber must be advised, and an incident report completed in line with local policy.

15.4.4 ADMINISTRATION OF MEDICATION IN THE PATIENT'S HOME

According to the Royal Pharmaceutical Society (RPS, 2019), organisational policies define who can administer medicines or when appropriate to delegate the administration of medicines within a particular setting. This means that according to the organisation or trust caring for the patient, policies and procedures will be in place to ensure the safe administration of medication to the patient and this will include prescription only medicines (POMs) and controlled drugs (CDs). Often patients can independently administer their medication, but in some cases, they may need assistance. Technology has brought user-friendly devices to aid the self-administration of many medications, but often assistance is sought from social care services for a range of different reasons such as lack of dexterity, sensory impairment and cognitive decline. Furthermore, pharmacists have facilities to provide multicompartment compliance aids such as blister packs or dosette boxes to aid the ease of safe self-administration of medication.

Nurses working in the community may need to delegate medicine administration to trained healthcare assistants or nurse associates. The RCN informs us that 'If a registrant delegates a task to a nonregistrant, they must ensure that they have the appropriate skills and competence. Nonregistrants should not accept a delegated task if they are not competent to carry it out' (RCN, 2020).

15.4.5 MEDICINES ADMINISTRATION RECORD (MAR) CHARTS

MAR charts are the formal record of the administration of medicine within the care setting and may be required to be used as evidence in clinical investigations and court cases. It is therefore important that they are clear, accurate and up to date (RPS, 2009). The use of a MAR chart is considered central to careful and effective documentation and record keeping practice for medicines administration. A MAR chart must be completed and stored in the patient-held record, and/or electronic records. The MAR chart must include the date and time of administration, route, frequency, site of administration and dose given. Staff must legibly sign the record. (Batch numbers and expiry date should also be recorded for vaccines.) If a patient declines the medication or if the medication is not administered for any reason, the prescriber must be informed. The name of the prescriber must be clearly documented as well as the discussion with the patient/carer, the reason for the omission and the outcome.

15.4.6 MANAGING ERRORS OR INCIDENTS IN THE USE OF MEDICINES

A medication error is a preventable incident or associated with the use of medicines that have resulted in harm or potential for harm to a patient (European Medicines Agency, 2024). The incident may relate to any step in the medicines use process, including prescribing, dispensing, administration, storage or transfer of medication information. Furthermore, nurses must also report any near misses or potential hazards relating to any part of the medicines management process (including potential or actual prescribing errors, medicines reconciliation discrepancies).

The well-being and safety of the patient are the prime concerns following a medication incident. The incident must be reported as soon as possible to a member of the medical staff, where a decision will be made regarding any further clinical action; in addition the local trust policy should be followed. Furthermore, the patient/carer should be informed that an error has occurred.

15.4.7 STORAGE OF DRUGS IN THE COMMUNITY

Depending on the setting, the safe storage of medication in the community varies. As described previously, care homes, residential homes and nursing homes will use lockable spaces to store medication. These may be locked cupboards for stock items of medication and drug trolleys for more immediate use. Some care facilities provide individual dwellings for residents, small flats including bathrooms, bedrooms and kitchens. To provide safe care in these settings, there may be a necessity to store medications in locked cupboards in the patient's home.

In private dwellings, patients should be encouraged to store medicines safely and appropriately including being out of the reach of children and pets and not in hot, steamy rooms such as bathrooms. Some medicines require storage in the fridge and vaccines are to be transported in the appropriate equipment such as cold bags, as recommended by the local policy and infection control specialist nurses.

15.4.8 CONTROLLED DRUGS

The use of stronger painkillers or analgesia such as opiate derived medications like diamorphine or fentanyl for patients who may be suffering from increased levels of pain is commonplace and extremely important for the continuity of comfort. In addition, if the dying patient decides to remain at home towards and during the end of their lives, the storage of controlled drugs needs to be considered carefully. In the community, administration of controlled drugs may be carried out by one registered nurse. However, precautions must be taken which include the stock of controlled drugs being checked, counted, reconciled and clearly recorded. If a discrepancy is identified, it must be reported in line with the local policy so that an investigation can be carried out.

The NICE (2016) published a guideline on Controlled Drugs: Safe Use and Management. This document outlines the requirements of individuals self-administering, administering or helping to administer controlled drugs in noncare settings, such as patient's own homes or in refugee or homeless hostels. Careful monitoring of the whereabouts and the storage of these medications is essential in maintaining safe environments, and prevention of allowing them to fall into the wrong hands leaving the prescriber accountable for their inappropriate use. In dwellings of multiple occupancy such as hostels and hotels, CDs are to be kept under lock and key and administered by the patient themselves or by trained staff. In a care setting the amount of medication used is checked, monitored and recorded on a daily basis to ensure that its distribution and administration is appropriate and managed.

15.4.8.1 Drug Reactions

Community nurses involved in the administration of medicines by injection undergo annual training in the treatment of anaphylaxis and are responsible for having immediate access to an in-date adrenaline pack at all times. The ambulance service should be contacted immediately following the administration of the adrenaline and another dose prepared to ensure readiness if the ambulance is delayed—the plasma half-life of adrenaline only lasts for 2–3 minutes. The patient should never be left alone during this time.

Occasionally, it is possible for other reactions to drugs to take place, which may not be as immediate or life-threatening as anaphylaxis. A good example of this may be a reaction or sensitivity to antibiotic therapy, which may be administered orally or via the intravenous therapy (IV) route. More common responses might involve skin rashes or nausea and diarrhoea. The best course of action is to stop the medication immediately, contact a senior colleague such as general practitioner, pharmacist or District nursing lead, all whilst ensuring local policy is followed.

15.4.9 DISPOSAL OF MEDICATION IN THE COMMUNITY

When medication expires in date or is no longer required, it should be carefully disposed of, in accordance with policies relating to the correct management of waste. Unwanted or unused medication should be taken to a pharmacy for disposal; the pharmacy will request that there are no sharps such as needles attached to syringes or blades included in the waste. This is then sent for incineration, so the waste items do not contaminate ground water, protecting the environment and preventing active ingredients from appearing in drinking water (Personal Health Services, 2022). Further information on the disposal of sharps can be found in Chapter 5.

15.5 Prescribing in the Community

This section of the chapter will focus primarily on nurses entering work in the community and those on the pathway to District nursing programmes. Specialist practitioner (District Nursing) programmes are taught in a multitude of approved education institutions (AEIs), and they all carry a module on medicine management or Independent Nurse Prescribing (V300) (NMC, 2023).

15.5.1 HISTORY

In 1986, Mrs Julia Cumberlege, now Baroness Cumberlege, was commissioned by the UK Department of Health and Social Security (DHSS) to investigate and write a report on recommendations for changes in the ways that community nurses should practise in the UK. The report 'Neighbourhood Nursing – A Focus for Care: Report of the Community Nursing Review' (DHSS, 1986) came about as a response to various changes taking place within nursing as well as socio-economic factors affecting healthcare and public health at the time.

The report states:

> *'The DHSS should agree a limited list of items and simple agents which may be prescribed by nurses as part of a nursing care programme, and issue guidelines to enable nurses to control drug dosages in well-defined circumstances'.*
>
> (KING'S FUND CENTRE, 1986)

Since these recommendations were made, the administration of medications to patients in the community, in clinics and in more acute settings by nursing staff has progressed widely. As well as prescribing from a Community Formulary and the British National Formulary (BNF), the use of Patient Group Directions (PGDs) and Patient Specific Directions (PSDs) was widely introduced across the healthcare sector.

Independent prescribing nurses are placed on the NMC register as an additional qualification. Independent prescribing, previously known as nonmedical prescribing, came about because of the recognition that nurses had a great deal more contact time with their patients, and as a result in a greater understanding of the patient need, particularly in relation to requirements of medication (DHSS, 1986).

In consideration of the Independent Prescribing Course, a relevant starting point would be to become familiar with the local trust policies around medicines management in the community settings. A national view of policies and procedures in medicines management can be found in a variety of places (some are listed in Box 15.3).

Independent prescribing courses are currently run as stand-alone modules or as part of other academic programmes for specialist nurses. Currently, nurses can be inducted into the Community Prescribers Programme, also known as the V150, or into the Independent Nurse Prescribers Programme, the V300. Successful practitioners are placed onto the NMC register as either a V150 or V300 prescriber.

Healthcare trusts nationally are provided with a training budget and may well look to one or more AEIs to purchase educational courses for their staff every financial year. This can be limiting for the learner who may find that the course the trust has purchased does not meet their educational needs.

CASE STUDY 15.1

Community staff nurse Christine has worked with the District nursing service as a junior nurse since she qualified 2 years ago. She enjoys her work in the community and can see the value of becoming a qualified District nurse. She would like to take a further step toward fulfilling her ambition of becoming a Specialist Practitioner. She notices that the chosen university for the trust is running a District nursing course; the prescribing module attached to the course is a V300. The course information very clearly points out that if the learner does not pass the V300, then the other modules of the course leading to a Specialist Practitioner qualification will also be null and void. Christine finds this off putting and decides not to apply for the course, informing her manager that she does not feel confident enough to complete the course and the V300 module at the same time.

What do you think Christine should do in this scenario? If you were Christine, would you know where and how to look for other options?

15.5.2 THE INDEPENDENT PRESCRIBER COURSE

During the programme, assignments will be set and deadlines given for completion. Understanding and clarifying what, how and why these are required are going to set you off on the best foot. Since 2016 the NMC has referred governance of nonmedical prescribers to the RPS. The RPS has a Competency Framework that all prescribers other than medical prescribers (medical doctors are by far the largest prescribing group in the UK health service) are required to complete and abide by.

The NMC requires the Independent Nurse Prescriber (INP) and the Supplementary Prescriber (SP) to successfully pass a pharmacology examination at 80% and a numeracy examination at 100% (NMC, 2023). In addition, and depending on the AEI chosen, a written case study and a reflection on practice are required to add a contextual aspect to the qualification.

BOX 15.3 ■ Useful Resources

The Nursing and Midwifery Council (NMC)

The regulatory body for nurses and midwives in the United Kingdom provides a set of standards for nurse prescribers to adhere to. On successful completion of a training programme, the name of the newly trained prescriber appears on the register. In addition, the NMC writes and regulates standards for prescribing programmes for AEIs.

https://www.nmc.org.uk/standards/standards-for-post-registration/standards-for-prescribers/

The Royal College of Nursing (RCN)

The world's largest nursing union provides guidance and advise for both supplementary, independent and community nurse prescribing.

https://www.rcn.org.uk/Get-Help/rcn-advice/non-medical-prescribers

Medicines and Healthcare Products Regulatory Agency (MHRA)

The Medicines and Healthcare Products Regulatory Agency is an executive agency of the Department of Health and Social Care in the United Kingdom which is responsible for ensuring that medicines and medical devices work and are acceptably safe.

https://www.gov.uk/government/organisations/medicines-and-healthcare-products-regulatory-agency

The Royal Pharmaceutical Society (RPS)

The RPS sets out a competency framework for prescribers and ensures governance around all independent prescribing.

https://www.rpharms.com/resources/frameworks/prescribing-competency-framework/competency-framework

15.5.3 LIMITATIONS OF PRESCRIBING AND THE SCOPE OF PRACTICE

On passing the prescribing module, there will be thoughts around the scope of practice, e.g., where to begin, should it be broad or within the speciality? Will it be right? To start, a Scope of Practice (SoP) is effectively a list of medications that are most usefully prescribed in the chosen workplace/speciality, together with the reasons for prescribing. The SoP also asks the practitioner to describe the methods by which knowledge of the medication on the SoP is relevant, current and up to date. This serves as a useful reminder about where to look for information once the initial SoP is written and how/when it can be added to as progression takes place.

Taking that first step into the world of prescribing is a decision that will have been no doubt thought about from the first day of the module. Firstly, there will be two groups of newly qualified prescribers: those that are raring to go and those that are like rabbits caught in headlights. Secondly, there will be those nursing and medical colleagues who will be calling upon you to support with issuing prescriptions and other health, social and pharmacy care practitioners who can not quite get their head around the purple prescription pad.

Taking it slowly and building up speed in accordance with competence, knowledge and confidence are a good place to start. Identify what is needed and be aware of before embarking on the prescription writing journey. Take time to investigate which local policies and protocols relating to independent prescribing are within the organisation.

REFLECTION

- Are there forums/mandatory updates that need to be attended/done?
- Is there protected time to do this?
- Within the service, are there any in-house meetings that take place?
- Is there an expectation or mandate to perform self-audits?
- How will you feedback about what is being prescribed be obtained?
- What is the procedure for adding to the SoP?

15.5.4 CONCLUSION

Community-based prescribing and medication management play a key part in keeping patients safe in their own homes. There are laws, policies and protocols that govern the delivery, storage, administration and disposal of these medications which can often prove challenging. It is anticipated that transfers of care will be seamless between hospital and home but this is sometimes not the case and community nurses will need to act swiftly to ensure there is no detriment to the patient. If errors or adverse reactions are experienced, immediate action must take place and advice is sought from relevant parties. The role of the community nurse has been extended so that it is common to find individuals who can prescribe. This requires additional training which can be quite extensive and the ongoing SoP has to be carefully considered.

References

Ajibade, B. (2021). Assessing the patient's needs and planning effective care. *British Journal of Nursing*, *30*(20). Available at: https://www.britishjournalofnursing.com/content/clinical/assessing-the-patients-needs-and-planning-effective-care/ Accessed 6/11/23.

Anandaciva, S. (2023). How does the NHS compare to the health care systems of other countries? [online] Available at: https://www.kingsfund.org.uk/sites/default/files/2023-06/How_NHS_compare_2023.pdf.

Best. (2023). NHS still reliant on paper patient notes and drug charts despite electronic upgrades, *The BMJ* finds. *BMJ*, *382*, 2050. https://doi.org/10.1136/bmj.p2050. PMID: 37704231.

Brooks, N. (2021). How to undertake effective record-keeping and documentation. *Nursing Standard*, *36*(4), 31–33. https://doi.org/10.7748/ns.2021.e11700. Epub 2021 Mar 15. PMID: 33719232.

Brown. (2022). Clinical negligence claims for pressure injuries from the perspective of a tissue viability medico-legal nurse expert. *British Journal of Community Nursing*, *27*(9), 14.

Care Quality Commission. (2022). *Duty of candour: Notifiable safety incidents*. Care Quality Commission. [online] www.cqc.org.uk. Available at: https://www.cqc.org.uk/guidance-providers/all-services/duty-candour-notifiable-safety-incidents.

Chaneliere, M., Koehler, D., Morlan, T., Berra, J., Colin, C., Dupie, I., & Michel, P. (2018). Factors contributing to patient safety incidents in primary care: A descriptive analysis of patient safety incidents in a French study using CADYA (categorization of errors in primary care). *BMC Family Practice*, *19*(1). https://doi.org/10.1186/s12875-018-0803-9.

Clayphan, B., Dixon, L., Biggs, S., Jordan, L., Pullyblank, A., Holden, K., et al. (2022). PreciSSIon: A collaborative initiative to reduce surgical site infections after elective colorectal surgery. *Journal of Hospital Infection*, *130*, 131–137. https://doi.org/10.1016/j.jhin.2022.08.012. ISSN 0195-6701.

DHSS. (1986). *Neighbourhood nursing: A focus for care (Cumberlege report)*. London: HMSO.

East London NHS Foundation Trust. (n.d.). *ELFT's quality management system*. Available at: https://qi.elft.nhs.uk/elfts-quality-management-system/.

Eden, A. (2023). *NHS delivery and continuous improvement review: recommendations.* How can improvement-led delivery enhance the quality of outcomes for our patients, communities and our health and care workforce?. NHS England. Available at: https://www.england.nhs.uk/wp-content/uploads/2023/04/B2137-nhs-delivery-and-continuous-improvement-review-recommendations-april-2023.pdf.

European Medicines Agency. (2024). Medication errors. Available at: https://www.ema.europa.eu/en/human-regulatory-overview/post-authorisation/pharmacovigilance-post-authorisation/medication-errors.

Greenhalgh, T., Howick, J., & Maskrey, N. (2014). Evidence based medicine: A movement in crisis? *BMJ*, 348. https://doi.org/10.1136/bmj.g3725. 2014.

Harper-McDonald, B. (2020). District nurses' experiences with a caseload profiling tool: A service evaluation. *British Journal of Community Nursing*, *25*(7), 318–326. https://doi.org/10.12968/bjcn.2020.25.7.318. PMID: 32614664.

Health Foundation. (2020). Pressure reduction through continuous monitoring in community settings (PROMISE). [online] Available at: https://www.health.org.uk/improvement-projects/pressure-reduction-through-continuous-monitoring-in-community-settings-promise.

Health Innovation Network West of England. (n.d.). PreciSSIon. [online] Available at: https://www.healthinnowest.net/our-work/transforming-services-and-systems/preventing-surgical-site-infections/precission/ [Accessed 15 Jan. 2024].

Hollnagel, E., Braithwaite, J., & Wears, R. L. (2013). *Resilient Health Care*. Ashgate.

Hollnagel, E., Wears, R. L., & Braithwaite, J. (2015). From safety-I to safety-II: A white paper. [online] Available at: https://www.england.nhs.uk/signuptosafety/wp-content/uploads/sites/16/2015/10/safety-1-safety-2-whte-papr.pdf.

Hon, R., & Hewitt, P. (2023). The Hewitt review: An independent review of integrated care systems. [online] Available at: https://assets.publishing.service.gov.uk/government/uploads/system/uploads/attachment_data/file/1148568/the-hewitt-review.pdf.

King's Fund Centre. (1986). Cumberlege report – neighbour nursing. https://archive.kingsfund.org.uk/concern/published_works/000003610?locale=en#?cv=9&xywh=226,795,1311,335&p=0.

Leatherman, S., & Sutherland, K. (2008). *The quest for quality: Refining the NHS reforms: A policy analysis and chartbook*. [online]. Available at: https://www.nuffieldtrust.org.uk/sites/default/files/2017-01/quest-for-quality-report-web-final.pdf.

Moldskred, P. S., Snibsøer, A. K., & Espehaug, B. (2021). Improving the quality of nursing documentation at a residential care home: A clinical audit. *BMC Nurs*, *20*, 103. https://doi.org/10.1186/s12912-021-00629-9.

Mutshatshi, T. E., Mothiba, T. M., Mamogobo, P. M., & Mbombi, M. O. (2018). Record-keeping: Challenges experienced by nurses in selected public hospitals. *Curationis*, *41*(1), e1–e6. https://doi.org/10.4102/curationis.v41i1.1931.

National Institute for Health and Care Excellence. (2016). *Controlled drugs: Safe use and management*. Available at https://www.nice.org.uk/guidance/ng46/resources/controlled-drugs-safe-use-and-management-pdf-1837456188613. Accessed 23/11/23.

National Institute for Health and Care Excellence. (2017). Managing medicines for adults receiving social care in the community. Available at: https://www.nice.org.uk/guidance/ng67/resources/managing-medicines-for-adults-receiving-social-care-in-the-community-pdf-1837578800581.

NHS England. (2013). Human factors in healthcare: A concordat from the national quality board. 3. Available at: https://www.england.nhs.uk/wp-content/uploads/2013/11/nqb-hum-fact-concord.pdf.

NHS England. (2019a). *The NHS patient safety strategy. Safer culture, safer systems, safer patients.* NHS England and NHS Improvement. [online] Available at: https://www.england.nhs.uk/wp-content/uploads/2020/08/190708_Patient_Safety_Strategy_for_website_v4.pdf.

NHS England. (2019b). NHS long term plan. Available at: https://www.longtermplan.nhs.uk/wp-content/uploads/2019/08/nhs-long-term-plan-version-1.2.pdf.

NHS England. (2021). *Information governance framework for integrated health and care: Shared care records*. NHS Transformation Directorate. https://transform.england.nhs.uk/information-governance/guidance/summary-of-information-governance-framework-shared-care-records/information-governance-framework-for-integrated-health-and-care-shared-care-records/.

NHS England. (2022a). Patient safety incident response framework. [online] Available at: https://www.england.nhs.uk/wp-content/uploads/2022/08/B1465-1.-PSIRF-v1-FINAL.pdf.

NHS England. (2022b). *Patient safety learning response toolkit*. [online] Available at: https://www.england.nhs.uk/publication/patient-safety-learning-response-toolkit/.

NHS England. (2023a). *National Quality Board*. Available at: https://www.england.nhs.uk/ourwork/part-rel/nqb/.

NHS England. (2023b). Patient safety. [online] Available at: https://www.england.nhs.uk/patient-safety/#:~:text=Patient%20safety%20is%20the%20avoidance.

NHS Improvement. (2018). Patient experience improvement framework. https://www.england.nhs.uk/wp-content/uploads/2021/04/nhsi-patient-experience-improvement-framework.pdf.

NHS Oversight Framework. (2022). Available at: https://www.england.nhs.uk/wp-content/uploads/2022/06/B1378_NHS-System-Oversight-Framework-22-23_260722.pdf.

NHS South West London. (2022). NHS South west London (SWL) interface prescribing policy. Appendix 5.1: Principles of shared care. Available at: https://swlimo.southwestlondon.icb.nhs.uk/wp-content/uploads/2022/10/20221020-Principles-of-Shared-Care-.pdf.

NHS. (2008). *High quality care for all: NHS next stage review final report*. The Stationery Office. [online]. Available at: https://assets.publishing.service.gov.uk/government/uploads/system/uploads/attachment_data/file/228836/7432.pdf.

NHS. (2023). *Why we're developing standards for nursing documentation*. NHS Transformation Directorate. https://transform.england.nhs.uk/blogs/why-were-developing-standards-for-nursing-documentation/.

NICE. (2015). *Medicines optimisation: The safe and effective use of medicines to enable the best possible outcomes*. . https://www.nice.org.uk/guidance/ng5/resources/medicinesoptimisation-the-safe-and-effective-use-of-medicinesto-enable-the-best-possible-outcomes-pdf-51041805253.

NICE. (2023). *Shared decision making. NICE guidelines. NICE guidance. Our programmes. What we do. About*. NICE. https://www.nice.org.uk/about/what-we-do/our-programmes/nice-guidance/nice-guidelines/shared-decision-making.

Nursing and Midwifery Council. (2018a). The code: Professional standards of practice and behaviour for nurses, midwives and nursing associates. *The Nursing and Midwifery*.

Nursing and Midwifery Council. (2018b). Professional standards of practice and behaviour for nurses, midwives and nursing associates. Available at: https://www.nmc.org.uk/standards/code/.

Nursing and Midwifery Council. (2022). Read the professional duty of candour. https://www.nmc.org.uk/standards/guidance/the-professional-duty-of-candour/read-the-professional-duty-of-candour/.

Nursing and Midwifery Council. (2023). Standards for prescribing programmes. https://www.nmc.org.uk/globalassets/sitedocuments/standards/2023-pre-reg-standards/new-vi/standards-for-prescribing-programmes.pdf Accessed 22/10/23.

Papanicolas, I., Mossialos, E., Gundersen, A., Woskie, L., & Jha, A. K. (2019). Performance of UK national health service compared with other high income countries: Observational study. *BMJ*, *367*(8224), l6326. https://doi.org/10.1136/bmj.l6326. [online].

Personal Health Services. (2022). Safe disposal of unwanted pharmaceuticals – a complete guide to best practices. Available at: https://www.phs.co.uk/about-phs/expertise-news/safe-disposal-of-unwanted-pharmaceuticals-a-complete-guide-to-best-practices/#:~:text=How%20to%20dispose%20of%20pharmaceutical,of%20separately%20and%20subsequently%20incinerated.

Pullyblank, A., Tavaré, A., Little, H., Redfern, E., le Roux, H., Inada-Kim, M., Cheema, K., & Cook, A. (2020). Implementation of the National Early Warning Score in patients with suspicion of sepsis: Evaluation of a system-wide quality improvement project. *British Journal of General Practice*, *70*(695). https://doi.org/10.3399/bjgp20x709349. bjgp20X709349.

QNI. (2023). Nursing in a digital age. https://qni.org.uk.

Rose, T. (2023). How can I design and implement a Quality Management System in my trust?. [online] Available at: https://www.youtube.com/watch?v=PFvJN-J8TTw. [Accessed 25 September 2023] Accessed.

Rose, T. J. (2023). *The Meaning of Quality and The Juran Trilogy*. Q Community. The Health Foundation. Available at: https://q.health.org.uk/blog-post/the-meaning-of-quality-and-the-juran-trilogy/.

Royal College of Nursing. (2020). Medicines management – an overview for nursing. Available at https://www.rcn.org.uk/clinical-topics/Medicines-management Accessed 22/11/23.

Royal College of Nursing. (2023). Record keeping: The facts. https://www.rcn.org.uk/Professional-Development/publications/rcn-record-keeping-uk-pub-011-016.

Royal Pharmaceutical Society. (2009). Principles of safe and appropriate production of medicine administration chart. https://www.rpharms.com/Portals/0/RPS%20document%20library/Open%20access/Hub/production-medicine-administration-charts.pdf. [Accessed 29 September 2023].

Royal Pharmaceutical Society. (2019). Professional guidance on the administration of medicines in health care settings. Available at https://www.rpharms.com/Portals/0/RPS%20document%20library/Open%20access/Professional%20standards/SSHM%20and%20Admin/Admin%20of%20Meds%20prof%20guidance.pdf Accessed 21/11/23.

Sewell-Jones, A. (2019). Making data count: Getting started: #plotthedots. Available at: https://www.england.nhs.uk/wp-content/uploads/2019/12/making-data-count-getting-started-2019.pdf.

The Health Foundation. (2020). *The case for building a quality management system*. [online]. Available at: https://q.health.org.uk/blog-post/the-case-for-building-a-quality-management-system/. [Accessed 25 September 2023].

The Shelford Group. (2019). The safer nursing care tool data. https://shelfordgroup.org/safer-nursing-care-tool/.

Williams, F. (2022). The use of digital devices by district nurses in their assessment of service users. *British Journal of Community Nursing*, *27*(7), 342.

World Health Organization. (2023). Patient safety. [online] Available at: https://www.who.int/news-room/fact-sheets/detail/patient-safety#:~:text=Patient%20safety%20is%20defined%20as.

CHAPTER 16

Introduction to Digital Health Management

Kumbi Kariwo ■ Lincoln Gombedza ■ Lesley Mills

LEARNING OUTCOMES

After reading this chapter you should be able to:

- Explore the potential of digital health tools in empowering patients
- Recognise the governance, ethical and practical considerations associated with implementing digital health tools
- Foster a mindset of lifelong learning through the utilisation of digital health tools

16.1 Introduction

In the rapidly evolving landscape of healthcare delivery, digital technologies have emerged as powerful tools to transform patient care and empower individuals to take an active role in their health management. The district nursing service, a vital component of community-based care within the National Health Service (NHS), is well positioned to leverage these digital innovations to enhance patient engagement, provide tailored health education and support self-management strategies. As digital healthcare technologies become more prevalent, it is important to understand patient and staff views and perspectives on their adoption and implementation (Brown & Hartley, 2021). Embracing digital tools has also become imperative, in coping with the rising demand and complexity of cases. The integration of digital health tools in nursing practice represents a paradigm shift in patient engagement, health education and self-management strategies. By leveraging these innovative technologies, nurses can empower patients to take an active role in their care, promote lifelong learning and stay ahead of evolving best practices. Nurses working in the community, as frontline caregivers, can provide valuable insights into workflow integration, user experience and patient preferences, ensuring that digital tools align with real-world clinical practices (Laranjo et al., 2018).

16.1.1 ENGAGING PATIENTS THROUGH DIGITAL TOOLS

Effective patient engagement is crucial for achieving better health outcomes, especially in community-based care settings where patients may experience challenges in accessing healthcare services. Community nurses can provide valuable insights into the needs of their patients, the challenges they face and the practicalities of using technology in their day-to-day work. Digital tools offer innovative ways to connect with individuals, facilitating two-way communication and fostering a collaborative approach to care.

Digital health tools, such as mobile applications, patient portals and wearable devices, have the potential to transform the way individuals interact with their health information and manage their conditions. These platforms allow individuals to securely access their health records, communicate with healthcare providers, schedule appointments and receive reminders and updates regarding their care plan. By providing real-time access to health records, educational resources and communication channels with healthcare providers, these tools can enhance engagement and promote self-management (Sawesi et al., 2016).

16.1.2 ELECTRONIC HEALTH RECORDS

The widespread adoption of electronic health records (EHRs) across the UK's NHS has been hailed as a transformative step towards modernising healthcare delivery. These digital repositories of client information promise to streamline clinical workflows, enhance data accessibility and improve care coordination. However, as nurses navigate this technological shift, the impact of EHRs on their practice remains a topic of debate, with both potential benefits and pitfalls emerging.

One of the most popular advantages of EHRs is their ability to provide nurses with comprehensive, up-to-date patient information at their fingertips, regardless of location or care setting (Cresswell et al., 2017). The concept of enhancing clinical decision-making, reducing medication errors, and facilitating more efficient care planning and delivery through accessibility is a well-discussed topic in healthcare. For instance, shared decision-making is a process that involves a person and their healthcare professional working together to reach a joint decision about care (Carmona et al., 2021). This approach respects patient autonomy and promotes client engagement (Elwyn et al., 2010). Additionally, EHRs offer the potential for improved communication and collaboration among healthcare professionals. By enabling real-time sharing of patient data, EHRs can foster better coordination between nurses, physicians and other members of the care team, ultimately leading to more integrated and cohesive individualised care (Vos et al., 2020). Moreover, the standardisation of documentation and data capture within EHRs can contribute to better quality control and enable more robust data analysis for research and population health initiatives (Cresswell et al., 2017). This data-driven approach aligns with the NHS's goals of delivering evidence-based, value-based care.

The implementation of EHRs has not been without its challenges, particularly for nurses on the frontline of client care. One of the most significant concerns is the potential for increased administrative burden and documentation workload (Moy et al., 2021). Nurses may find themselves spending more time entering data into EHRs, detracting from the time available for direct client care and potentially contributing to burnout and job dissatisfaction. Furthermore, the usability and user-friendliness of EHR systems have been widely criticised, with nurses often citing cumbersome interfaces, navigation challenges and a lack of intuitive design (Chen et al., 2023). These usability issues can lead to frustration, inefficiencies and potential errors, undermining the intended benefits of EHRs. Additionally, concerns have been raised about the potential for EHRs to disrupt the nurse–patient relationship and compromise the human element of care (Chen et al., 2023). Nurses may find themselves spending more time focused on data entry and screen interactions, potentially diminishing their ability to provide compassionate, person-centred care.

As the NHS continues to invest in and expand the use of EHRs, it is crucial to address these challenges head-on. Ongoing training and support for nurses in using EHR systems effectively and efficiently are essential. Moreover, involving nurses in the design and implementation processes can help ensure that EHR interfaces and workflows are tailored to their specific needs and work patterns (Moy et al., 2021). Equally important is striking a balance between the digitisation of healthcare and the preservation of the human touch that is integral to nursing practice. While EHRs offer the potential for improved data accessibility and care coordination, they should not come at the expense of the nurturing, compassionate care that patients expect and deserve.

As the healthcare landscape continues to evolve, nurses must adapt and embrace technological advancements while remaining steadfast in their commitment to delivering high-quality, patient-centred care. By addressing the pitfalls and capitalising on the benefits of EHRs, nurses can play a pivotal role in shaping a healthcare system that seamlessly integrates technology with the art and science of nursing.

16.1.3 VIRTUAL WARDS

The COVID-19 pandemic has accelerated the adoption of digital health technologies across the UK's NHS, with virtual wards emerging as a game-changing innovation. These remote monitoring systems enable healthcare professionals, particularly nurses, to provide care for patients in their homes, transforming the traditional model of nursing practice.

Virtual wards leverage digital tools like wearable devices, apps and video conferencing to monitor individuals vital signs, symptoms and overall health status remotely (NHS England, 2021). Nurses can track conditions, adjust care plans and intervene promptly if needed, without requiring hospital admission (Ajibade, 2021). The benefits of this approach are multifaceted. Firstly, virtual wards help alleviate pressure on overcrowded hospitals by enabling home-based care, freeing up beds for those with acute needs (Vindrola-Padros et al., 2021). This is invaluable in the aftermath of the pandemic's strain on healthcare systems. Secondly, virtual wards promote client autonomy and self-management of chronic conditions by actively involving people in monitoring and reporting their health status (Shi et al., 2024). This patient empowerment aligns with the NHS's goals of delivering person-centred care. Moreover, virtual wards offer significant cost savings by reducing hospital admissions and associated costs, such as those related to hospital-acquired infections (Hakim, 2023). This financial advantage is crucial in the face of limited healthcare budgets and rising demand.

However, the implementation of virtual wards is not without challenges. Ensuring equitable access to digital healthcare services is a major concern, as certain population groups, such as the elderly or those from lower socioeconomic backgrounds, may face barriers to adopting and effectively utilising virtual ward technologies due to limited digital literacy or access to devices and internet connectivity (NHS England, 2022). Additionally, there are valid concerns about the potential erosion of the personal, human connection between nurses and individuals. While virtual wards offer convenience and efficiency, some patients may feel disconnected from their healthcare providers, potentially impacting their overall care experience and satisfaction (Lasserson et al., 2023). Furthermore, the reliance on digital technologies raises questions about data privacy, security and the potential for technical glitches or system failures, which could compromise patient safety and continuity of care (Quach et al., 2022).

As with any transformative healthcare innovation, the successful implementation of virtual wards requires a careful balance between embracing technological advancements and preserving the fundamental principles of compassionate, patient-centred care. Nurses, as the frontline providers of care, play a pivotal role in this transition. Continuous training and upskilling are essential to ensure that nurses are proficient in using virtual ward technologies while maintaining their ability to build meaningful relationships with their case load, even in a remote setting. Effective communication, empathy and a deep understanding of each patient's unique needs remain paramount (NHS England, 2022). Moreover, robust protocols and safeguards must be in place to address issues related to digital inclusion, data privacy and technical support, ensuring that virtual wards do not inadvertently exacerbate existing health disparities or compromise patient safety (Hakim, 2023).

As the NHS continues to explore and expand the use of virtual wards, it is crucial to involve nurses, clients and other stakeholders in the decision-making process. Their insights and experiences will shape the future of this innovative care model, ensuring that it truly serves the best interests of those individuals who we care for while supporting the evolving role of nurses in the digital age.

16.1.4 THE NATIONAL HEALTH SERVICE APP

The National Health Service (NHS) App, launched in 2019, is a prime example of a digital tool designed to empower patients and improve their healthcare experience. This mobile application provides a range of features, including the ability to book appointments, order repeat prescriptions, access medical records and receive personalised health advice. By integrating the NHS App into their practice, community nurses can encourage people to actively participate in their care, fostering a sense of ownership and responsibility.

16.1.5 TELEHEALTH AND REMOTE MONITORING

Telehealth and remote monitoring technologies have gained significant traction in the NHS, particularly during the COVID-19 pandemic. These digital tools enable community nurses to conduct virtual consultations, monitor patients' vital signs and symptoms remotely and provide timely interventions without the need for in-person visits, reducing the burden on healthcare systems.

The Attend Anywhere platform, adopted by several NHS Trusts, offers secure video consultation capabilities, allowing community nurses to conduct virtual appointments with people in their homes. This initiative has proven particularly beneficial for those with mobility challenges, those living in remote areas or during periods of increased infection control measures, ensuring continuity of care while minimising risks.

REFLECTION

The NHS Diabetes Prevention Programme (NHS DPP) incorporates digital coaching tools to support individuals at risk of developing type 2 diabetes. The NHS has piloted the use of wearable devices and remote monitoring technologies for chronic condition management, such as the Diabetes Digital Coach and the COPD Remote Monitoring Service (Ross et al., 2022). Through these tools, patients receive tailored lifestyle advice, goal-setting assistance and regular encouragement, empowering them to make positive changes and adopt healthier behaviours.

- In your practice area, have any new remote monitoring devices been introduced?
- What are the benefits and disadvantages?

16.1.6 PATIENT ONLINE LEARNING MODULES AND EDUCATIONAL RESOURCES

Online learning modules and educational resources have become increasingly valuable in healthcare, offering accessible and engaging platforms for patients to acquire knowledge about their conditions, treatment plans and healthy lifestyle practices.

The NHS Choices website, now integrated into the NHS.UK platform, provides a wealth of information on various health topics, conditions and treatments. Community nurses can direct people to trusted online resources, ensuring they receive accurate and reliable information. Additionally, condition-specific websites, such as Diabetes UK and the British Heart Foundation, offer tailored educational materials and resources for patients with specific health conditions.

16.1.7 DIGITAL COACHING AND SUPPORT SYSTEMS

Digital coaching and support systems leverage artificial intelligence and machine learning algorithms to provide personalised guidance, feedback and motivation to patients as they navigate their self-management journeys. Mobile applications, for instance, can offer personalised goal setting, medication reminders and symptom tracking, enabling patients to take an active role in their care (Zhao et al., 2016). Public portals facilitate secure communication with healthcare teams, access to test results and the ability to request prescription refills, reducing barriers to care (Ammenwerth et al., 2012). Moreover, wearable devices and remote monitoring technologies can provide valuable insights into people's health status, enabling early intervention and tailored care plans (Dobkin & Dorsch, 2011).

It is important to note that the implementation and adoption of digital solutions may vary across different regions and healthcare organisations within the UK. Additionally, new solutions and initiatives are constantly emerging to enhance healthcare delivery and client experiences.

Incorporating data analytics into district nursing care aligns with the broader goals of the NHS Long Term Plan, which emphasises a shift towards proactive, preventive and personalised care, as well as the integration of services across different healthcare settings. By leveraging these data-driven approaches, district nurses can play a crucial role in improving health outcomes, reducing health inequalities and delivering high-quality care tailored to the needs of local populations in England; see Box 16.1 for more specific examples.

16.2 Digital Inclusion and Exclusion

Digital inclusion and exclusion are important issues in England, especially when it comes to accessing essential services like healthcare. The NHS has recognised the challenges posed by digital exclusion and has implemented various strategies and initiatives to ensure digital inclusion and equity. One notable example is the NHS Digital Inclusion Strategy, which was launched in 2021 with the aim of ensuring that everyone, regardless of their circumstances, has the skills, motivation, and means to access digital services safely and confidently. The strategy outlines several key areas of focus, including:

BOX 16.1 ■ Data Analytics

Incorporating data analytics and population health insights into district nursing care in England is crucial for several reasons.

Proactive and preventive care: data analytics can help identify population health trends, risk factors and patterns of illness or disease within specific communities or geographic areas. By analysing these data, community nurses can tailor their care strategies to address the unique health needs of the populations they serve. This proactive approach enables early intervention, prevention of health issues and better management of chronic conditions.

Resource allocation and optimisation: data analytics can provide valuable insights into the utilisation of healthcare resources, such as district nursing services, within different regions or populations. This information can help healthcare providers and policymakers optimise resource allocation, ensuring that district nursing services are distributed equitably and efficiently based on the actual needs of the local populations.

Personalised and targeted care: by integrating population health data with individual patient records, community nurses can gain a comprehensive understanding of each patient's health status, risk factors and unique circumstances. This enables them to provide more personalised and targeted care plans, tailored to the specific needs of each patient within the context of their community.

Evidence-based practice: data analytics and population health insights can inform evidence-based practices in district nursing care. By analysing data on treatment outcomes, intervention effectiveness and patient responses, community nurses can make more informed decisions and adopt best practices that have been proven to yield positive results for specific populations or health conditions.

Collaboration and coordination: population health data can facilitate better collaboration and coordination among different healthcare providers and stakeholders involved in district nursing care. By sharing insights and data, community nurses can work more effectively with primary care providers, specialists, social services and community organisations to deliver holistic and integrated care for their patients.

Quality improvement and performance monitoring: by tracking population health indicators and monitoring the outcomes of district nursing interventions, healthcare organisations can continuously evaluate and improve the quality of care provided. Data analytics can help identify areas for improvement, measure the impact of new initiatives, and ensure that district nursing services are meeting the evolving needs of the communities they serve.

- Building digital skills and confidence: the NHS has committed to providing digital skills training and support to both staff and patients, recognising that a lack of digital literacy can be a significant barrier to accessing online services.
- Improving access to digital devices and connectivity: the NHS has partnered with organisations and charities to provide affordable or free devices and internet access to those who cannot afford them, ensuring that everyone has the means to go online.
- Enhancing digital service design: the NHS is working to ensure that its digital services are designed with accessibility and inclusivity in mind, adhering to best practices and guidelines for making online platforms user-friendly and accessible to all.

One example of this is through the NHS Widening Digital Participation Programme, which was launched in 2013 and aimed to improve digital inclusion for people with learning disabilities, autism and other neurodevelopmental conditions. The programme involved providing tailored digital skills training and support, as well as working with service providers to ensure that their digital platforms and resources were accessible and user-friendly for these populations (NHS Digital, 2018).

It is important to note that while these initiatives and strategies have made progress in addressing digital inclusion and equity, digital exclusion remains a significant

BOX 16.2 ■ Example in Practice

Enhancing Wound Care Equity With Digital Visual Solutions

Background

Birmingham Community Healthcare NHS Foundation Trust (BCHC) provides a wide range of community and integrated care services across Birmingham and the West Midlands region. One of the key challenges faced by BCHC's tissue viability and wound care teams was the difficulty in accurately identifying and detecting pressure ulcers in patients with dark skin tones. Traditional methods of visual inspection and manual documentation often failed to capture the subtle colour changes and early signs of tissue damage in these patients, leading to potential delays in diagnosis and treatment (Kariwo, Chapman, M & Oozageer Gunowa, N., 2023).

The Procurement Process

Recognising the need for a more equitable and effective approach to wound management, BCHC initiated a procurement process to explore digital visual solutions that could enhance their existing practices. The health inequities lead collaborated closely with the Research and Innovation Team, clinical stakeholders, including tissue viability nurses, District nurses, IT, information governance and other specialists, to identify the specific requirements for the new digital solution. Key considerations include:

- Functional requirements and capabilities
- Usability and user experience
- Interoperability and data integration
- Security and privacy
- Vendor reputation and support
- Total cost of ownership
- Regulatory compliance and certification
- Stakeholder involvement and acceptance

Implementation and Impact

After an extensive evaluation process, BCHC selected an appropriate and personalised digital wound management platform that leveraged advanced imaging techniques. The implementation of the digital visual solution was a collaborative effort. Comprehensive training sessions were conducted to ensure that nurses and healthcare professionals were proficient in using the new platform and understood its potential benefits.

Evaluation

Since its implementation, the digital visual solution has transformed BCHC's approach to wound management and pressure ulcer prevention. Clinical staff now have access to high-quality, standardised visual documentation of wounds and skin conditions. The organisation has gone on to deploy the digital app into other clinical areas that require visual monitoring and recording of episodes of patient care.

Summary

This case study highlights the importance of inclusive procurement processes that prioritise the diverse needs of patient populations and the potential of digital solutions to address healthcare disparities and promote health equity.

challenge in England, particularly for certain groups such as older adults, those with disabilities and those living in areas with limited internet connectivity or access to digital devices. Additionally, equitable access to digital resources should be a priority, as disparities in digital literacy and access to technology may exacerbate existing health inequities (Berner et al., 2021) (Box 16.2).

16.3 Challenges of Implementing Digital Healthcare Technologies

The implementation of digital healthcare technologies can bring numerous benefits, but it also presents several potential pitfalls that organisations should be aware of and address proactively. Here are some common pitfalls in the implementation of digital healthcare.

16.3.1 INADEQUATE STAKEHOLDER ENGAGEMENT AND USER RESISTANCE

Failing to involve key stakeholders, such as community nurses, patients and IT staff, in the planning and decision-making process can lead to resistance and low user adoption. Lack of understanding or consideration for user needs, workflows and preferences can result in technologies that are poorly aligned with practical requirements and contribute to user frustration and rejection.

16.3.2 INSUFFICIENT ORGANISATIONAL READINESS AND CHANGE MANAGEMENT

Insufficient organisational readiness and change management can significantly hinder the success of new initiatives and transformations within companies. This issue arises when organisations fail to adequately prepare their structures, processes, and people for impending changes (Weiner, 2009). It often manifests as resistance from employees, lack of necessary skills or resources, and misalignment between the change goals and existing organisational culture. Effective change management requires a systematic approach that includes clear communication, stakeholder engagement, and ongoing support throughout the transition process (Kotter, 1996). Without proper readiness and change management strategies, organisations risk project failures, decreased productivity, and increased employee turnover during periods of significant change.

16.3.3 INTEROPERABILITY AND DATA INTEGRATION ISSUES

Failure to ensure interoperability and data integration with existing healthcare information systems, EHRs and other relevant technologies can result in data silos, inefficiencies and potential patient safety risks (Watts et al., 2021). Noncompliance with industry standards and data exchange protocols can further exacerbate interoperability challenges and hinder seamless data sharing (Benson & Grieve, 2016).

16.3.4 PRIVACY, SECURITY, AND REGULATORY COMPLIANCE CONCERNS

Inadequate data privacy and security measures can lead to data breaches, compromising patient confidentiality and trust (Kruse et al., 2017). Noncompliance with relevant regulations, such as Health Insurance Portability and Accountability Act (HIPAA), General Data Protection Regulation (GDPR) and Food and Drug Administration (FDA) approvals, can expose organisations to legal and financial risks (Cohen & Mello, 2019).

16.3.5 DISRUPTION TO CLINICAL WORKFLOWS AND INEFFICIENCIES

Failure to assess and address the impact of digital technologies on existing clinical workflows can lead to disruptions, inefficiencies and increased workloads for healthcare professionals (Betten et al., 2020). Lack of user-centred design and integration into daily routines can hinder technology adoption and undermine potential productivity gains (Varghese et al., 2018).

16.3.6 INSUFFICIENT EVALUATION AND CONTINUOUS IMPROVEMENT

The absence of clear metrics and performance indicators can make it challenging to measure the success and impact of digital health technologies (Mandl & Kohane, 2020). Lack of ongoing evaluation and monitoring can result in missed opportunities for improvement, leading to suboptimal outcomes and potential technology abandonment (Ash et al., 2019).

16.3.7 LACK OF LEADERSHIP AND SUSTAINED COMMITMENT

Insufficient leadership support and commitment to digital health initiatives can undermine implementation efforts and long-term success (Topol, 2019). Inadequate resource allocation and funding for implementation, training and ongoing maintenance can impede effective adoption and sustainability of digital technologies (Kano et al., 2021).

By proactively addressing these potential pitfalls and adopting a comprehensive and user-centred approach, healthcare organisations can increase the likelihood of successful digital healthcare implementation and realisation of the intended benefits for individuals care, operational efficiency and overall healthcare delivery.

16.4 Governance

When implementing digital technologies in healthcare settings, several important considerations must be made to ensure successful integration and adoption. When designing digital strategies and systems for healthcare, it is crucial to establish a robust governance system and structure to ensure effective oversight, accountability and alignment with organisational goals and regulatory requirements.

While digital health tools offer numerous benefits, their implementation and adoption must be guided by robust governance frameworks and ethical principles. Ensuring data privacy, security and individual confidentiality is paramount, as digital tools often involve the collection and sharing of sensitive health information (Crico et al., 2021). Informed consent processes should be transparent, addressing potential risks and benefits and empowering individuals to make informed decisions about their participation (Parker et al., 2018).

16.5 Cultivating a Mindset of Lifelong Learning and Adaptability

As digital technologies continue to evolve rapidly, it is essential for community nurses to embrace a mindset of lifelong learning and adaptability. This mindset involves actively seeking out new knowledge, embracing change and continuously updating skills to stay aligned with best practices and emerging digital innovations.

Engaging in continuous professional development (CPD) is crucial for district nurses and community nurses to stay current with the latest advancements in digital healthcare technologies. CPD opportunities, such as online courses, webinars and conferences, can provide valuable insights into emerging digital tools, their applications and best practices for integrating them into nursing practice. Additionally, fostering a culture of innovation within healthcare organisations can encourage nurses to explore and experiment with new technologies, while providing platforms for sharing experiences and lessons learned (Wolfe & Bjordahl, 2018). By actively participating in the development and evaluation of digital health tools, nurses can play a pivotal role in shaping the future of client-centred care.

16.5.1 NATIONAL HEALTH SERVICE DIGITAL ACADEMY

The NHS Digital Academy offers a range of online courses and resources specifically designed to enhance the digital capabilities of healthcare professionals. District nurses can leverage these resources to upskill in areas such as data analytics, virtual consultations and digital health technologies, equipping themselves with the knowledge and skills needed to fully harness the potential of digital innovations.

Fostering and embracing a culture of innovation and collaboration within District nursing teams is essential for driving the successful adoption and implementation of digital tools. By encouraging open dialogue, sharing best practices and seeking input from colleagues and interdisciplinary teams, district nurses can collectively identify opportunities for digital transformation and overcome challenges more effectively.

16.5.2 NATIONAL HEALTH SERVICE DIGITAL INNOVATION HUBS

The NHS has established Digital Innovation Hubs across the country, designed to foster collaboration and facilitate the development and implementation of digital solutions. District nurses and community nurses can actively participate in these hubs, sharing their experiences, contributing ideas and learning from the successes and challenges encountered by others, fostering a collaborative approach to digital innovation in healthcare.

16.5.3 NETWORKS AND FORUMS

In the ever-evolving digital landscape, the significance of digital networking forums cannot be overstated. The QNI report (2023) shows that nurses have a high level of digital literacy, but there are missed opportunities for those who are using digital technology every day in their work to be involved in its development and implementation (Leary & Bushe, 2023). Digital networking communities bring together individuals with shared interests, professions or goals and have become invaluable platforms for collaboration, knowledge sharing and professional growth. At their core, digital networking forums provide a space for individuals to connect, exchange ideas and learn from one another's experiences (Ellison & Vitak, 2015). In an increasingly globalised and interconnected world, these forums break down geographical barriers, enabling professionals from diverse backgrounds and locations to engage in meaningful discourse and build valuable networks.

One of the key advantages of digital networking forums is their ability to facilitate knowledge exchange and foster continuous learning (Chiu et al., 2006). Participants can pose questions, share insights and access a wealth of information curated by their peers, fostering an environment of collective knowledge building (Wenger et al., 2002). This democratisation of knowledge not only benefits individuals but also contributes to the advancement of entire industries and disciplines (Faraj et al., 2011). Furthermore, digital networking forums serve as powerful platforms for professional development and career growth (Donelan, 2016). By engaging with like-minded individuals, professionals can gain exposure to new opportunities, stay updated on industry trends and receive valuable mentorship and guidance (Skeels & Grudin, 2009). These forums can also facilitate collaboration on projects, research or initiatives, opening doors to new partnerships and collaborations.

Beyond their professional applications, digital networking forums also play a vital role in fostering a sense of community and support. Individuals with shared experiences or challenges can find solace and understanding within these online spaces, forming meaningful connections and receiving emotional support when needed (Walther & Boyd, 2002).

16.5.4 NATIONAL DIGITAL SHARED DECISION-MAKING COUNCIL

In recognition of the growing importance of digital technologies in healthcare delivery, Helen Crowther and Ann Gregory established the National Digital Shared Decision-Making Council in March 2019. This council brings together nurses and midwives and digital health experts to provide strategic guidance on the development and implementation of digital tools and platforms that support shared decision-making between clients and their care providers. The council's main objectives include ensuring that digital shared decision-making solutions are designed to be accessible, user-friendly and aligned with patient needs and preferences. Additionally, the council plays a crucial role in promoting the adoption of these digital tools across the NHS, fostering a culture of patient empowerment and collaborative care planning. By incorporating diverse perspectives and expertise, the Digital Shared Decision-Making Council aims to harness the potential of digital technologies to enhance patient engagement, improve health outcomes and deliver personalised, person-centred care within the English healthcare system.

16.5.5 REGIONAL COUNCILS

There are seven regional Digital councils which feed into the National Council, East of England, London, Midlands, North East and Yorkshire, North West, South East, South West.

16.5.6 SHURI NETWORK

The Shuri Network is an initiative that was founded by Dr Shera Chok and Sarah Amani in 2019. They realised that over the last decade, there had only been a handful of women of colour in similar roles, as Chief Clinical Information Officers. They recognised that 'diverse teams are more creative, productive, attract the most talented people and are associated with better patient experience, we decided to change the balance'.

The Network is aimed at increasing digital literacy and access to digital careers for women from minority ethnic backgrounds. Named after the brilliant princess and technological genius from the Marvel Black Panther films, the Shuri Network provides mentorship, training and work experience opportunities in digital health and technology roles within the NHS. The programme partners with NHS England, Digital Health, NHS Providers, the NHS Confederation and many others to engage women interested in STEM fields, offering them a pathway to develop digital skills, gain hands-on experience through fellowships, networking opportunities, podcasts and bursaries, that enables the participants to explore diverse career options in healthcare technology and informatics. By nurturing home-grown digital talent from diverse communities, the Shuri Network aims to promote digital inclusion, address workforce gaps and foster innovation in the delivery of digitally enabled healthcare services that meet the needs of the UK's diverse population.

16.5.7 FLORENCE NIGHTINGALE FOUNDATION INNOVATION AND ENTREPRENEURSHIP SUBJECT EXPERT GROUP

The Florence Nightingale Foundation established the Innovation and Entrepreneurship Subject Expert Group to drive change and promote innovative thinking within nursing and midwifery in the UK. This group comprises leading nurses, midwives and interdisciplinary experts who collaborate to identify opportunities for innovation that can enhance patient care, service delivery and professional development. The Subject Expert Group serves as a catalyst for entrepreneurial ideas, supporting nurses and midwives in turning their novel concepts into practical solutions. They provide guidance on navigating the innovation landscape, securing funding and overcoming barriers to implementation. Additionally, the group plays a crucial role in knowledge sharing, disseminating best practices and successful case studies to inspire and empower healthcare professionals to embrace an entrepreneurial mindset. By fostering a culture of innovation and entrepreneurship, the Florence Nightingale Foundation aims to position nurses and midwives as key drivers of transformative change within the healthcare system.

16.5.8 DIGITAL HEALTH NETWORKS CHIEF NURSING INFORMATION OFFICER NETWORK

The Digital Health Networks CNIO Network is a collaborative initiative that brings together chief nursing information officers (CNIOs) from across the regional Digital Health Networks in England. These networks, established by NHSX (now NHS England's Transforming Health Systems Team), aim to drive digital transformation and foster collaboration among healthcare organisations within their respective regions. The CNIO Network serves as a platform for nursing informatics leaders to share insights, best practices and strategies for leveraging digital technologies to enhance nursing practice and improve patient care. Through regular meetings and knowledge-sharing sessions, CNIOs can learn from each other's experiences, discuss challenges and collectively shape the digital health agenda within their regions. The network also provides opportunities for collaboration on projects, pilots and initiatives that promote the adoption of user-friendly, clinically relevant digital tools tailored to the unique needs and workflows of nurses. By amplifying the voice of nursing informatics professionals, the Digital Health Networks CNIO Network ensures that nurses' perspectives are integrated into the design, development and implementation of digital health solutions across England's regional healthcare ecosystems.

16.6 Conclusion

To address the challenges posed by digital connectivity issues, healthcare provider organisations, commissioners and policymakers must conduct thorough reviews of Wi-Fi internet accessibility in all service delivery areas. Understanding the impact of connectivity on nurses delivering care in communities is crucial for optimising service delivery. Furthermore, scheduling tools and related apps should be developed and used in alignment with nursing principles, professional judgment and personalised care, ensuring individual needs remain central. Additionally, healthcare providers should designate experienced nurses to lead the integration and utilisation of digital technology within their organisations.

District nursing stands at the forefront of innovation in the dynamic digital landscape, poised to harness technology for enhanced patient engagement, education and self-management support. District nurses can foster closer connections between those we care for and healthcare professionals by adopting digital solutions such as patient portals, telehealth platforms, online educational resources and mobile applications. By empowering people to participate in their healthcare journey actively, nurses facilitate a shift towards person-centred care, promoting autonomy and accountability among individuals.

References

Ajibade, B. (2021). Assessing the patient's needs and planning effective care. *British Journal of Nursing*, *30*(20). https://www.britishjournalofnursing.com/content/clinical/assessing-the-patients-needs-and-planning-effective-care (Accessed 6/7/2024).

Ammenwerth, E., Schnell-Inderst, P., & Hoerbst, A. (2012). The impact of electronic patient portals on patient care: A systematic review of controlled trials. *Journal of Medical Internet Research*, *14*(6), e162.

Ash, J. S., Duan, R., Ryan, P. B., & Wright, A. (2019). Improving healthcare and health. *Journal of the American Medical Informatics Association*, *26*(3), 261–267.

Benson, T., & Grieve, G. (2016). *Principles of health interoperability: SNOMED CT, HL7 and FHIR*. Springer.

Berner, J., Rennemark, M., Karlsson, M., & Berglund, J. (2021). Factors influencing Internet use among patients in Sweden. *Informatics for Health and Social Care*, *46*(1), 1–18.

Betten, A. W., Hoyt, R. E., Wiggins, A. T., Bankar, S. P., Callan, G. L., & Jain, P. (2020). Improving healthcare operations using digital transformation: A systematic review. *Healthcare*, *8*(4), 459.

Brown, A., & Hartley, K. (2021). Digital transformation in community nursing. *British Journal of Community Nursing*, *26*(9). https://www.britishjournalofcommunitynursing.com/content/professional/digital-transformation-in-community-nursing/ (Accessed 6/7/2024).

Carmona, C., Crutwell, J., Burnham, M., & Polak, L. (2021). Shared decision-making: Summary of NICE guidance. *BMJ*, *373*, n1430. https://doi.org/10.1136/bmj.n1430

Chen, Z., Liang, N., Zhang, H., et al. (2023). Harnessing the power of clinical decision support systems: Challenges and opportunities. *OpenHeart*, *10*, e002432. https://doi.org/10.1136/openhrt-2023-002432

Chiu, C. M., Hsu, M. H., & Wang, E. T. G. (2006). Understanding knowledge sharing in virtual communities: An integration of social capital and social cognitive theories. *Decision Support Systems*, *42*(3), 1872–1888. https://doi.org/10.1016/j.dss.2006.04.001

Cohen, I. G., & Mello, M. M. (2019). The digital health revolution and regulation. *JAMA*, *321*(14), 1359–1360.

Cresswell, K., Williams, R., & Sheikh, A. (2017). Developing and applying a formative evaluation process for health information technology implementations: Qualitative investigation. *Journal of Medical Internet Research*, *19*(6):e175.

Crico, C., Neumann, P. J., Blumenthal, R. S., & Morgan-Bathke, M. (2021). Digital health data governance: Outlining a governance framework for digital health data. *Digital Medicine*, *4*(1), 1–11.

Dobkin, B. H., & Dorsch, A. (2011). The promise of mHealth: Daily activity monitoring and outcome assessments by wearable sensors. *Neurorehabilitation and Neural Repair*, *25*(9), 788–798.

Donelan, H. (2016). Social media for professional development and networking opportunities in academia. *Journal of Further and Higher Education*, *40*(5), 706–729. https://oro.open.ac.uk/42255/

Ellison, N. B., & Vitak, J. (2015). Social network site affordances and their relationship to social capital processes. In S. S. Sundar (Ed.), *The handbook of the psychology of communication technology*. https://doi.org/10.1002/9781118426456.ch9

Elwyn, G., Laitner, S., Coulter, A., Walker, E., Watson, P., & Thomson, R. (2010). Implementing shared decision making in the NHS. *BMJ*, *341*, c5146. https://doi.org/10.1136/bmj.c5146

Faraj, S., Jarvenpaa, S. L., & Majchrzak, A. (2011). Knowledge collaboration in online communities. *Organization Science*, *22*(5), 1224–1239. https://ssrn.com/abstract=2536138

Fitz-Gerald, M., & Gemmel, P. (2021). Organizational readiness for digital health: A systematic review. *Journal of Medical Internet Research*, *23*(9):e28777.

Hakim, R. (2023). *Realising the potential of virtual wards. Exploring the critical success factors for realising the ambitions of virtual wards*. NHS Confederation. https://www.nhsconfed.org/publications/realising-potential-virtual-wards (Accessed 6/7/2024).

Kano, M., Klvanec, J., Shamekhi, A., Murray, P. J., Petersen, C., & Sevick, S. (2021). Vendor selection criteria for healthcare information technology: A literature review. *Health Services Research*, *56*(1), 153–165.

Kariwo, K., Chapman, M., & Oozageer Gunowa, N. (2023). How does skin tones affect staff confidence when dealing with pressure ulcers. *Wounds International*, *14*(2), 21–27.

Kotter, J. P. (1996). *Leading change*. Harvard Business School Press.

Kruse, C. S., Frederick, B., Jacobson, T., & Monticone, D. K. (2017). Cybersecurity in healthcare: A systematic review of modern threats and trends. *Technology and Health Care*, *25*(1), 1–10.

Laranjo, L., Dunn, A. G., Tong, H. L., Kocaballi, A. B., Chen, J., Bashir, R., ... Coiera, E. (2018). Conversational agents in healthcare: A systematic review. *Journal of the American Medical Informatics Association*, *25*(9), 1248–1258. https://doi.org/10.1093/jamia/ocy072

Lasserson, D., & Cooksley, T. (2023). Virtual wards: Urgent care policy must follow the evidence. *BMJ*, *380*. https://doi.org/10.1136/bmj.p343

Leary, A., & Bushe, D. (2023). *The QNI: Nursing in the digital age 2023. Using technology to support patients in the home*. The Queen's Nursing Institute, International Community Nursing Observatory. https://qni.org.uk/wp-content/uploads/2023/02/Nursing-in-the-Digital-Age-2023.pdf (Accessed 6/7/2024).

Mandl, K. D., & Kohane, I. S. (2020). A 21st-century health IT system: Creating a real-world information system to help patients and professionals. *Journal of the American Medical Informatics Association*, *27*(2), 178–182.

Moy, A. J., Schwartz, J. M., Chen, R., Sadri, S., Lucas, E., Cato, K. D., & Rossetti, S. C. (2021). Measurement of clinical documentation burden among physicians and nurses using electronic health records: A scoping review. *Journal of the American Medical Informatics Association*, *28*(5), 998–1008. https://doi.org/10.1093/jamia/ocaa325

NHS Digital. (2018). *Widening Digital Participation Programme helps patients improve their health. Two pilot projects are proving that digital technology helps people to better manage their health.* https://digital.nhs.uk/news/2018/widening-digital-participation (Accessed 6/7/2024).

NHS Digital. (2022). *Digital services for integrated care.* https://digital.nhs.uk/services/digital-services-for-integrated-care

NHS England. (2020). *Diabetes digital coach.* https://www.england.nhs.uk/aac/what-we-do/how-can-the-aac-help-me/test-beds/diabetes-digital-coach/

NHS England. (2021). *A guide to setting up technology-enabled virtual wards - Key tools and information - NHS Transformation Directorate*, Published 21 December 2021. (england.nhs.uk). https://transform.england.nhs.uk/key-tools-and-info/a-guide-to-setting-up-technology-enabled-virtual-wards/ (Accessed 6/7/2024).

NHS England. (2022). *Supporting information for ICS leads. Enablers for success: Virtual wards including hospital at home.* Version 1, 25 April 2022, Publication approval reference: PAR1382. https://www.england.nhs.uk/wp-content/uploads/2022/04/B1382_supporting-information-for-integrated-care-system-leads_enablers-for-success_virtual-wards-including-hos.pdf (Accessed 6/7/2024).

Parker, L., Karliychuk, T., Gillies, D., Mintzes, B., Raven, M., & Grundy, Q. (2018). A health app developed for parents of children newly diagnosed with leukemia: Ethical challenges and solutions. *JMIR mHealth and uHealth*, *6*(8):e9216.

Quach, S., Thaichon, P., Martin, K. D., Weaven, S., & Palmatier, R. W. (2022). Digital technologies: Tensions in privacy and data. *Journal of the Academy of Marketing Science*, *50*, 1299–1323. https://doi.org/10.1007/s11747-022-00845-y

Ross, JAD., Barron, E., McGough, B., Valabhji, J., Daff, K., Irwin, J., Henley, W. E., Murray, E. (2022). Uptake and impact of the English National Health Service digital diabetes prevention programme: observational study. *BMJ Open Diabetes Research and Care*, *10*:e002736. https://doi.org/10.1136/bmjdrc-2021-002736

Sawesi, S., Rashrash, M., Phalakornkule, K., Carpenter, J. S., & Jones, J. F. (2016). The impact of information technology on patient engagement and health behavior change: A systematic review of the literature. *JMIR Medical Informatics*, *4*(1):e1.

Shi, C., Dumville, J., Rubinstein, F., Norman, G., Ullah, A., Bashir, S., … Vardy, E. R. (2024). Inpatient-level care at home delivered by virtual wards and hospital at home: A systematic review and meta-analysis of complex interventions and their components. *BMC Medicine*, *22*, 145. https://doi.org/10.1186/s12916-024-03312-3

Skeels, M., & Grudin, J. (2009). When social networks cross boundaries: A case study of workplace use of facebook and linkedin. In *Proceedings of the ACM 2009 international conference on supporting group work* (pp. 95–104). Sanibel Island. https://doi.org/10.1145/1531674.1531689. http://dl.acm.org/citation.cfm?id=1531689

Topol, E. (2019). *The Topol review: Preparing the healthcare workforce to deliver the digital future.* London: NHS.

Vos, J.F.J., Boonstra, A., Kooistra, A. Seelen.m., van Offenbeek.M.A.G. (2020). The influence of electronic health record use on collaboration among medical specialties. *BMC Health Serv Res*, *20*, 676. https://doi.org/10.1186/s12913-020-05542-6

Varghese, J., Sandrev, S. S., Varghese, S. A., & Mavally, A. P. (2018). Workflow issues in healthcare provider practices and its impact on meaningful use of health information technology. *Computers in Biology and Medicine*, *100*, 70–84.

Vindrola-Padros, C., Singh, K. E., Sidhu, M. S., et al. (2021). Remote home monitoring (virtual wards) for confirmed or suspected COVID-19 patients: A rapid systematic review. *EClinicalMedicine*, *37*. https://doi.org/10.1016/j.eclinm.2021.100965

Walther, J. B., & Boyd, S. (2002). Attraction to computer-mediated social support. In C. A. Lin, & D. Atkin (Eds.), *Communication technology and society: Audience adoption and uses* (pp. 153–188). Cresskill, NJ: Hampton Press.

Watts, A. D., Craven, T., Chisholm, E., Moser, E., & Oppenheimer, R. (2021). Evaluating digital health capabilities for improved stakeholder engagement in clinical trials. *BMC Medical Informatics and Decision Making*, *21*(1), 1–14.

Weiner, B. J. (2009). A theory of organizational readiness for change. *Implementation Science*, *4*, 67. https://doi.org/10.1186/1748-5908-4-67

Wenger, E., McDermott, R. A., & Snyder, W. (2002). *Cultivating communities of practice: A guide to managing knowledge*. Harvard Business Press.

Wolfe, A., & Bjordahl, J. (2018). Innovation in nursing education: Building digital talent for a digital era. *Nursing Administration Quarterly*, *42*(3), 225–231.

Zhao, J., Freeman, B., & Li, M. (2016). Can mobile phone apps influence people's health behavior change? An evidence review. *Journal of Medical Internet Research*, *18*(11), e287.

CHAPTER 17

Nursing Research in the Community

Jacqui Scrace Lee Tomlinson Hayley Thrumble

LEARNING OUTCOMES

After reading this chapter you should be able to:

- Understand the opportunities for research in the community
- Appreciate how community nurses can get involved in research
- Recognise the importance of research dissemination

17.1 Introduction

There is an ever-increasing emphasis on quality and excellence in healthcare, with key guidelines, including the National Institute for Health and Care Excellence (NICE) guidelines, providing information to support up-to-date, best practice. Consequently, evidence-based practice is a recognised requirement within health and life sciences (Timmins, 2015). Historically, key information was passed down to passive audiences through a linear knowledge pipeline, absorbed and followed without critical appraisal from healthcare staff implementing it into practice (Rafi et al., 2021). However, the knowledge pipeline was extensively criticised for its simplicity and lack of insight into how real-world complexities affect patients, practitioners and healthcare systems (Greenhalgh et al., 2016). This prompted a transition from knowledge exchange via traditional theory and anecdote to research-supported, evidence-based practice (Dagne & Beshah, 2021). The use of research-driven practice demonstrates benefits for professional development, patient outcomes and reduction of costs associated with the healthcare systems (Moule, 2021). This highlights the importance for nurses to recognise the contribution of research and ensure it is woven into clinical practice (Moule, 2021). However, the application of research into practice remains slow and inconsistent, with estimated timelines of around 17 years for scientific research to translate into practice (Churruca et al., 2019).

Research is responsible for the analysis of increasing demands on healthcare systems and resources as a result of the increasing complexity of healthcare due to continually changing, diverse populations (Timmins, 2015). It promotes positive challenge of current practices and values within healthcare and often leads to policy updates and subsequent practice change. It is crucial that nurses are equipped with the skills required to access, understand, critically appraise and disseminate information acquired through research to ensure the implementation of positive change in practice (Dagne & Beshah, 2021). Development of these research skills has a positive effect on standards of care, with practitioners being able to assess the appropriateness and validity of current practices while contributing to identification of ongoing research priorities, ensuring continual development of evidence-based practice (Moule, 2021). Community-based research is a core strategic aim, placing the development of both community-based workforce and research infrastructure as national priorities (National Institute for Health Research (NIHR), 2024). The scale, diversity and importance of community nursing present a huge source of opportunity and potential, not only in the delivery of excellent care but in the development of the care of future (Badley et al., 2022).

In 2020 Dame Ruth May, the Chief Nursing Officer (CNO) for England, appointed two Heads of Nursing Research; these were new national nursing roles in NHS England. Their roles worked toward ensuring that evidence-based research was at the heart of the nursing profession and individual nursing careers (Ford, 2020) and their appointment showed commitment toward this aim from the CNO office. In November 2021 they launched Making Research Matter, Chief Nursing Officer for England's Strategic Plan for Research (National Health Service, 2021). The ambitious plan indicated investment and support for nurses to lead, participate in and deliver research across all settings in health and social care.

Release of the plan has supported individual and strategic conversations to enable the growth of research involving nurses. There is a growing community of nurses and nurse researchers building evidence for out-of-hospital care. There are national communities of practice pulling together to make ambitions a reality and provide connections and a network for sharing ideas and plans. In addition, research managers from out-of-hospital settings have pulled together in an alliance: Community Healthcare Alliance for Research Trusts (CHART). In the 2023 CNO Summit, there was strong recognition of the contribution from all nurses and nursing associates from all settings with an emphasis on social care and the voluntary sector.

DEFINITION

When using the word 'delivery' in research, it refers to the conduct of the study to gather the information needed, be that through recruiting people or conducting a survey to establish the outcome of the research.

17.2 Funding Streams

17.2.1 THE NATIONAL INSTITUTE FOR HEALTH AND CARE RESEARCH (NIHR)

The NIHR is the research arm of the Department of Health and Social Care (DHSC); the latest iteration was set up by Chris Whitty in 2019. It funds research to enable and deliver high-quality, world leading health and social care research to improve the health and well-being of the population. The NIHR publishes documents such as *Best Research for Best Health: The Next Chapter* (2021) to outline strategic areas of priority and focus in health and care research. It enables its ambitions through supportive opportunities to people working in health and care. Go to the NIHR website and have a look around: https://www.nihr.ac.uk/

17.2.2 FUNDING PROGRAMMES

These programmes are usually nationally competitive to secure large grants to develop a research study. It is usual that a group of academic, health and care colleagues come together to submit a bid jointly. There are many different funds to apply for and themed calls that may be specific to a population group.

17.2.3 INVESTING IN INFRASTRUCTURE

The NIHR holds the Clinical Research Network (CRN), made up of 15 regional networks to support the delivery of research in the NHS.

These CRNs have been replaced by new Regional Research Delivery Networks (RRDNs) as of October 1, 2024. There is an appreciation in the development of the RRDNs for the differences experienced in different settings for research. This is a positive move from the historical medicalised model of research and the participant residing in a hospital bed; there will be increased support for delivery of research in out-of-hospital settings, be that in a prison, someone's home, a hospice or community centre for example.

The NIHR also funds local collaborations called Applied Research Collaboratives (ARCs). These are to support applied health research and the implementation of health and care evidence in day-to-day practice. Again, there are 15 ARCs and they map the same geography as the RRDNs, they bring together NHS providers, universities, charities, local authorities and innovation networks. The ARCs provide different opportunities to progress research ideas or to implement evidence into practice, in response to local population needs (Fig. 17.1). They act as a great resource for connection across the NHS and academia and can support mentorship and pulling a team together (Box 17.1).

The NIHR also supports the setup and development of world leading research facilities including Clinical Trials Units and Biomedical Research centres.

17.2.4 DELIVERING NATIONAL RESEARCH STUDIES

The easiest way to get involved in research is to support the delivery of a national portfolio study. These studies have been developed through a team elsewhere in the country applying and being successful in achieving a research grant to deliver their planned study. Most of these studies require additional sites to support with recruitment; this not only ensures that the output from the study is generalisable but also ensures that different populations and individuals are represented in the study findings. There are many roles needed for these studies in local communities such as the principal investigator or local lead. Sometimes, studies will need blinded assessors, or a specialist, to carry out an intervention or identify suitable potential participants. These roles cannot be underestimated; if a study does not open in a particular area, the local population has not had an opportunity to contribute their perspective. We have a duty as community nurses to support the inclusion of as many and different individuals and groups into research studies as possible.

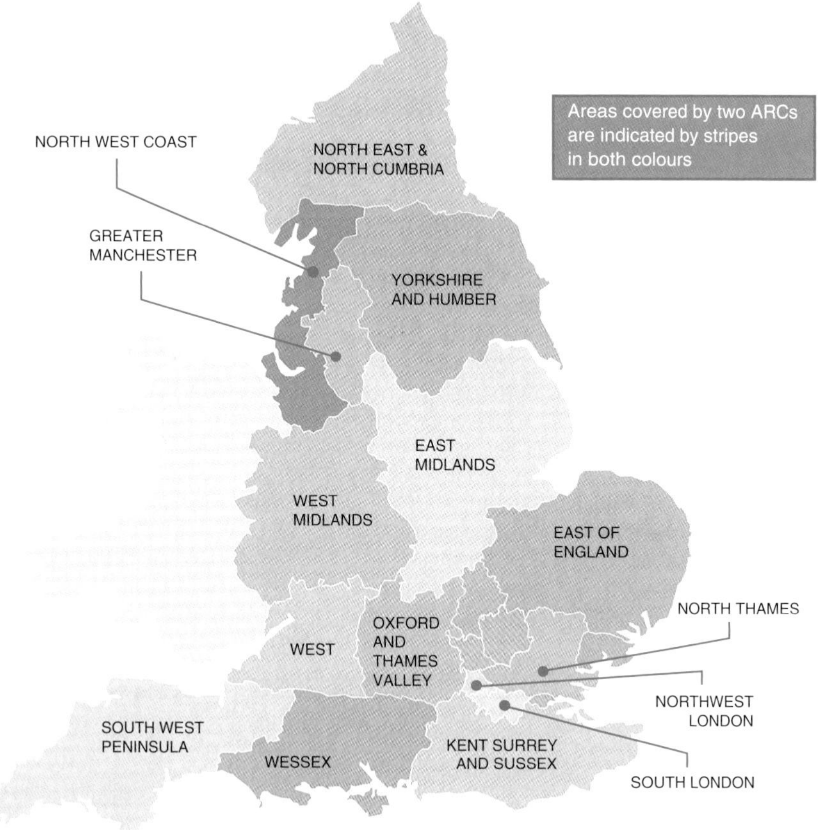

Fig. 17.1 The 15 Applied Research Collaboratives (ARCs). (From NIHR. (2023). The 15 ARCs. Retrieved from www.nihr.ac.uk/explore-nihr/support/collaborating-in-applied-health-research.htm#two.)

BOX 17.1 ■ Involvement in Research

Consider reaching out to Regional Research Delivery Networks and letting them know the area and service you work in to see if there are any opportunities for you to support the delivery of research.

17.2.5 ENGAGING AND PARTNERING WITH THE PUBLIC

Working with patients and the public to ensure that their experiences and perspectives shape the design and delivery of a study is a priority for NIHR and other research funders. To ensure that studies are written with the intended population in mind means that the representatives from that group need to be involved in the design, to make sure it works for them. When a study is open, it is possible that some people will not get the

BOX 17.2 ■ Community Nursing Top 10 Research Priorities

Community Nursing Top 10

1. How can community nurse teams better meet the complex needs of patients with multiple health conditions?
2. How can community nurses promote shared care/self-care amongst patients, and support carers to provide some aspects of care (e.g., changing dressings)?
3. How can community nurse teams best contribute to the management of acutely ill patients at home? What difference does this make to hospital admissions?
4. What are the best ways for community nurses to involve unpaid carers/relatives/friends in decisions about their loved one's treatment and care?
5. How can community nurse teams work effectively with social services and care services to improve the quality of patient care?
6. How has community nursing changed in response to COVID-19? Are any of the changes (e.g., timed visits, new skills and working from home) worth keeping?
7. Does seeing the same community nurse(s) over time make a difference to the quality of patient care?
8. How can community nurses work effectively with other health professionals in hospitals and specialist community services to improve patient care?
9. What are the stresses on community nurses and what impact does this have on their health and well-being? How can this be improved?
10. How can nurses be encouraged to become community nurses and to stay in the profession?

Community Nursing Top 10 list of research priorities, JLA. www.jla.nihr.ac.uk.

opportunity to participate, to give their perspective or to have the opportunity to try a new recovery method. This is often because some individuals will not reside in the usual place, or access services through the usual route or routinely attend check-ups in health clinics. It is important that research is inclusive of everyone and includes as wide a population as possible (Brett et al., 2017). To achieve this, research teams need to consider different routes of access and to have these conversations with people to understand how they could be involved. A way in which this has been achieved is through the James Lind Alliance (JLA) to determine the top 10 research priorities for community nursing. These were achieved following a well-defined process led by the JLA with patients, family members and community nurses (Henshall et al., 2022). The result is inclusive priorities for teams to build research questions from Box 17.2.

17.3 Community Nurses and Research

Community nurses are best placed to know what research, evidence and innovation will benefit their communities; they are also best placed to lead it (Badley et al., 2022). However, a rapid appraisal was undertaken in 2022, where community nurses, Band 5–8, were invited to share their experiences of the current use of research, evidence and innovation in practice which highlighted the following key themes shown in Box 17.3.

BOX 17.3 ■ Key Themes

- Unrelenting pressure of clinical service delivery impacts upon the opportunities to be involved in research.
- Commissioning of services prioritises performance and clinical efficiency, leaving little time for research and improvement activities.
- In comparison to allied health professionals (AHPs) and medics, where research forms part of the professional expectation, the professional nursing culture does not lend itself to nurses being involved in research.
- Limited scope to absorb activities beyond clinical care.
- Limited expectation of research and improvement activities within nursing roles, particularly for more junior nurses.
- Advanced clinical practitioners did recognise the need for research and improvement activities within their role, but lacked competence and confidence in these areas in comparison to the other pillars of advanced practice.
- Lack of visibility of career options and limited community nursing role models in research.

REFLECTION

- What does research and evidence mean to you?
- How might you be able to influence this in your practice?

Nurses often shy away from research; however, when thinking about evidence-based practice, or evidence-based nursing, nurses do naturally engage with research, as there is a sense of ownership, it means something, it means that what is being done, is correct, current and is hopefully 'best practice' (Finney, 2022). If considering clinical variation or clinical uncertainty in some areas of practice, nurses are very aware of lots of research questions with this focus.

17.3.1 EMBEDDED IMPLEMENTATION RESEARCH AND COPRODUCTION

The use of embedded implementation in research differs from more traditional approaches which typically demonstrate disparate roles and rigid protocols (Churruca et al., 2019). Traditional research methods usually have an external researcher to provide evidence and conduct summative evaluations which are disseminated to relevant teams (Churruca et al., 2019). Embedded implementation research challenges these traditional paradigms and recognises multiple forms of knowledge, by utilising an experienced researcher working with or within the team responsible for the proposed improvement, supporting adoption and implementation into practice (Churruca et al., 2019). The primary advantage of this is that frontline staff who can identify gaps in evidence-based practice and have the capacity to influence change can collaborate with researchers who possess the knowledge and expertise to provide empirical evidence for the need for such change (Rycroft-Malone et al., 2016).

In an environment in which public scrutiny of research processes and findings is commonplace, dissemination of research in this way can foster a culture of trust and partnership between researchers, healthcare professionals, patients and stakeholders ensuring that all relevant parties can understand the overarching priorities—thus

TABLE 17.1 **Key Benefits to Parties Involved in the Implementation of Research**

Researcher Benefit	Implementer Benefit
Access and buy-in Motivation for change and participation in research and its evaluation are more likely to be sustained with researchers embedded in the team.	**Exposure to new skills and knowledge** Researchers bring empirical knowledge, research skills and experience to implementers which are transferable beyond the initial research project.
System learning Implementers can provide researchers with 'real-world' insights which contextualises research and expands knowledge base and theories, supporting researchers to ask the right questions.	**Enhance the improvement effort** Implementers can feedback findings to relevant communities more efficiently and adapt the improvement effort accordingly.
Ongoing improvement The partnerships built between implementers and researchers through research collaboration form the basis for further improvement initiatives, benefitting future quality improvement projects.	

creating a more unified approach to quality improvement (Hagan et al., 2017). Table 17.1 describes some of the key benefits to parties involved in embedded implementation of research.

One way to bring nurses to the forefront of new research is to support them to identify research questions and to engage them in the search, critique and implementation processes of best evidence via the use of the critically appraised topic (CAT).

17.3.2 CRITICALLY APPRAISED TOPICS

CATs provide a summary of the best available evidence to answer a clinical question (Finney, 2022). The question for a CAT group is identified by the nurses themselves, supported by a clinical academic and derived from a specific patient situation or problem that has arisen in clinical practice. It aims to present research in an accessible way, allowing findings to be easily transferable and to support the implementation of a change in practice, where necessary (Finney et al., 2020).

CASE STUDY 17.1

The CAT methodology, which had proved so successful for general practice nurses and allied health practitioners, was successfully piloted with a group of children's community nurses, following an area of practice that was highlighted as a particular clinical issue with wide variation across the UK: troubleshooting nasogastric (NG) tubes for babies, children and young people to avoid hospital attendance or admission to confirm placement. The group was supported by a clinical academic based within a university who was also a children's nurse. Through the CAT process, the group identified that there was, in fact, limited research and evidence on troubleshooting nasogastric tubes for babies, children and young people in the community, so went beyond the CAT group to reexamine and reevaluate the evidence base together and produce new, updated guidance on the care of NG tubes in the community.

(From Tatterton, M., Mulcahy, J., Mankelow, J., Harding, M., Scrace, J., Fisher, M., & Bethell, C. (2023). Nasogastric tube safety in children cared for in the community: a re-examination of the evidence base. *Nursing Children and Young People*. doi: https://doi.10.7748/ncyp.2023.e1493.)

Bringing together community nurses and clinical academics in this way enables the cross-fertilisation of knowledge and skills, allowing the clinical academic to remain up to date with current practice issues, and nurses to improve their literature searching, evidence interpretation and appraisal skills, to translate evidence into practice (Finney et al., 2016).

17.3.3 TRAINING RESEARCHERS

Good Clinical Practice (GCP) is a set of internationally recognised ethical and scientific quality requirements that must be followed when designing, conducting, recording and reporting clinical trials that involve people. It is a legal requirement that people working on studies that involve drugs or devices are GCP trained. It is good practice for staff within teams to have completed their training so that they are aware of the governance requirements for research.

17.3.4 APPLICABILITY TO COMMUNITY NURSING

The NIHR also has personal development awards available to nurses. In 2023 Professor Ruth Endacott, The Director of Nursing and Midwifery for NIHR, secured £30 million funding a year to support and enable the growth of research careers for healthcare professionals. With the promotion and support of nursing research, the historical and now outdated medical model for research is being challenged. Nurses, midwives and allied health professionals are leading the direction for evidence-based care.

There are now multiple opportunities for nurses to increase their skills and knowledge in research. This can be through the traditional academic route in pursuit of a clinical academic post for example. Such funded opportunities through the NIHR include internships, predoctoral fellowships through to PhD and beyond. There are similar opportunities for progression in research delivery through academic study and leadership opportunities to lead on strategy locally and nationally, increasing the sphere of influence through networking and development opportunities.

17.3.5 DISSEMINATION OF RESEARCH

Dissemination of research is a fundamental aspect of any study (Hagan et al., 2017). It informs developments within the field of research, demonstrates the benefits of the study's findings to those it is relevant to and promotes public examination of the methods used and conclusions drawn from the study (Hagan et al., 2017).

REFLECTION

- How have you seen research findings disseminated in your practice?
- What sorts of forums and materials are used?
- How do the staff you work with find out about research findings?
- How do you keep yourself abreast of current practice?

17.3.6 DISSEMINATION PLANS

As part of the dissemination process when applying for research funding, funding bodies like the NIHR request researchers to provide a dissemination plan. These plans identify

BOX 17.4 ■ Components of a Dissemination Plan

- What needs to be disseminated?
- Who is the audience for dissemination and who will apply it in practice?
- Who are your dissemination partners—who else might be involved?
- What materials or methods of dissemination might you use to convey research outcomes?
- Will you evaluate how effectively the dissemination plan worked—how will you do this?
- What resources are available and are needed to execute the plans?

(From Carpenter, D., Nieva, V., Albaghal, T., & Sorra, J. (2005). Development of a planning tool to guide research dissemination. In K. Henriksen, J. B. Battles, E. S. Marks, & I. S. Lewin (Eds.), *Advances in patient safety: From research to implementation (volume 4: Programs, tools, and products)*. Rockville (MD): Agency for Healthcare Research and Quality (US). Available from: https://www.ncbi.nlm.nih.gov/books/NBK20603/.)

how the researcher intends to disseminate their research and help to ensure that research findings are accessible to a range of audiences (Moule et al., 2017). The researcher must consider their target audience carefully as this will determine the most appropriate method of dissemination. There are several tools available to support researchers in developing dissemination plans; an example available from Carpenter et al. (2005) demonstrates the components and considerations of a good quality dissemination plan and can be used as a guideline (Box 17.4).

17.4 Conclusion

The ever-increasing spotlight and support for nursing research at a national level and, in particular, growing community-based activity signals an exciting time for community nurses. It is important that community nursing is recognised, and the value seen in an increasing evidence base built through research. The results are evident both in terms of improving patient outcomes and standards of care through to leading changes to policy.

This chapter outlines the current infrastructure in place to enable community nurses to engage in research activity. By definition, community nurses are best placed to understand how and what research will be of benefit to the communities they are part of and they must ensure that their patients are invited to contribute their perspectives or data wherever possible. With the move forward from a historic medical model of research to recognising the multidisciplinary approaches to leading research, there are increased opportunities for community nurses to build their confidence and engage at many different levels and time points in the research process. Research needs to be embedded in daily practice and viewed as a priority alongside clinical care, a professional expectation across all levels of community nursing. This shift in focus, away from the traditional medical model of research, brings a huge opportunity for community nurses to lead the way for evidence-based care.

References

Badley, A., Tomlinson, L., Scrace, J., & Williams, S. (2022). *Nurses in the community. A rapid appraisal of research, evidence and innovation in practice.* The Academy of Research and Improvement, Solent NHS Trust. https://www.academy.solent.nhs.uk.

Brett, J., Staniszewska, S., Simera, I., Seers, K., Mockford, C., Goodlad, S.,.... Tysall, C. (2017). Reaching consensus on reporting patient and public involvement (PPI) in research: methods and lessons learned from the development of reporting guidelines. *BMJ Open*, 7(10):e016948 pmid:29061613.

Carpenter, D., Nieva, V., Albaghal, T., & Sorra, J. (2005). Development of a planning tool to guide research dissemination. In K. Henriksen, J. B. Battles, E. S. Marks, & I. S. Lewin (Eds.), *Advances in patient safety: From research to implementation (volume 4: Programs, tools, and products)*. Rockville (MD): Agency for Healthcare Research and Quality (US). Available from: https://www.ncbi.nlm.nih.gov/books/NBK20603/.

Churruca, K., Ludlow, K., Taylor, N., et al. (2019). The time has come: Embedded implementation research for health care improvement. *Journal of Evaluation in Clinical Practice*, *25*(3), 373–380. https://doi.org/10.1111/jep.13100. [Accessed 20 October 2023].

Dagne, A. H., & Beshah, M. H. (2021). Implementation of evidence based practice: The experience of nurses & midwives. *PLoS One*, *16*(8), E0256600. Available at: https://www.ncbi.nlm.nih.gov/pmc/articles/PMC8396772/. [Accessed 6 September 2023].

Finney, A. (2022). Promoting true evidence-based practice using critically appraised topics (CATs). Evidence-Based Nursing blog (bmj.com).

Finney, A., Harper, C., Viggars, R., & Edwards, J. (2020). Integrating 'best evidence' into general practice nursing. *Practice Nurse Nov*, *20*, 26–29.

Finney, A., Johnson, K., Edwards, J., Duffy, H., & Dziedzic, K. (2016). Critically appraised topics (CATs): A method of integrating best evidence into general practice nursing. Practice Nurse, 46(3), 32.

Ford, S. (2020). Nottingham nurse appointed to national role to boost nursing research. Nursing Times. https://www.nursingtimes.net/news/leadership-news/nottingham-nurse-appointed-to-national-role-to-boost-nursing-research-04-07-2020/.

Greenhalgh, T., Jackson, C., Shaw, S., & Janamian, T. (2016). Achieving research impact through co–creation in community–based health services: Literature review and case study. *Milbank Q*, *94*(2), 392–429.

Hagan, T. L., Schmidt, K., Ackison, G. R., et al. (2017). Not the last word: Dissemination strategies for patient-centred research in nursing. *J Res Nurs*, *22*(5), 388–402. https://doi.org/10.1177/1744987117709516. Epub 2017 Jun 26. PMID: 29081824; PMCID: PMC5659264.

Henshall, C., Jones, L., Armitage, C., & Tomlinson, L. (2022). Identifying the top ten unanswered questions in community nursing: A James Lind Alliance priority setting partnership in community nursing. *Advances in Public Health*. https://doi.org/10.1155/2022/2213945. Article ID 2213945, 10 pages, 2022.

James Lind Alliance. Community Nursing Top 10 (nihr.ac.uk)

Moule, P. (2021). *Making sense of research in nursing, health and social care*. London, Los Angeles: SAGE.

Moule, P., Aveyard, H., & Goodman, M. (2017). *Nursing research: An introduction*. Los Angeles: SAGE.

National Health Service. (2021). Making research matter. *Chief Nursing Officer for England's strategic plan for research*. https://www.england.nhs.uk/wp-content/uploads/2021/11/B0880-cno-for-englands-strategic-plan-fo-research.pdf.

NIHR. (2023). The 15 ARCs. Image. Available online: www.nihr.ac.uk/explore-nihr/support/collaborating-in-applied-health-research.htm#two.

NIHR. (2024). Our areas of strategic focus. Available at: https://www.nihr.ac.uk/about-us/our-key-priorities/.

Rafii, F., Nasrabadi, A. N., & Tehrani, F. J. (2021). How nurses apply patterns of knowing in clinical practice: A grounded theory study. *Ethiopian Journal of Health Science*, *31*(1), 139–146. Available at: https://www.ncbi.nlm.nih.gov/pmc/articles/PMC8188100/. [Accessed 17 November 2023].

Rycroft–Malone, J., Burton, C. R., Bucknall, T., et al. (2016). Collaboration and co–production of knowledge in healthcare: Opportunities and challenges. *International Journal of Health Policy and Management*, *5*(4), 221–223.

Timmins, F. (2015). Disseminating nursing research. *Nursing standard*, *29*(48), 34–39. https://doi.org/10.7748/ns.29.48.34.e8833. PMID: 26219810.

CHAPTER 18

Health and Well-being of District and Community Nurses

Karen Storey Julia Fairhall Nathan Illman Heather Lane

LEARNING OUTCOMES

By reading this chapter nurses will be able to:

- Understand the importance of their own and other colleagues' health and well-being
- Comprehend the term 'psychological well-being'
- Appreciate why self-care is important in maintaining nurses' mental health and well-being
- Recognise tools to help nurses manage their mental health and well-being, including support systems for individuals who identify as neurodivergent

18.1 Introduction

Community nursing plays a crucial role in delivering exceptional healthcare to individuals within their residences and communities. Given the rising number of elderly individuals with multiple long-term conditions, the demand for community nursing has grown, placing strain on both capacity and resources. Consequently, maintaining consistent, high-quality care for community populations becomes challenging, and this challenge takes a toll on the psychological well-being of the staff.

The National Health Service (NHS) Workforce Plan (NHS, 2023a) identifies well-established evidence indicating a connection between the health and well-being of staff and patient outcomes. There is a recognition of the need for a cultural shift to empower nurses to proactively manage their own health and well-being. It underscores the imperative for enhancements in NHS leadership to provide comprehensive support for the physical and mental health of NHS staff. Notably, it encourages NHS staff to prioritise discussions about their health and well-being in conversations with managers, teams and during staff appraisals.

In district and community nursing, nurses will certainly cultivate a deep sense of meaning and purpose as they pursue their careers. Providing care within the confines of people's homes allows nurses to gain access to their world. This privilege grants nurses the chance to establish profound connections and impact patients, often leading to the extension or preservation of lives. Nurses in this field will encounter levels of pride, joy, gratitude, connectedness and love that surpass the experiences of most individuals. However, there is a downside to this, as the immense responsibility also brings the possibility of negative emotions and inner turmoil for nurses. Mistakes can have serious consequences, leading to a significant impact on the mind. Resource constraints and organisational policies may force nurses into situations that test their internal sense of morality and ethics. Nurses might encounter choices where there is no ideal solution, leading to self-doubt or self-judgment or becoming entangled in endless cycles of thought and worry. Nurses may find themselves dealing with a combination of stress and challenging emotions like never before. In the healthcare sector, this can be the emotional toll of being deeply invested in our profession.

It is commonly asserted that nurses excel in caring for others but often struggle with self-care reference. Engaging in self-care can seem self-indulgent, especially when the daunting task of managing domestic responsibilities appears overwhelming. While there is limited research specifically addressing the impact of this issue on community nurses, there is evidence suggesting that the emotional demands of nursing affect caregivers. In a study primarily focused on hospital nurses, Sawbridge and Hewison (2013) found a lack of widespread support systems for staff dealing with the emotional aspects of their work. This deficiency was identified as a factor contributing to nurses delivering substandard care.

Currently, there is a broader discourse on staff health and well-being. Recently, the Royal College of Nursing (RCN) (2023) has released several documents stressing the significance of nurses setting personal boundaries that allow them to prioritise their own health and well-being. This approach is essential for ensuring they can consistently deliver excellent care to patients.

In the following sections, there are a range of resources and advice that will help nurses in developing this crucial self-care mindset.

18.2 Community Nursing and Psychological Well-being

Prior to and throughout the pandemic, community nurses have consistently worked in fluctuating environments which have consisted of increased daily pressures, financial constraints, complexity of patients and increased public demands for service provision as well as working with ever-changing community demographics, leaving the profession feeling in heightened stress at times and at risk of burn out (Wallbank, 2013a, 2013b). Therefore for those working within these environments, the importance of looking after themselves and nursing teams is paramount.

During the COVID-19 pandemic, the role of professional nurse advocate (PNA) was introduced by the Chief Nursing Officer in March 2021 when universities were commissioned to provide an academic programme to both educate and support the embedment of PNAs within organisations across the UK. This has proved to be a pivotal role in raising the profile of the importance of the health and well-being of nurses (NHS England (NHSE), 2023c). The PNA programme recognises the importance of reflective practice and supporting nurses through restorative clinical supervision. The model, although structured, recognises the value of those opportune ad hoc opportunities which can start a health and well-being conversation but then lead to a structured more in-depth restorative supervision session.

The importance of pausing, taking a breath, taking protected time, having the space to think and reflect. Professional nurse advocacy gives an opportunity to share ideas in a psychologically safe environment, with a trusted colleague to consider alternative approaches whether that be with dealing with teams or reviewing patient care. However, for this change to be embedded, a culture shift in caring for self and team needs to be prioritised.

Community nurses are compassionate, caring people who deliver care in the most challenging and often isolated of situations. Nursing is a safety-critical profession founded on four pillars: clinical practice, education, research and leadership (RCN, 2023). Registered nurses use evidence-based knowledge and professional and clinical judgement to assess, plan, implement and evaluate high-quality person-centred nursing care (RCN, 2023). Community visits are primarily undertaken alone and since the COVID-19 pandemic there has been a reduction in human connection and face-to-face interaction with teams, which can impact one's sense of value and belonging. Following the peak of COVID, some teams now only meet virtually with very little face-to-face contact; the long-term implications of this are yet unknown. Community nurses are involved in complex, traumatic and emotional care interventions with patients and their families. The care delivered by nurses can have a personal impact on a nurse's health and well-being. In practice, sometimes, the smallest of events can open a personal drawer full of emotion that has been carried for days, months or years and this can be overwhelming. The professional nurse advocacy role is pivotal in stopping that custom and practice and encouraging bravery in sharing when support is needed.

18.3 Advocating for Education and Quality Improvement Model

Professional nurse advocacy follows a model referred to as Advocating for Education and Quality Improvement (A-EQUIP) model (NHSE, 2023c) (Fig. 18.1). The model provides opportunities to help nurses stop, slow down and reflect on experiences through honest and open reflection. The A-EQUIP model stems from the three functions of clinical supervision (MacDondald, 2019) which include three components: normative, formative and restorative (NHSE, 2023c). NHS England added a fourth function: personal action and quality improvement (McCormack & McCance, 2017), which resulted in the further development of the A-EQUIP model for use in professional nursing leadership and clinical supervision, and for use by PNAs. Through restorative supervision, a community nurse can challenge thinking in a supportive environment and consider viewing situations from different perspectives this supports future decision-making.

18.3.1 THE FOUR KEY ASPECTS TO THE A-EQUIP MODEL EXPLAINED

18.3.1.1 Restorative Clinical Supervision

This function of the model has benefits for staff to feel supported, develop personally and, professionally, feel less isolated and experience less stress and could potentially lead to fewer work absences. This in turn has a positive impact on emotional and physical well-being and focuses on staff individually or in teams building toolkits to mitigate workforce stresses. Organisations will then find they have staff groups who have community staff who are developing themselves, improving and monitoring and developing best practices but more importantly feeling motivated and experiencing joy in their roles. Staff who have experienced restorative clinical supervision have been found to show slightly increased levels of compassion and role contentment which has been regarded as a protective barrier to individual stress and burnout (Rouse, 2019).

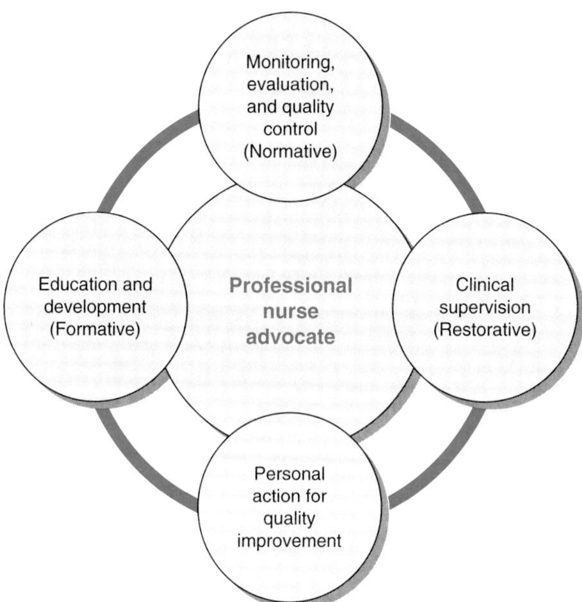

Fig. 18.1 The four functions of A-EQUIP. (Adapted from NHS England. (2023). *Professional nurse advocate A-EQUIP model: a model of clinical supervision for nurses.* https://www.england.nhs.uk/long-read/pna-equip-model-a-model-of-clinical-supervision-for-nurses/.)

18.3.1.2 Personal Action for Quality Improvement

This links to the importance of nurses being familiar with and contribute to quality improvement to improve patient care. This methodology can be quantified, measured and analysed to demonstrate improved patient outcomes.

18.3.1.3 Education and Development

This aspect is intrinsically linked to restorative clinical supervision and focuses on learning development and knowledge components from experiences, competence and influencing positive change (NHSE, 2023c).

18.3.1.4 Monitoring Evaluation and Quality Control

This aspect promotes professional accountability, involvement in quality improvement and effectiveness and supports services improvements, leading to improve patient care.

18.3.2 ROLE OF PROFESSIONAL NURSE ADVOCATES

PNAs can be full time but are predominately PNAs as part of their substantive role. Their role is primarily support, adhering to supervision confidentiality. In terms of reporting, activity is reported in the numbers of sessions carried out by a PNA and consists of broad themes such as burnout. In Box 18.1, there are examples of support available to community nurses.

BOX 18.1 ■ Examples of Support

PNA support is always offered during work hours. Examples of support provided can be:

- Planned 1-1 sessions
- Planned group sessions
- Career advice and support
- Development advice and support
- Drop-in clinics
- Walk and talk

BOX 18.2 ■ Examples of How Staff Have Impacted Self and Team Health and Well-Being

- Guardian Angel: A scheme originating in schools whereby staff members are allocated someone to look out for them, give them time to talk, listen to any concerns or worries and show them recognition for the work they are doing. However, your guardian angel is unknown to you.
- Health and well-being boxes
- Colouring wall promoting conversation
- Investing in our environments—plants
- Quiet spaces
- Health and well-being team check-in meetings—not work related
- Book clubs

Nurses need to prioritise and take responsibility for how they look after themselves and each other to provide high-quality patient-centred care. Box 18.2 showcases examples of support systems in place.

18.4 The Power of Self-compassion

The certainty of district nursing that was outlined earlier is the honest recognition of the pain that can arise in one's role. While community nurses will receive valuable social support from colleagues, friends and family, it remains crucial to cultivate a robust and supportive internal relationship with oneself. After all, a significant portion of a person's time is spent in solitude, within the confines of their own thoughts. This constructive and nurturing connection is commonly referred to as self-compassion.

In this section/part, an overview of what self-compassion entails, why it holds significance and methods for its cultivation will be presented. The aim is to facilitate the ability to navigate through life's challenges with resilience, wisdom and courage. The process involves forgiving oneself for errors, replacing self-doubt and judgment with inner kindness and motivation and, ultimately, embracing self-compassion.

To begin, it is helpful to define the term 'self-compassion'. One prominent definition states that it is 'a sensitivity to suffering…with a commitment to alleviate it' (Gilbert, 2017). Suffering may arise from challenging thoughts, memories, distressing emotions such as shame and anxiety or physical pain from illness. The essence of self-compassion lies in attentiveness to internal experiences and responding with kindness and care. This response may manifest through compassionate self-talk or outward actions, such as taking rest when fatigued.

BOX 18.3 ■ Using Compassion for Another to Understand Self-Compassion

Imagine a nursing friend is going through a difficult time. They've been run down with multiple colds lately, have a young child and are as overloaded at work as you are.

They recently made a small error in their notes, and you know they're being hard on themselves and feeling stressed. You've overheard them saying things like 'I never get things right!' and you can see the stress through the tension in their body. This is evidently a moment of suffering for them.

As a kind and caring friend, what would you say to them?

- How would you say it? What would you do to support them?
- Would you lay a hand on them and project a soft, caring facial expression to comfort and reassure them?
- Would you remind them of the fact that, 'we all make mistakes at times' and let them know how well they're doing apart from this one tiny error?

Self-compassion is simply these kinds of gestures, words and intentions directed inwardly toward ourselves. It is a kind and friendly attitude. It is a capacity and willingness to forgive oneself. It is a supportive and motivational inner voice. It is a turning toward our emotions and asking ourselves 'What is it I most need right now?' And then giving ourselves what we need, be it rest, food, connection or some other form of action.

A fundamental approach to grasping self-compassion is to initially envision extending compassion to someone else and then contemplate how this empathetic perspective can be turned inward on oneself (see Box 18.3).

18.4.1 WHY IS SELF-COMPASSION IMPORTANT FOR NURSES?

The presence of stress is a certainty within the nursing role. Nevertheless, individuals with elevated levels of self-compassion and self-forgiveness exhibit enhanced regulation of the stress response in the body. This correlation is underscored by findings indicating that those who cultivate high self-compassion experience lower rates of mental ill health (Neff, 2023), report better health status (Sirois, 2020) and enjoy heightened levels of well-being (Zessin et al., 2015). Notably, among nurses, a study revealed that those with higher self-compassion had lower rates of burnout, improved sleep and increased job satisfaction (Vaillancourt & Wasylkiw, 2020). In summary, acquiring the skill of self-compassion is conducive to leading a healthier and more contented life

18.4.2 DEVELOPING THE SKILLS OF SELF-COMPASSION AND SELF-FORGIVENESS

It is essential to note that the components of self-compassion and self-forgiveness encompass various micro skills that can be acquired through learning. For instance, the ability to recognise and dissect individual emotions requires practice and often necessitates guidance. Developing the skill to replace self-criticism with a more compassionate and supportive inner dialogue is also crucial. Hence, nurses should approach the learning process of self-compassion and self-forgiveness with the same mindset applied to acquiring other skills—namely, with a growth mindset. Focusing on practicing one skill at a time and committing to experimentation with subsequent feedback is encouraged.

BOX 18.4 ■ Exercise 1: How Do I Know If I Am Self-Compassionate or Not?

Answer the following questions in your mind.

1. When I make a mistake or fall short in some way, do I frequently and intensely berate myself?
2. Would I say I can quickly move on from mistakes and forgive myself?
3. Can I motivate myself through kindness and positive support, rather than through criticism and intense pressure?
4. Do I allow myself to feel my emotions, or do I cut myself off or avoid how I'm feeling?
5. Do I prioritise my own needs regularly?

Remember, be kind to yourself in this moment. Avoid the urge to be self-critical about the fact that you might not be self-compassionate!

Read on for some practical tools to start developing self-compassion.

BOX 18.5 ■ Exercise 2: Self-Compassion in Action: 'Permission to Feel'

A core aspect of self-compassion is giving yourself permission to feel your emotions fully.

When we disown our feelings, we disown ourselves. Without a full acknowledgment of the emotions in your body, your body will hold tightly onto things and present repercussions later on.

Take the time you need to go through the following questions:

Permission to feel.

What is an area that has been causing me stress lately?

What am I resisting feeling in this moment?

If I gave myself full permission to feel my body, where do I notice tension?

If I gave myself full permission to feel all the emotions that are present, what is present?

In which part of my body do I feel this?

Upon mastering several self-compassion tools through regular practice, individuals will have them readily available. These tools can be employed as effortlessly as retrieving a stethoscope. Two exercises, with the first aimed at enhancing a core skill of self-compassion—identifying and regulating emotions (Box 18.4). The second exercise involves the intentional cultivation of self-forgiveness (Box 18.5).

18.4.3 SELF-FORGIVENESS

The focus of this section is specifically on self-forgiveness. The experience of not achieving perfection or making errors is a familiar aspect of the nursing profession (or any other role in life). Generally, when mistakes occur or shortcomings arise, they tend to fade from consciousness over time, albeit after an initial period of distress. Instead of relying solely on the passage of time as a healing mechanism, engaging in reflection and deliberate self-forgiveness can be a transformative process. This practice has the potential to foster enhanced self-awareness and personal growth.

Through the conscious practice of self-forgiveness, the cultivation of self-compassion becomes possible, enabling individuals to navigate beyond errors without succumbing to intense self-judgment, worry, guilt and shame. In Box 18.6, a simple yet effective practice is outlined.

BOX 18.6 ■ Self-Forgiveness in Action: A Simple Script for Developing Forgiving Self-Talk

Self-Forgiveness Journaling Exercise

What is a situation I am being hard on myself for (some perceived or actual error or mistake)?

What is hard about this situation for me?

Why do I care? What does that say about what is important to me?

What am I feeling?

Now say the following to yourself out loud:

'May I forgive myself for this mistake. May I be kind. I am only human'.

Notice what it feels like to say this, then repeat it again and really *feel* into the words.

Now you have forgiven yourself, what do you want to focus on moving forward? Do you need to change your behaviour? Take more care with something? Or simply just be kinder to yourself?

18.4.4 TAKING THINGS FORWARD

The cultivation and maintenance of self-compassion requires consistent attention. Like a garden requiring continual nurturing, neglect of the self-relationship results in a deterioration of the inner world. A commitment to some form of daily self-compassion practice becomes essential for this reason. This practice can be as simple as a brief, conscious attempt to introspect and apply the questions detailed above.

By practicing self-compassion, it will be far easier to navigate and overcome the stress, negative emotion and self-doubt that your role may bring. Self-compassion will also open up a broad range of positive emotions too, such as joy, pride and satisfaction. Altogether, having a self-compassion practice in your toolkit will leave you feeling resilient and empowered to take on the challenges of district nursing.

18.5 Practical Support for Your Mental Health and Well-Being

There is a saying, 'You can't pour from an empty cup'. Essentially, the saying means that to effectively take care of others, we must first take care of ourselves. It has taken many years for nurses to realise how important self-care is, and often nurses are the last to realise that their own 'emotional cup' has only had a few drops left in it.

Undoubtedly, the psychological well-being of nurses was impacted by the COVID-19 pandemic, as evidenced by *the Impact of COVID-19 on the Nursing and Midwifery Workforce* (ICON) study (Couper et al., 2022). The study highlighted that a blend of pre-existing workforce challenges, swift alterations to professional routines and practices, the emotional toll of handling elevated patient mortality rates, the personal risk of illness to both the nurse and their family and the response of healthcare organisations to the pandemic could have a significant and observable psychological impact on the nursing and midwifery workforce in the UK.

The most recent sickness rates of NHS Hospital and Community Health Services (HCHS) staff have reported slightly lower numbers than in previous years; however, they do report that the reasons for sickness and absence are mainly related to anxiety, stress and depression (NHS England, 2023b). The King's Fund (2020) and The Queen's Nursing Institute (QNI) (2022) share the same opinion that high levels of stress and

BOX 18.7 ■ How Are You Feeling in This Present Moment?

Exercise

Self-care allows us as humans to maintain balance and continue functioning like a well-oiled machine that increases our ability to help care for others. Just as you would not expect your car to run continuously for miles without stopping for petrol or having its oil changed, you too cannot expect that of yourself! Running on empty eventually leads to a machine that no longer functions.

It is important to recognise that as nurses we are human, and we cannot continually keep giving to others without thinking of ourselves. Recognising that you cannot pour from an empty cup is the first step in self-care.

Take a few moments to check in with yourself and ask: how are you feeling in this present moment?

- How full is your emotional cup? Or, how full is your petrol tank right now?
- Do you need to stop and fill up?
- What resources do you currently use to help?
- If you don't do anything, why not? What's stopping you?
- Do you prioritise your own self-care?

burnout impact negatively on staff well-being in district nursing and, in turn, on the safety and quality of care being provided to patients.

A concerning report from the Samaritans (2021) highlighted healthcare workers as one of five groups whose risk of suicide may be heightened due to the pandemic. The report detailed the challenges faced by healthcare workers, including feelings of anxiety, trauma and mental exhaustion stemming from their work during the pandemic. Additionally, it emphasised the impact of being consistently exposed to serious illness and death at unprecedented levels, often without sufficient support and resources.

It is acknowledged that nurses excel in caring for others but may struggle to prioritise caring for themselves. Nursing as a profession is both physically and emotionally demanding, with nurses dedicating a significant part of their physical and emotional well-being to both patients and their families. Unfortunately, self-care often takes a backseat. Hochschild (2012), a pioneer in the study of emotional labour, emphasised that emotional labour is essential, challenging work that requires experience, yet often goes unrecognised as part of the job. Emotional labour involves managing or suppressing emotions to maintain an external appearance that elicits appropriate mental states and a sense of comforting care in a secure environment. Continually presenting a composed front by suppressing personal emotions can lead to emotional exhaustion, self-defence mechanisms and eventual burnout (RCN, 2020).

The introduction of the PNA role which focuses on leadership, advocacy, guiding and supporting staff aims to help develop a strong work team culture that encourages colleagues to talk through difficult issues to avoid burnout from happening. PNAs encourage learning and positive behaviours and aim to motivate individuals and teams to promote change, all of which lead to improved care and outcomes for patients (Nash, 2021).

Individually, we can take the initiative to seek resources that support our physical and mental well-being, potentially resulting in enhanced mental health and overall well-being. It is also up to each of us as individuals to instigate these changes, beginning with self-awareness: understanding how we care for ourselves and cultivating the practice of self-care (Box 18.7).

Self-care is what people do for themselves to establish and maintain health and to prevent and deal with illness (WHO, 2020). It is crucial for nurses to prioritise self-care as a prerequisite for performing their roles effectively and providing optimal care to their patients. As mentioned earlier, the nursing profession is physically and emotionally demanding, leading many nurses to face burnout due to the overwhelming load of caregiving responsibilities. Nurses can only allocate a limited amount of their physical and emotional energy to their patients and families.

Nurses need to understand that practicing self-care is not a selfish act. Engaging in self-care is a vital aspect of maintaining balance and ensuring that we can function effectively, much like a well-maintained machine. Just as you would not anticipate your car to run endlessly without refuelling or having its oil changed, it is unrealistic to expect the same from yourself. Operating on empty eventually results in a breakdown, and the machine ceases to function.

Since the onset of the pandemic, significant efforts have been made to alleviate the stigma surrounding mental health, characterised by fear of repercussions or concerns about others' opinions. However, the reduction of stigma within nursing has only recently seen progress, particularly with the introduction of initiatives such as the NHS (2020) People Plan, which suggests that if health professionals feel engaged and satisfied in their work, then this can result in positive well-being (Kinman et al., 2020).

Additional strides in enhancing mental health and well-being among nurses have been propelled by staff-focused initiatives in the NHS, and nursing charities like the QNI. Notably, the QNI established a 'listening line' during the pandemic, offering a secure space for nurses in community, primary and social care to share their experiences and receive emotional support from trained listeners.

18.5.1 STRESS FACTORS

The factors that lead to stress differ from person to person; typically, feelings of stress arise when individuals lack the resources to effectively handle the challenges they are confronting. Stressful feelings may originate from work-related issues, challenges in home life or unexpected life events.

It is crucial for nurses to identify common stress symptoms in themselves and be conscious of when they are experiencing stress. Taking the time to recognise and acknowledge their feelings in the moment, and determining the appropriate actions to alleviate stress, is essential.

Numerous self-help apps are accessible in the market to alleviate stress and enhance mental health and well-being. However, many of them come with associated costs. The ShinyMind app, developed in collaboration with NHS Nurses and Midwives, is offered at no charge to all nurses, midwives, health care support workers and nursing associates (Box 18.8).

18.5.2 NEURODIVERGENCE

Neurodivergent people make up approximately 15%–20% of the global population (Lexxic, 2023). Neurodivergence is an umbrella term for people who have a neurodevelopmental or learning difference, including Autism, Attention Deficit Hyperactivity

BOX 18.8 ■ The ShinyMind Mental Health and Well-Being App

The ShinyMind app is a mental health and well-being app that is free for all NHS nurses, midwives, healthcare support workers and nursing associates and anyone who has an nhs.net email address. Nurses who do not have an NHS email address can contact ShinyMind on the following hello@shinymind.co.uk to enquire about access.

The nursing and midwifery version of the ShinyMind app has been coproduced with NHS staff; it is based in psychotherapy, and contains over 150 interactive exercises and resources that aim to empower nurses and others to take control over their own mental health and well-being and prioritise self-care. We know that the mind affects the body, and the body affects the mind and one way that we can control this is to become more attuned to the way we think. Daily use of the app can help the user to develop positive habits that can improve our physical and mental health and well-being.

ShinyMind is designed to make us more aware of how we think, why we think a certain way, to become more aware of our thoughts, feelings and behaviours and manage these thoughts more effectively and choose whether we continue to think this way or choose a different way to think and behave.

Disorder (ADHD), Dyslexia, Dyspraxia, Dyscalculia and Tourette's (ADHD Aware, 2023). The terminology is changing rapidly, as neurodiversity means 'brain different', which as individuals process information and interact with our surroundings differently. However, neurodivergence refers to the brain difference that sets someone apart from societal norms and those who are not neurodivergent (Ellis et al., 2023). In 2022, there were almost 705,000 nurses on the Nursing and Midwifery Council register (NMC, 2022). It is not known how many nurses are neurodivergent, but the nursing role does lend itself to the skill set of those with ADHD, autism, dyslexia and dyspraxia with problem solving, pattern recognition, photographic memory, compassion, ability to think outside the box, attention to detail, strong communication skills, hyper focused, animated, passionate, kind, sensitive, empathetic and energetic to name a few strengths (RCN, 2023).

Those who identify as neurodivergent have many strengths but there are many challenges too that require strategies, tools and various approaches to help support and overcome the barriers that may be encountered at work. The Equality Act (2010) outlines the legal obligations to protect those with a long-term physical or cognitive disability that affects their day-to-day life. Employers have a responsibility to put reasonable adjustments in place for employees who have disclosed a neurodivergent diagnosis. However, this relies on a deficit model rather than a holistic universal strength-based approach that enables equity for all (Ellis et al., 2023). Employers are gradually becoming more accommodating of neurodivergent needs, but there is still more that can be done to destigmatise, increase awareness and ensure a level playing field for all. However, a neurodivergent diagnosis does not need to be disclosed to an employer, although it may be difficult receiving support if they are not aware. Nurses can access their occupational health provider for support, where the consultation is confidential.

There are many strategies that can be deployed to support community nurses who are neurodivergent to enable greater success with meeting their workload responsibilities. Most of the neurodivergent conditions affect executive functioning abilities to varying degrees. Undertaking different approaches can support a person's cognition and

BOX 18.9 ■ Top Tips

- Use of an analogue clock face to help visualise segments of time
- Having a clock in every room
- Use mobile devices to set alarms, reminders and timers

Note: Always explain to the patient and set time boundaries, so your intentions are clear at the start of the visit.

goal-directed behaviours that affect emotional regulation and mental flex ability to plan, organise, time manage, initiate and problem solve (Neff, 2023).

To support working memory and help organise tasks, it is useful to carry a notebook. Writing key information down will support brain unloading to manage thought holding, which can be exhausting and will improve cognitive efficiency needed to stay on task and support memory recall. Most individuals with ADHD or autism are visual learners who need visual stimulation and reminders, as out of sight out of mind! Using a white board and writing to do lists can help, but they need to be realistic and achievable to enable reward and success. Colour coding can reinforce information uptake and aid novelty and creativity which are necessary for reward and cognitive engagement. Colourful Post-it notes can support with information urgency and enable prioritisation of tasks (Pierce, 2022).

Time blindness is the difficulty to perceive the passing of time, which is common with neurodivergence, especially ADHD (Laub, 2022). It is important to understand that time blindness is not a choice but is attributed to differences in several areas of the brain (Sosnoski, 2022). Therefore time management strategies are essential. Community nurses need to identify how to quantify and keep track of time. In Box 18.9, you may find some helpful tips.

18.5.3 INCLUSIVE WORKSPACE

Music and exercise have been proven to improve executive functioning and reduce anxiety, depression and stress (Applewhite et al., 2022). Parking further away from home visits or taking a walk during the lunch break can help to break up daily tasks and promote movement which increases endorphins and neurotransmitters such as dopamine and serotonin (Lin & Kuo, 2013). Regular physical exercise will promote better physical and mental health, which is beneficial for individuals who are neurodivergent (Mehren et al., 2020). Listening to 'pleasurable' music in the car between visits, via ear pods or having a radio on in the background in the work environment can support cognitive productivity, focus and increase neurotransmitters (Rodgers, 2023). Individuals who are sensory sensitive may benefit from using noise-cancelling headphones or earplugs in a busy office environment to reduce noise aversion or distraction. Having access to a quiet space in the work environment, if possible, can be beneficial for some neurodivergent employees to reduce stimulation and distractibility and promote calmness. There is a need for environmental flexibility to enable an inclusive workspace for all. This might include standing desks, sound-reducing partitions, visual aids like clear signage, colour coding visual information and decluttering workspace (Insightful Environments, 2020).

Everyone's neurodivergent 'spiky profile' is different, as most neurodivergent conditions coexist with others on the spectrum with an overlap of traits in varying degrees (Do It, 2023). There are some similarities within conditions like ADHD, ASC and dyslexia, but each individual is affected differently as their condition manifests with different strengths and challenges on the neurodivergent spectrum. Understanding and accepting neurodivergence will promote self-awareness; this is essential for the individual to manage their condition or difference successfully to enable better control and utilisation of supportive strategies. Self-awareness is necessary to articulate the need for support and communicate challenges or barriers within the workplace (Rosqvist et al., 2023). The government has an 'Access to Work' scheme to support individuals who are neurodivergent in the workplace. However, this is only available for those diagnosed with a disability or health condition, which includes neurodivergence (Gov.UK, 2023). Promoting an inclusive culture and equity within community nursing is essential to ensure neuro-inclusive practices that enable all to thrive, meet their full potential and destigmatise neurodivergence.

18.6 Conclusion

Embarking on a career as a district or community nurse brings a profound sense of meaning and purpose. It provides the privilege of forming deep connections with patients and making a positive impact on their lives. However, it also entails potential emotional challenges and inner turmoil due to the substantial responsibility of caring for others.

The practice of self-compassion and self-forgiveness plays a crucial role in supporting nurses' resilience and their ability to navigate the challenges they may encounter. This practice regulates stress responses, builds emotional strength and contributes to improved mental health and well-being. Nurses should extend the same compassion and care towards themselves as they do towards their patients.

Fostering a strong team culture, seeking support from PNAs, participating in restorative clinical supervision and utilising resources such as the ShinyMind app can enhance the overall well-being of community nurses. As you progress in your community nursing journey, remember the importance of self-care, self-compassion and the significance of nurturing your relationship with yourself. While caring for others, do not forget to prioritise your own health and well-being, as doing so can result in a lasting and positive impact on the lives of those you care for.

References

ADHD Aware. (2023). What is neurodiversity? Available at: https://adhdaware.org.uk/what-is-adhd/neurodiversity-and-other-conditions/. [Accessed: 8/4/23].

Applewhite, B., Cankaya, Z., Heiderscheit, A., & Himmerich, H. (2022). A systematic review of scientific studies on the effects of music in people with or at risk for Autism Spectrum Disorder. *International Journal of Environmental Research and Public Health, 19*, 5150. https://www.ncbi.nlm.nih.gov/pmc/articles/PMC9100336/. [Accessed: 30/12/23].

Couper, K., Blake, H., Kelly, D., Kent, B., Maben, J., Rafferty, A, … Harris, R. (2022). The impact of COVID-19 on the wellbeing of the UK nursing and midwifery workforce during the first pandemic wave: A longitudinal survey study. *International Journal of Nursing Studies*. https://doi.org/10.1016/j.ijnurstu.2021.104155. Elsevier.

Do It. (2023). *Do It Profiler*. https://doitprofiler.com/. [Accessed: 30/12/23].

Ellis, R., Williams, K., Brown, A., Healer, E., & Grant, A. (2023). A realist review of health passports for Autistic adults. *PLoS ONE*, *18*(9):e0279214. https://doi.org/10.1371/journal.pone.0279214.

Equality Act. (2010). London: Department of Health. Gov.UK. Available at: https://www.gov.uk/guidance/equality-act-2010-guidance. [Accessed: 8/4/23].

Gilbert, P. (2017). Compassion: Definitions and controversies. In P. Gilbert (Ed.), *Compassion: Concepts, research and applications* (pp. 3–15). Routledge/Taylor & Francis Group. https://doi.org/10.4324/9781315564296-1.

Gov.UK. (2023). Access to Work: get support if you have a disability or health condition. https://www.gov.uk/access-to-work. [Accessed: 30/12/23].

Hochschild, A. (2012). *The managed heart*. University of California Press. Taylor Francis.

Insightful Environments. (2020). The neurodiverse workspace: A space for all to thrive. https://www.ie-uk.com/blog/the-neurodiverse-workplace [Accessed: 30/12/23].

King's Fund. (2020). The courage of compassion: Supporting nurses and midwives to deliver high-quality care. https://www.kingsfund.org.uk/publications/courage-compassion-supporting-nurses-midwives.

Kinman, G., Teoh, K., & Harriss, A. (2020). *The mental health and wellbeing of nurses and midwives in the United Kingdom*. London: The Society of Occupational Medicine. https://www.som.org.uk/sites/som.org.uk/files/The_Mental_Health_and_Wellbeing_of_Nurses_and_Midwives_in_the_United_Kingdom.pdf.

Laub, E. (2022). Time blindness: What is it? And how to overcome it? https://www.choosingtherapy.com/time-blindness/. [Accessed: 3/12/23].

Lexxic. (2023). The leading neurodiversity experts in the UK. Available at: https://www.lexxic.com/. [Accessed: 8/4/23].

Lin, T. W., & Kuo, Y. M. (2013 Jan 11). Exercise benefits brain function: The monoamine connection. *Brain sciences*, *3*(1), 39–53. https://doi.org/10.3390/brainsci3010039. PMID: 24961306; PMCID: PMC4061837.

MacDondald, B. (2019). Professional restorative clinical supervision: A reflection. *British Journal of Midwifery*, *27*(4). https://doi.org/10.12968/bjom.2019.27.4.258.

McCormack, B., & McCance, T. (2017). Person-centred practice in nursing and health care, theory and practice (2nd ed.). Oxford: Blackwells.

Mehren, A., Reichert, M., Coghill, D., Müller, H. O., Braun, N., & Philipsen, A. (2020). Physical exercise in attention deficit hyperactivity disorder – Evidence and implications for the treatment of borderline personality disorder. *Borderline Personality Disorder and Emotion Dysregulation*, *7*, 1. https://www.ncbi.nlm.nih.gov/pmc/articles/PMC6945516/. [Accessed: 30/12/23].

Nash, K. (2021). Improving the culture of care. *British journal of midwifery*, *29*(9), 486–488. https://doi.org/10.12968/bjom.2021.29.9.486

Neff, M. (2023). *Neurodivergent insights*. https://neurodivergentinsights.com/mentalhealthresources/executive-function-helpers. [Accessed: 2/12/23].

NHS. (2020). We are the NHS: People Plan 2020/21 – Action for us all. https://www.england.nhs.uk/wp-content/uploads/2020/07/We-Are-The-NHS-Action-For-All-Of-Us-FINAL-March-21.pdf.

NHS England. (2023a). NHS long term workforce plan. https://www.england.nhs.uk/ltwp/.

NHS England. (2023b). NHS sickness absence rates. https://digital.nhs.uk/data-and-information/publications/statistical/nhs-sickness-absence-rates/july-2023-provisional-statistics.

NHS England. (2023c). Professional nurse advocate: Role and responsibilities checklist. Available from https://www.england.nhs.uk/long-read/role-and-responsibilities-checklist/.

NMC. (2022). Our latest information about nursing and midwifery in the UK. April 2021 to March 2022. Available at: https://www.nmc.org.uk/globalassets/sitedocuments/data-reports/march-2022/nmc-register-data-march-2022-easy-read.pdf. [Accessed: 23/9/23].

Pierce, R. (2022). 14 tips for managing ADHD and neurodivergence at work. *Life Skills Advocate*. https://lifeskillsadvocate.com/blog/14-tips-for-managing-adhd-and-neurodivergence-at-work/ [Accessed: 12/1/24].

QNI. (2022). The role of the professional nurse advocate in primary care. https://qni.org.uk/the-role-of-professional-nurse-advocates-in-primary-care/.

RCN. (2020). Parliamentary submission: Workforce Burnout and resilience in the NHS & social care. https://www.rcn.org.uk/about-us/our-influencing-work/policy-briefings/CONR-9320.

RCN. (2023). What is neurodiversity? Available at: https://www.rcn.org.uk/Get-Help/Member-support-services/Peer-support-services/Neurodiversity-Guidance/What-is-Neurodiversity [Accessed: 23/9/23].

Rodgers, A. (2023). Music therapy: Sound medicine for ADHD. *ADDitude*. https://www.additudemag.com/music-therapy-for-adhd-how-rhythm-builds-focus/ [Accessed: 30/12/23].

Rosqvist, H., Hultman, L., & Hallqvist, J. (2023). Knowing and accepting oneself: Exploring possibilities of self-awareness among working autistic young adults. *Autism*. https://journals.sagepub.com/doi/pdf/10.1177/13623613221137428 [Accessed: 30/12/23].

Rouse, S. (2019). The role of the PMA and barriers to the successful implementation of restorative clinical supervision. *British Journal of Midwifery*, *27*(6), 381–386. http://www.rcn.org.uk/nursingpractice.

Samaritans. (2021). COVID 1 year on report. https://media.samaritans.org/documents/Samaritans_Covid_1YearOn_Report_2021_BJCM8rI.pdf.

Sawbridge, Y., & Hewison, A. (2013). Thinking about the emotional labour of nursing – Supporting nurses to care. *Journal of Health Organization and Management*, *27*(1), 127–133. https://doi.org/10.1108/14777261311311834

Sirois, F. M. (2020). The association between self-compassion and self-rated health in 26 samples. *BMC Public Health*, *20*(1). https://doi.org/10.1186/s12889-020-8183-1

Sosnoski, K. (2022). How does ADHD affect your time perception? https://psychcentral.com/adhd/cutting-down-on-chronic-lateness-for-adults-with-adhd [Accessed: 3/12/23].

Vaillancourt, E. S., & Wasylkiw, L. (2020). The intermediary role of burnout in the relationship between self-compassion and job satisfaction among Nurses. *The Canadian Journal of Nursing Research*, *52*(4), 246–254. https://doi.org/10.1177/0844562119846274

Wallbank, S. (2013a). Maintaining professional resilience through group restorative supervision. *Community Practitioner*, *86*(8), 26–28.

Wallbank, S. (2013b). Reflecting on leadership in health visiting and the restorative model of supervision. *Journal of Health Visiting*, *2013*(3), 173–176.

WHO. (2020). Self-care for health and well-being (who.int).

Zessin, U., Dickhäuser, O., & Garbade, S. (2015). The relationship between self-compassion and well-being: A meta-analysis. *Applied Psychology: Health and Well-Being*, 7(3), 340–364. https://doi.org/10.1111/aphw.12051

Note: Page numbers followed by f indicate figures, t indicate tables and b indicate boxes.

E

F

G

H

I

Q

R